D1755794

Decision Making in Small Animal Soft Tissue Surgery

Veterinary Titles

Binnington, Cockshutt:
    Decision Making in
    Small Animal Soft Tissue Surgery

Farrow:
    Decision Making in
    Small Animal Radiology

Horney:
    Decision Making in
    Large Animal Alimentary Tract Surgery

Sumner-Smith:
    Decision Making in
    Small Animal Orthopaedic Surgery

Decision Making in Small Animal Soft Tissue Surgery

Allen G. Binnington, D.V.M., M.Sc., Diplomate A.C.V.S.
Associate Professor
Department of Clinical Studies
Ontario Veterinary College
University of Guelph
Guelph, Ontario, Canada

Joanne R. Cockshutt, D.V.M., M.Sc.
Assistant Professor
Department of Clinical Studies
Ontario Veterinary College
University of Guelph
Guelph, Ontario, Canada

1988
B.C. Decker Inc • Toronto • Philadelphia

Publisher

B.C. Decker Inc
3228 South Service Road
Burlington, Ontario L7N 3H8

B.C. Decker Inc
320 Walnut Street
Suite 400
Philadelphia, Pennsylvania 19106

Sales and Distribution

United States and Possessions	**The C.V. Mosby Company** 11830 Westline Industrial Drive Saint Louis, Missouri 63146
Canada	**The C.V. Mosby Company, Ltd.** 5240 Finch Avenue East, Unit No. 1 Scarborough, Ontario M1S 4P2
United Kingdom, Europe and the Middle East	**Blackwell Scientific Publications, Ltd.** Osney Mead, Oxford OX2 OEL, England
Australia	**Harcourt Brace Jovanovich** 30–52 Smidmore Street Marrickville, N.S.W. 2204 Australia
Japan	**Igaku-Shoin Ltd.** Tokyo International P.O. Box 5063 1-28-36 Hongo, Bunkyo-ku, Tokyo 113, Japan
Asia	**Info-Med Ltd.** 802-3 Ruttonjee House 11 Duddell Street Central Hong Kong
South Africa	**Libriger Book Distributors** Warehouse Number 8 "Die Ou Looiery" Tannery Road Hamilton, Bloemfontein 9300
South America (non-stock list representative only)	**Inter-Book Marketing Services** Rua das Palmeriras, 32 Apto. 701 222-70 Rio de Janeiro RJ, Brazil

Decision Making in Small Animal Soft Tissue Surgery   ISBN 0-941158-68-3

© 1988 by B.C. Decker Incorporated under the International Copyright Union. All rights reserved. No part of this publication may be reused or republished in any form without written permission of the publisher.

Library of Congress catalog card number: 87-71765

CONTRIBUTORS

BRIAN C. BUCKRELL, D.V.M., M.Sc., Diplomate A.C.T.
> Assistant Professor, Department of Population Medicine, Ontario Veterinary College, University of Guelph, Guelph, Ontario, Canada

SUSAN M. COCHRANE, B.Sc., M.Sc., D.V.M.
> Department of Clinical Studies, Ontario Veterinary College, University of Guelph, Guelph, Ontario, Canada

DORIS H. DYSON, B.Sc., D.V.M., D.V.Sc., Diplomate A.C.V.A.
> Assistant Professor, Department of Clinical Studies, Ontario Veterinary College, University of Guelph, Guelph, Ontario, Canada

CINDY L. FRIES, D.V.M.
> Department of Clinical Studies, Ontario Veterinary College, University of Guelph, Guelph, Ontario, Canada

DAVID L. HOLMBERG, D.V.M., M.V.Sc., Diplomate A.C.V.S.
> Associate Professor, Department of Clinical Studies, Ontario Veterinary College, University of Guelph, Guelph, Ontario, Canada

DENNIS A. JACKSON, D.V.M., M.S., Diplomate A.C.V.S.
> Veterinary Referral Services Ltd, Vancouver, British Columbia, Canada

WALTER H. JOHNSON, D.V.M., M.V.Sc., Diplomate A.C.T.
> Associate Professor, Department of Population Medicine, Ontario Veterinary College, University of Guelph, Guelph, Ontario, Canada

ELIZABETH J. LAING, B.S., D.V.M., D.V.Sc.
> Department of Clinical Studies, Ontario Veterinary College, University of Guelph, Guelph, Ontario, Canada

KAROL A. MATHEWS, D.V.M., D.V.Sc.
> Department of Clinical Studies, Ontario Veterinary College, University of Guelph, Guelph, Ontario, Canada

CRAIG W. MILLER, D.V.M., M.V.Sc., Diplomate A.C.V.S.
> Assistant Professor, Department of Clinical Studies, Ontario Veterinary College, University of Guelph, Guelph, Ontario, Canada

JOANE PARENT, B.Sc., D.V.M., M.V.Sc., Diplomate A.C.V.I.M.
> Associate Professor, Department of Clinical Studies, Ontario Veterinary College, University of Guelph, Guelph, Ontario, Canada

PETER J. PASCOE, B.V.Sc., D.V.A., Diplomate A.C.V.A.
> Associate Professor, Department of Clinical Studies, Ontario Veterinary College, University of Guelph, Guelph, Ontario, Canada

HOWARD B. SEIM III, D.V.M., Diplomate A.C.V.S.
> Associate Professor, Department of Clinical Sciences, Colorado State University, Fort Collins, Colorado, U.S.A.

LAURA L. SMITH-MAXIE, D.V.M., M.Sc.
> Associate Professor, Department of Clinical Studies, Ontario Veterinary College, University of Guelph, Guelph, Ontario, Canada

BERNHARD M. SPIESS, D.V.M., Diplomate A.C.V.O.
> Visting Professor, Department of Clinical Studies, Ontario Veterinary College, University of Guelph, Guelph, Ontario, Canada

ELIZABETH A. STONE, D.V.M., M.S., Diplomate A.C.V.S.
> Associate Professor, Department of Companion Animals and Special Species Medicine, School of Veterinary Medicine, North Carolina State University, Raleigh, North Carolina, U.S.A.

GEOFF SUMNER-SMITH, B.V.Sc., M.Sc., F.R.C.V.S.

    Professor, Department of Clinical Studies, Ontario Veterinary College, University of Guelph, Guelph, Ontario, Canada

DAVID C. TWEDT, D.V.M., Diplomate A.C.V.I.M.

    Associate Professor, Department of Clinical Sciences, Colorado State University, Fort Collins, Colorado, U.S.A.

MELANIE M. WILLIAMS, D.V.M., Diplomate A.C.V.O.

    Assistant Professor, Department of Clinical Studies, Ontario Veterinary College, University of Guelph, Guelph, Ontario, Canada

PREFACE

When Walter Bailey of B.C. Decker approached us about editing a decision-making book on small animal surgery, the task appeared simple and straightforward. However, as our enthusiasm for the project grew so did our realization that the production of a logical and concise medical algorithm is no simple matter.

The purpose of a medical algorithm is to provide a logical plan of attack for solving a problem and, in some instances, to provide a rational therapeutic plan. Each chapter is designed to stand alone, but occasionally, an umbrella chapter has been used to tie several chapters together.

Decision Making in Small Animal Soft Tissue Surgery is intended to complement, not to replace, existing textbooks. It will serve to jog the memory of the practicing veterinarian and may prevent tunnel vision. For the veterinary student it will promote logical thinking and suggest alternatives when approaching problems in small animal surgery.

Contributing authors were selected on the basis of special expertise in their fields; each chapter represents an individual approach and judgment on a specific problem. The editors, however, have striven to maintain a uniform style while allowing individual approaches to show through.

It is our hope that readers will contact us if their approaches or conclusions differ from ours.

ACKNOWLEDGEMENT

We would like to thank Brian Decker and Walter Bailey of B.C. Decker for their support and encouragement during this project. A special thank you goes to Agnes McIvor, Associate Medical Editor, whose guidance was essential in the construction of high quality surgical algorithms. We also wish to thank Muriel Burke and Mary Sinclair for their patience in typing and retyping the algorithms and text, and Lloy Osburn for her illustrations.

Allen G. Binnington
Joanne R. Cockshutt

CONTENTS

GASTROINTESTINAL DISORDERS

Benign Oral Neoplasia 2
Howard B. Seim III

Malignant Oral Neoplasia 4
Howard B. Seim III

Tonsillar Abnormality 6
Howard B. Seim III

Salivary Mucocele 8
Howard B. Seim III

Caustic Ingestion 10
Howard B. Seim III

Cricopharyngeal Achalasia 12
Howard B. Seim III

Cervical Esophageal Foreign Body 14
Howard B. Seim III

Thoracic Esophageal Foreign Body 16
Howard B. Seim III

Megaesophagus 18
Howard B. Seim III

Esophageal Stricture 20
Howard B. Seim III

Vomiting 22
Howard B. Seim III

Gastric Dilatation-Volvulus 24
Howard B. Seim III

Obstruction of the Small Intestine 26
Howard B. Seim III

Intussusception 28
Howard B. Seim III

Linear Intestinal Foreign Body 30
Howard B. Seim III

Intestinal Perforation 32
Howard B. Seim III

Colonic Obstruction 34
Howard B. Seim III

Rectal Prolapse 36
Howard B. Seim III

Rectal Polyp 38
Howard B. Seim III

Perianal Neoplasia 40
Howard B. Seim III

Imperforate Anus 42
Howard B. Seim III

Anal Sac Abscess 44
Howard B. Seim III

Perianal Fistula 46
Howard B. Seim III

Acute Diarrhea 48
David C. Twedt

Chronic Diarrhea 50
David C. Twedt

Acute Liver Trauma 52
Karol A. Mathews

Hepatic Mass 54
Karol A. Mathews

Biliary Tract Trauma 56
Karol A. Mathews

Bile Duct Obstruction 58
Howard B. Seim III

xi

Pancreatitis 60
Howard B. Seim III

Pancreatic Neoplasia 62
Elizabeth J. Laing

Respiratory Disorders

Coughing 64
Dennis A. Jackson

Nasal Discharge 66
Dennis A. Jackson

Epistaxis 68
Dennis A. Jackson

Airway Obstruction 70
Dennis A. Jackson

Pleural Filling Defects 72
Dennis A. Jackson

Pulmonary Mass 74
Dennis A. Jackson

Thoracic Trauma 76
Dennis A. Jackson

Thoracic Wall Disease 78
Dennis A. Jackson

Cardiovascular Disorders

Common Differentials for Congenital
Cardiac Defects 80
David L. Holmberg

Patent Ductus Arteriosus 82
David L. Holmberg

Pulmonic Stenosis 84
David L. Holmberg

Aortic Stenosis 86
David L. Holmberg

Ventricular Septal Defect 88
David L. Holmberg

Tetralogy of Fallot 90
David L. Holmberg

Vascular Ring Anomaly 92
David L. Holmberg

Artificial Cardiac Pacemaker 94
David L. Holmberg

Pericardial Effusion Tamponade 96
David L. Holmberg

Arteriovenous Fistula 98
David L. Holmberg

Acute Vascular Embolism 100
David L. Holmberg

Canine Heartworm 102
David L. Holmberg

Portosystemic Shunt 104
Karol A. Mathews

Urinary Disorders

Urinary Tract Infection 106
Elizabeth A. Stone

Hematuria 108
Elizabeth A. Stone

Canine Urethral Obstruction 110
Elizabeth A. Stone

Feline Urethral Obstruction 112
Elizabeth A. Stone

Uroperitoneum 114
Elizabeth A. Stone

Neurogenic Urinary Incontinence 116
Elizabeth A. Stone

Nonneurogenic Urinary Incontinence 118
Elizabeth A. Stone

Reproductive Disorders

Infertility in the Cyclic Bitch 120
Brian C. Buckrell
Walter H. Johnson

Infertility in the Acyclic Bitch 122
Brian C. Buckrell
Walter H. Johnson

Infertility in the Dog 124
Brian C. Buckrell

Canine Dystocia 126
Brian C. Buckrell

Vaginal Protrusion 128
Brian C. Buckrell

Vaginitis 130
Brian C. Buckrell

Pyometra 132
Brian C. Buckrell

Prostatic Disease 134
Brian C. Buckrell

NEUROLOGIC DISORDERS

Lesion Localization in Spinal
Cord Disease 136
Joane Parent

Neck Pain 138
Joane Parent
Susan M. Cochrane

Cervical Intervertebral Disc Disease 140
Joane Parent

Thoracolumbar Intervertebral Disc
Disease 142
Joane Parent
Laura L. Smith-Maxie

Peripheral Nerve Disease
(Mononeuropathy) 144
Joane Parent
Susan M. Cochrane

Head Tilt 146
Joane Parent

OPHTHALMOLOGIC DISORDERS

Deep Red Eye 148
Melanie M. Williams
Bernhard M. Spiess

Superficial (Extraocular) Red Eye 150
Melanie M. Williams
Bernhard M. Spiess

Intraocular Red Eye 152
Melanie M. Williams
Bernhard M. Spiess

Cloudy Eye 154
Melanie M. Williams
Bernhard M. Spiess

Conjunctivitis 156
Melanie M. Williams
Bernhard M. Spiess

Ulcerative Keratitis 158
Melanie M. Williams
Bernhard M. Spiess

Wet Eye 160
Bernhard M. Spiess
Melanie M. Williams

Chronic Purulent Ocular Discharge 162
Bernhard M. Spiess
Melanie M. Williams

Protruding Eye 164
Bernhard M. Spiess
Melanie M. Williams

Blindness 166
Melanie M. Williams
Bernhard M. Spiess

INTEGUMENTARY DISORDERS

Acute Full-Thickness Wound 168
Craig W. Miller

Chronic Full-Thickness Wound 170
Craig W. Miller

Wound Reconstruction 172
Craig W. Miller

Thermal Burn 174
Craig W. Miller

Skin Tumors 176
Elizabeth J. Laing

Canine Mammary Tumor 178
Elizabeth J. Laing

Feline Mammary Gland Tumor 180
Elizabeth J. Laing

Anesthesiology and Critical Care

Hypotension 182
  Doris H. Dyson

Apnea Associated with Anesthesia 184
  Doris H. Dyson

Intraoperative or Postoperative Pain 186
  Peter J. Pascoe

Poor Recovery 188
  Doris H. Dyson

Fluid Therapy 190
  Doris H. Dyson

Cardiac Arrest: Dog or Cat 192
  Peter J. Pascoe

Post Cardiopulmonary Resuscitation:
Circulatory Resuscitation 194
  Peter J. Pascoe

Post Cardiopulmonary Resuscitation: Rate and
Arrhythmia Control 196
  Peter J. Pascoe

Post Cardiopulmonary Resuscitation:
Cerebral Resuscitation 198
  Peter J. Pascoe

Miscellaneous Considerations

Neoplasia 200
  Elizabeth J. Laing

Choosing a Suture Material 202
  Cindy L. Fries

Abdominal Fluid 204
  Karol A. Mathews

Chylous Ascites 208
  Karol A. Mathews

Septic Peritonitis 210
  Karol A. Mathews

Splenic Disorder 212
  Cindy L. Fries

Pinna Discomfort 214
  Geoff Sumner-Smith

External Ear Canal Disease 216
  Geoff Sumner-Smith

Middle Ear Disease 218
  Geoff Sumner-Smith

Conditions of Growing Teeth 220
  Geoff Sumner-Smith

Malocclusion 222
  Geoff Sumner-Smith

Diseases of Periodontal Tissue 224
  Geoff Sumner-Smith

Diseases of the Teeth 226
  Geoff Sumner-Smith

INTRODUCTION

Decision Making in Small Animal Soft Tissue Surgery is divided into ten sections, each based upon body systems. Within each section are chapters consisting of an algorithm and explanatory comments. The algorithmic heading may be a patient's symptom (urinary incontinence), clinical sign (epistaxis), or presumptive diagnosis (suspicion of megaesophagus). Some sections contain an introductory algorithm, which is intended to simplify a complex subject or to provide a starting point in the initial diagnostic plan; from this the reader may proceed to a more specific algorithm.

Each algorithm flows downward. The path branches when a specific feature is characterized that is important in the decision-making sequence. This point may be a sign or symptom, clinical finding, or test result. Each branch leads ultimately to a diagnostic or therapeutic end point.

Arrows entering the algorithm signify information obtained from the history taking and physical examination, specific tests, and diagnostic procedures. Therapeutic recommendations are enclosed in boxes. Surgical procedures and invasive diagnostic procedures are written in capital letters.

Some algorithms provide a variety of possible conclusions. Occasionally a reevaluation of the patient or of test results is recommended, a list of differential diagnoses may be offered, or the reader may be referred to another algorithm.

Where special emphasis or explanation is required, a letter is placed to the left of the item in question referring the reader to a corresponding paragraph on the opposite page. These comments are referable only to the algorithm; the text is not designed to be read in continuity. References have been provided as a source of detailed information, and their use is strongly recommended.

BENIGN ORAL NEOPLASIA

Howard B. Seim III

A. Patients with oral neoplasia generally present with any one or a combination of the following signs: difficulty in eating, anorexia, foul breath, oral bleeding, oral swelling, dysphagia, facial deformity, and loose dentition.

B. Visual oral examination generally results in a presumptive diagnosis of oral neoplasia. Digital palpation to assess the presence or absence of bony involvement should be done. Palpation of regional lymph nodes is recommended to assess possible involvement.

C. Masses that appear to involve the bone should be radiographed to verify the presence of bony invasion and to assess the margins.

D. Incisional or excisional biopsy of any oral mass is mandatory in order to definitively diagnose the lesion. Even the most benign-looking mass may be malignant, thus dramatically changing the treatment and prognosis. Biopsy results generally dictate the extent and/or combination of treatment procedures necessary to effect a cure.

E. Canine oral papillomatosis is a viral disease of young dogs that is seen occasionally. If only a few papillomas are present, they require no treatment and can be expected to regress. Multiple tumors or large tumors that interrupt normal occlusion, mastication, swallowing, or respiration should be excised using scalpel excision, electrocautery, or cryosurgery. An autogenous vaccine may be used.

F. Epulides are tumors of the periodontal ligament and are the most common benign oral tumors in dogs. Three types of epulides are recognized: fibromatous epulis, ossifying epulis, and acanthomatous epulis. Fibromatous epulides are noninvasive and respond favorably to local and deep excision. This tumor is often called an epulis, gingival hypertrophy, or gingival hyperplasia. Recurrence is common after superficial resection. Osseous epulides are similar to fibromatous epulides except for the presence of osteoid, and treatment and biologic behavior are identical. Acanthomatous epulides tend to be more invasive and often involve bone. Partial mandibulectomy or partial maxillectomy is required for control. Prognosis for epulides is excellent, provided complete excision is performed.

G. Tumors of dental laminar epithelium are rare in dogs and include ameloblastoma and odontoma. These tumors often invade bone and must be evaluated radiographically prior to treatment. Surgical excision (partial mandibulectomy or partial maxillectomy), cryotherapy after curettage of the tumor cavity, or radiation have proven to be the most rewarding forms of therapy. The prognosis is favorable if complete excision is performed.

References

Norris AM, Withrow SJ, Dubielzig RR. Oropharyngeal neoplasms. In: Harvey CE, ed. Veterinary dentistry. Philadelphia: WB Saunders, 1985:123.

Richardson RC, Jones MA, Elliott GS. Oral neoplasms in the dog: a diagnostic and therapeutic dilemma. Comp Cont Ed 1983; 5(6):441.

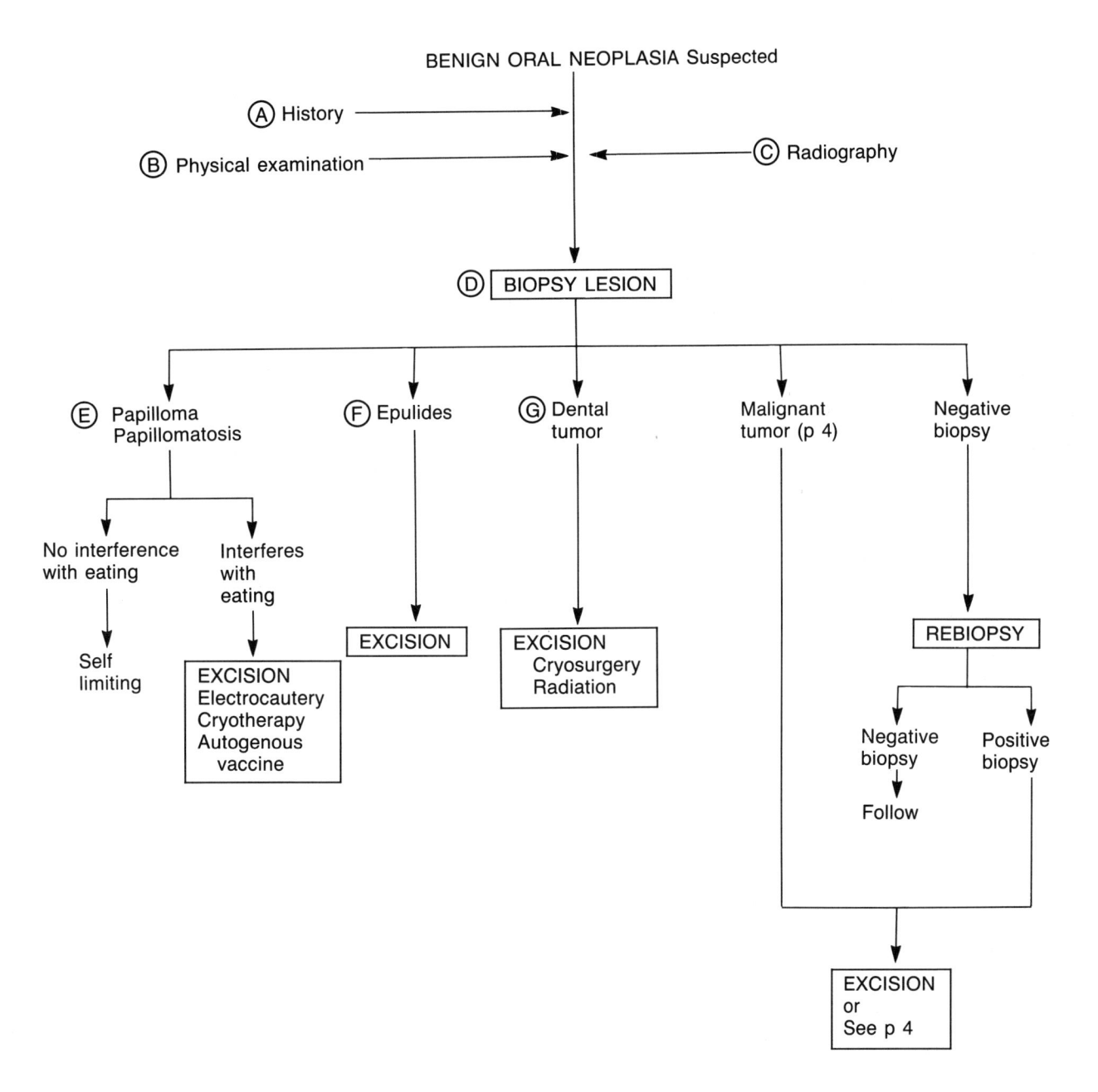

BENIGN ORAL NEOPLASIA Suspected

- (A) History
- (B) Physical examination
- (C) Radiography

↓

(D) **BIOPSY LESION**

Branches:

- (E) Papilloma / Papillomatosis
  - No interference with eating → Self limiting
  - Interferes with eating → **EXCISION** / Electrocautery / Cryotherapy / Autogenous vaccine
- (F) Epulides → **EXCISION**
- (G) Dental tumor → **EXCISION** / Cryosurgery / Radiation
- Malignant tumor (p 4) → **EXCISION or See p 4**
- Negative biopsy → **REBIOPSY**
  - Negative biopsy → Follow
  - Positive biopsy → **EXCISION or See p 4**

3

MALIGNANT ORAL NEOPLASIA

Howard B. Seim III

Generally, therapy and prognosis for malignant oral neoplasia is dictated by the histologic tumor type, location of the primary tumor, extent of its involvement, and the condition of the patient. The most common malignant oral neoplasms in the dog are malignant melanoma, fibrosarcoma, squamous cell carcinoma, and primary bone tumor. In the cat, squamous cell carcinoma, and fibrosarcomas are the most prevalent oral neoplasms.

A. Patients with oral neoplasia generally present with any one or a combination of the following signs: difficulty in eating, anorexia, foul breath, oral bleeding, oral swelling, dysphagia, facial deformity, and loose dentition.

B. Presumptive diagnosis of oral neoplasia can often be made during the initial physical examination. Visualization of a mass, erosion or ulceration in the oral cavity may be an early sign of neoplastic disease. As the neoplasm grows, facial deformity, oral bleeding, fetid odor, and palpable, enlarged regional lymph nodes may be observed.

C. A complete series of skull radiographs should be taken including ventrodorsal, lateral, right and left lateral obliques, skyline, and open mouth views. It is important to assess the presence or absence of bony involvement in order to better define the necessary treatment.

D. An incisional or excisional biopsy, if possible, is performed to assess the histologic tumor type. Fine needle or Tru Cut samples are also of diagnostic value. This information, coupled with accurate radiographic assessment and lymph node biopsy, will help dictate definitive therapy.

E. Primary bone tumors involving the oral cavity are relatively rare in dogs. These tumors respond best to local excision.Partial or hemimandibulectomy and partial maxillectomy are the treatment of choice depending upon the location of the tumor.

F. Malignant melanoma of the oral cavity is a rapidly growing, locally invasive tumor that metastasizes rapidly. Treatment consists of early local control through excision, cryosurgery, electrocautery, hyperthermia, and/or radiation, as well as systemic treatment with appropriate chemotherapeutic drugs to control metastases. The prognosis for long-term survival is unfavorable. If metastasis is present at the time of diagnosis, the prognosis is grave.

G. Fibrosarcoma is a rapidly growing, extensive, invasive tumor with a high recurrence rate. Metastasis at the time of diagnosis is frequent. Treatment consists of early local tumor control by wide excision as described for malignant melanoma. The prognosis for patients that present with fibrosarcoma is unfavorable. Patients that have distant metastases at the time of diagnosis have a grave prognosis.

H. Squamous cell carcinoma generally is characterized as locally invasive, particularly to bone, yet with little tendency for distant metastasis. Treatment is by local control of the tumor. The prognosis for early and complete removal of squamous cell carcinoma is guarded to unfavorable. The radiosensitive nature of squamous cell carcinomas may make local control by radiation more successful. Malignant oral neoplasms in general have an unfavorable prognosis. Although at present most of the treatment regimens are palliative, various combination treatments carry the most hope for local and systemic control.

References

Harvey HJ, MacEwen FB, Brown D, et al. Prognostic criteria for dogs with oral melanoma. JAVMA 1980; 178(6):580.

Hoyt RF Jr, Withrow SJ. Oral malignancy in the dog. JAAHA 1984; 20:83.

Thrall DE. Orthovoltage radiotherapy of oral fibrosarcomas in dogs. JAVMA 1981; 179:159.

Todoroff RJ, Brodey RS. Oral and pharyngeal neoplasia in the dog: a retrospective survey of 361 cases. JAVMA 1979; 175(6):567.

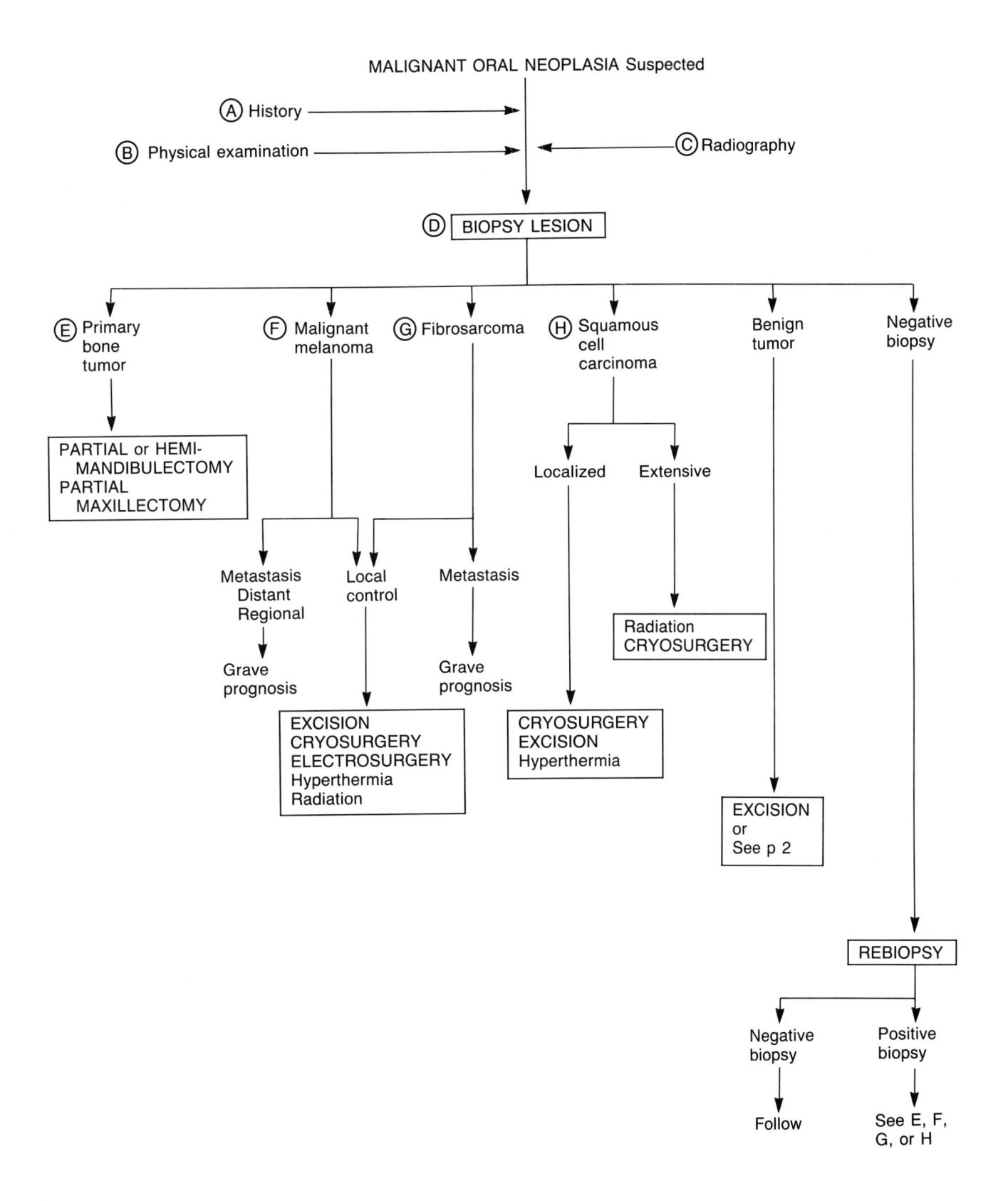

MALIGNANT ORAL NEOPLASIA Suspected

- (A) History
- (B) Physical examination
- (C) Radiography

↓

(D) **BIOPSY LESION**

Branches:

- (E) **Primary bone tumor** → PARTIAL or HEMI-MANDIBULECTOMY / PARTIAL MAXILLECTOMY
- (F) **Malignant melanoma**
  - Metastasis Distant Regional → Grave prognosis
  - Local control → EXCISION / CRYOSURGERY / ELECTROSURGERY / Hyperthermia / Radiation
- (G) **Fibrosarcoma**
  - Local control → EXCISION / CRYOSURGERY / ELECTROSURGERY / Hyperthermia / Radiation
  - Metastasis → Grave prognosis
- (H) **Squamous cell carcinoma**
  - Localized → CRYOSURGERY / EXCISION / Hyperthermia
  - Extensive → Radiation / CRYOSURGERY
- **Benign tumor** → EXCISION or See p 2
- **Negative biopsy** → REBIOPSY
  - Negative biopsy → Follow
  - Positive biopsy → See E, F, G, or H

TONSILLAR ABNORMALITY

Howard B. Seim III

A. Patients with disorders of the tonsils often present with an acute history of gagging, retching, drooling, and dysphagia. As the tonsillar disorder progresses, signs such as anorexia, depression, and oral bleeding may occur.

B. A thorough physical examination with emphasis on the oral cavity should be performed. Localized or generalized oral inflammation, fetid odor to the breath, and unilateral or bilateral tonsillar enlargement and eversion of the tonsil from the tonsillar crypt may be seen.

C. Tonsillitis, as a primary disease entity in the dog and cat, is rare. It is more likely associated with a systemic disorder or local involvement (e.g., neoplasia, foreign body). Further investigation of the patient that presents with tonsillitis is mandatory in order to establish a definitive diagnosis.

D. Patients with bilateral tonsillar involvement are evaluated as to the presence of a noninflammatory or inflammatory process. Noninflammatory tonsillar enlargement implies metastatic neoplasia or a systemic disorder. Biopsy of an affected tonsil allows definitive diagnosis of neoplastic disease or reveals a nonspecific response if a systemic disorder is present. Tonsillar biopsy is also recommended for patients presenting with inflammatory disorders (e.g., foreign body, infection, trauma) causing bilateral tonsillar enlargement. Histopathologic evidence of specific disease entities may help to determine an appropriate treatment regimen.

E. Patients with unilateral tonsillar involvement are also evaluated for the presence of an inflammatory or noninflammatory process. Differential diagnosis requires tonsillar biopsy. Histopathologic results dictate the appropriate treatment regimen. The most common primary tumor of tonsillar origin is squamous cell carcinoma that arises from the tonsillar crypt. Other tumor types, such as lymphosarcoma, rarely originate from the tonsil.

F. Primary inflammatory disease of the tonsil is rare. When present, it generally occurs secondary to external trauma or foreign objects (grass awn, porcupine quill) lodged in the tonsillar crypt. Tonsillar inflammation is generally secondary to systemic disorders, such as canine distemper and upper respiratory infections, or secondary to chronic coughing.

G. Treatment of inflammatory disorders of the tonsil is dictated by the etiology. In primary tonsillitis, the tonsillar crypts should be carefully examined for the presence of a foreign object. Removal of the foreign object generally results in a cure.

H. Patients that have chronic recurrences of primary tonsillitis with no evidence of a foreign body may be helped by tonsillectomy. In cases of secondary tonsillitis, treatment of the underlying systemic disorder generally results in resolution of the tonsillar involvement.

I. Peroral tonsillectomy is performed by grasping the tonsil with an Allis tissue forcep, everting the tonsil from its crypt, placing a Kelly or Carmalt hemostat across the base of the tonsil, excising the tonsil, and oversewing the tissue that remains in the clamp. This technique allows complete removal of lymphoid tissue as well as primary suturing of pharyngeal mucosa to control hemorrhage.

References

Brodey RS. Differentiating tonsillar lesions in the dog. Mod Vet Pract 1966; 47:58.

Dulisch MC. The tonsils. In: Slatter DH, ed. Textbook of small animal surgery. Philadelphia: WB Saunders, 1985:1219.

MacMillan R, Withrow SJ, Gillette EL. Surgery and regional irradiation for treatment of canine tonsillar squamous cell carcinoma: retrospective review of eight cases. JAAHA 1982; 18:311.

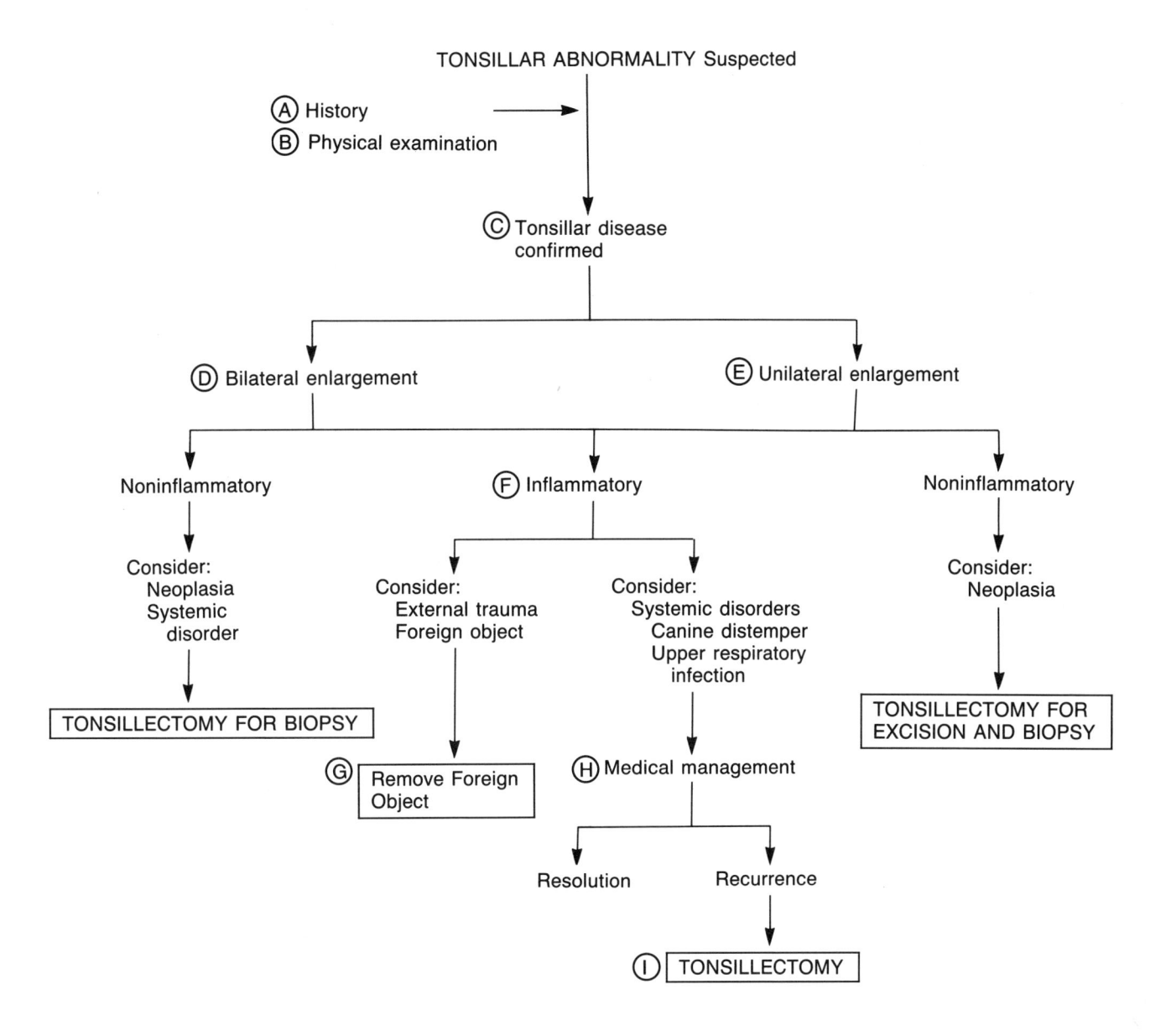

TONSILLAR ABNORMALITY Suspected

- (A) History
- (B) Physical examination

↓

(C) Tonsillar disease confirmed

├── (D) Bilateral enlargement
│   ├── Noninflammatory
│   │   └── Consider: Neoplasia, Systemic disorder
│   │   └── **TONSILLECTOMY FOR BIOPSY**
│   └── (F) Inflammatory
│   ├── Consider: External trauma, Foreign object
│   │   └── (G) Remove Foreign Object
│   └── Consider: Systemic disorders, Canine distemper, Upper respiratory infection
│   └── (H) Medical management
│   ├── Resolution
│   └── Recurrence
│   └── (I) **TONSILLECTOMY**
└── (E) Unilateral enlargement
    └── Noninflammatory
        └── Consider: Neoplasia
            └── **TONSILLECTOMY FOR EXCISION AND BIOPSY**

SALIVARY MUCOCELE

Howard B. Seim III

A. Patients that present with a nonpainful, fluctuant mass in the intermandibular space, pharyngeal region, or base of the tongue should be considered to have a salivary mucocele. The most commonly affected salivary glands are the mandibular and sublingual, with the sublingual gland being the most frequent source of saliva. Diagnosis is based on history, physical examination, palpation, and aspiration and cytology.

B. Aspiration of a neoplastic mass may produce little or no fluid, with the occurrence of an occasional neoplastic cell on cytologic evaluation. Aspiration of an abscess generally produces purulent fluid with neutrophils and bacteria on cytology. Aspiration of a salivary mucocele reveals a viscous, serosanguineous to straw colored fluid with occasional neutrophils and macrophages on a proteinaceous background. Sialography may be attempted for diagnostic purposes, but is time consuming and often gives questionable results. Differential diagnoses include neoplasia (salivary gland adenocarcinoma, thyroid adenocarcinoma, or squamous cell carcinoma) and cervical abscess.

C. There are three major classifications of salivary mucoceles, categorized according to their anatomic locations: pharyngeal mucoceles, cervical mucoceles, and ranulas.

D. Salivary mucoceles are occasionally found in the pharyngeal region. These pharyngeal mucoceles appear as a fluctuant, smooth, dome-shaped swelling in the lateral pharyngeal wall. Initial treatment consists of opening and draining the mucocele, partially excising the overlying pharyngeal mucosa, and suturing the cut edges of the mucosa to the adjacent pharyngeal wall (marsupialization). If this fails, mucocele marsupialization and ipsilateral resection of the mandibular and sublingual salivary glands should be performed.

E. Cervical mucoceles are generally located on the ventrolateral aspect of the head and neck from the level of the mandibular and sublingual salivary glands to the intermandibular space. The majority of patients present with mucoceles in the intermandibular space. Determination of the side involved (right versus left) can be accomplished by the following: historical evaluation; oral examination for a ranula or pharyngeal mucocele; placing the patient in dorsal recumbency and gently forcing saliva to the right or left side (saliva tends to migrate to the side of origin); or sialography. Treatment of a cervical mucocele with the side of origin known is accomplished by ipsilateral mandibular and sublingual salivary gland removal. Because of the intimate anatomic association of the mandibular and sublingual salivary glands, both glands are removed together. An intracapsular dissection of the glands is preferred; this facilitates complete dissection of both glands, as well as visualization of the major blood supply present on the dorsomedial surface of the glands. Careful dissection of the portion of the sublingual gland that follows the duct is important to ensure complete gland resection. The duct is ligated and transected to complete the resection. A communication of the mucocele and duct may be found during dissection. This helps to confirm that the correct side has been operated on. The saliva that has accumulated ventrally is removed, and ventral drainage is established by making a stab incision and placing a latex rubber drain. The saliva is drained ventrally for 2 to 3 days. If the side of origin of a cervical mucocele is unknown, treatment is accomplished by bilateral mandibular and sublingual salivary gland resection. Since dogs have eight salivary glands, bilateral resection of the mandibular and sublingual salivary glands does not have a detrimental effect on the ability of the patient to produce adequate saliva.

F. Ranulas are formed by an accumulation of saliva along the base of the tongue. Marsupialization is the treatment of choice. If the ranula recurs, or if it is associated with a cervical mucocele, an ipsilateral resection of the mandibular and sublingual salivary glands, should be performed along with marsupialization of the ranula.

References

Harvey CE. The salivary glands - diseases. In: Slatter DH, ed. Textbook of small animal surgery. Philadelphia: WB Saunders, 1985: 645.

Harvey HJ. Pharyngeal mucoceles in dogs. JAVMA 1981; 178(12):1282.

SALIVARY MUCOCELE Suspected

- (A) History
- Physical examination

↓

(B) Aspiration and Cytology

- Neoplasia (See p 200) → **INCISIONAL OR EXCISIONAL BIOPSY**
- Salivary mucocele → (C) Location
- Cervical abscess → Ventral Drainage / Antibiotics / Remove Foreign Body

(C) Location:

- (D) Pharyngeal mucocele → **MARSUPIALIZATION**
  - Recurrence → **MARSUPIALIZATION AND SALIVARY GLAND EXCISION**
  - Resolution

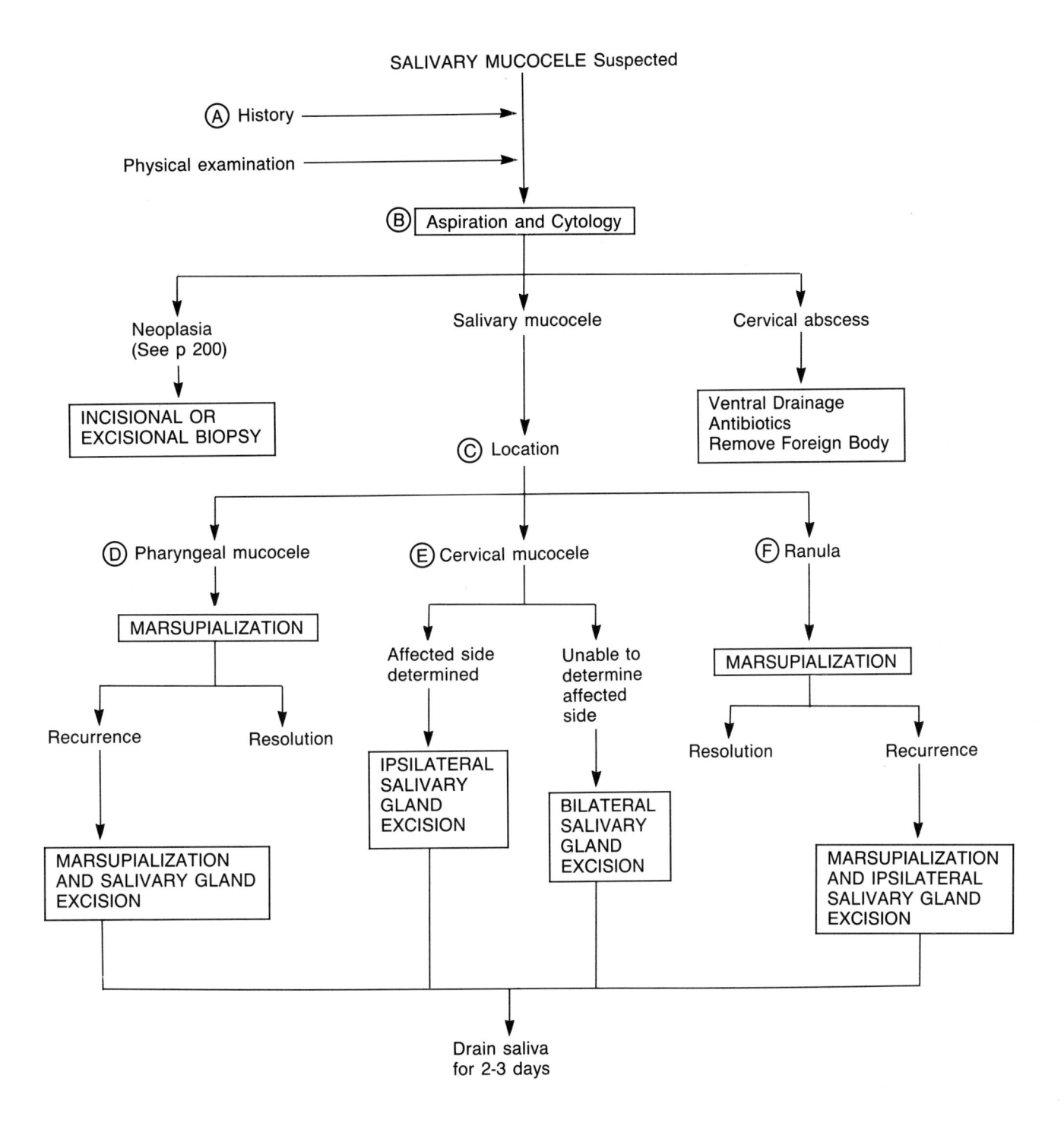

- (E) Cervical mucocele
  - Affected side determined → **IPSILATERAL SALIVARY GLAND EXCISION**
  - Unable to determine affected side → **BILATERAL SALIVARY GLAND EXCISION**

- (F) Ranula → **MARSUPIALIZATION**
  - Resolution
  - Recurrence → **MARSUPIALIZATION AND IPSILATERAL SALIVARY GLAND EXCISION**

↓

Drain saliva for 2-3 days

CAUSTIC INGESTION

Howard B. Seim III

A. An accurate history of the type and amount of toxic material ingested and the time from ingestion to presentation helps to dictate early specific therapy.

B. Careful physical examination of the oral cavity for evidence of erythema, erosions, and ulcers gives some idea of the caustic nature of the ingested chemical. The patient should also be examined for burns involving the face, mouth, and eyes. Upper airway obstruction secondary to inflammation and edema must be recognized and treated immediately by endotracheal intubation or tracheostomy.

C. Early supportive therapy should be instituted and includes systemic antibiotics, intravenous maintenance and replacement fluids, anti-inflammatory medications (steroids), nothing by mouth, and maintenance of an open airway.

D. Examination of the esophageal mucosa by esophagography or endoscopy allows critical evaluation of the extent of mucosal damage and dictates the aggressiveness of therapy.

E. Patients with evidence of severe mucosal erosion or ulceration (particularly if 360 degrees of the esophageal mucosa is involved) should receive aggressive medical therapy to decrease the chance of stricture formation. The rationale for therapy is as follows: cimetidine and antacids to decrease gastric acid formation and thus decrease reflux esophagitis, dietary restriction to decrease mechanical irritation, antibiotics to protect against secondary bacterial infection and possible abscessation, steroids to decrease fibrous protein synthesis, and lidocaine viscous for pain relief. Treatment should continue for 10 to 14 days. Severely debilitated patients may benefit from placement of a gastrostomy tube to deliver maintenance caloric needs. Pharyngostomy tubes are contraindicated owing to added mechanical irritation.

F. Esophagography should be performed 2 to 3 weeks after treatment to assess the degree of esophageal stricture. If the stricture is so severe that signs of regurgitation occur, esophageal dilation (bougienage) or esophageal reconstruction should be considered.

G. Graduated sizes of bougies are inserted through the esophageal stricture until appropriate esophageal dilation is accomplished. Concurrent treatment with steroids may increase the long-term efficacy of bougienage.

H. If esophageal dilation fails, an esophageal reconstructive procedure is necessary. Longitudinal incision with a transverse closure, longitudinal incision with a vascular pedicle graft of muscle to serve as a patch (sternothyroideus for the cervical esophagus or diaphragm for the distal esophagus, p 20), or resection and anastomosis are several available techniques. The surgical procedure is dictated by the location and extent of the stricture.

References

Clifford DH. The esophagus. In: Gourley IM, Vasseur PB, eds. General small animal surgery. Philadelphia: JB Lippincott, 1985: 285.

Harvey CE. Esophageal stricture; conservative treatment of acquired esophageal stricture. In: Slatter DH, ed. Textbook of small animal surgery. Philadelphia: WB Saunders, 1985:661.

CAUSTIC INGESTION Suspected

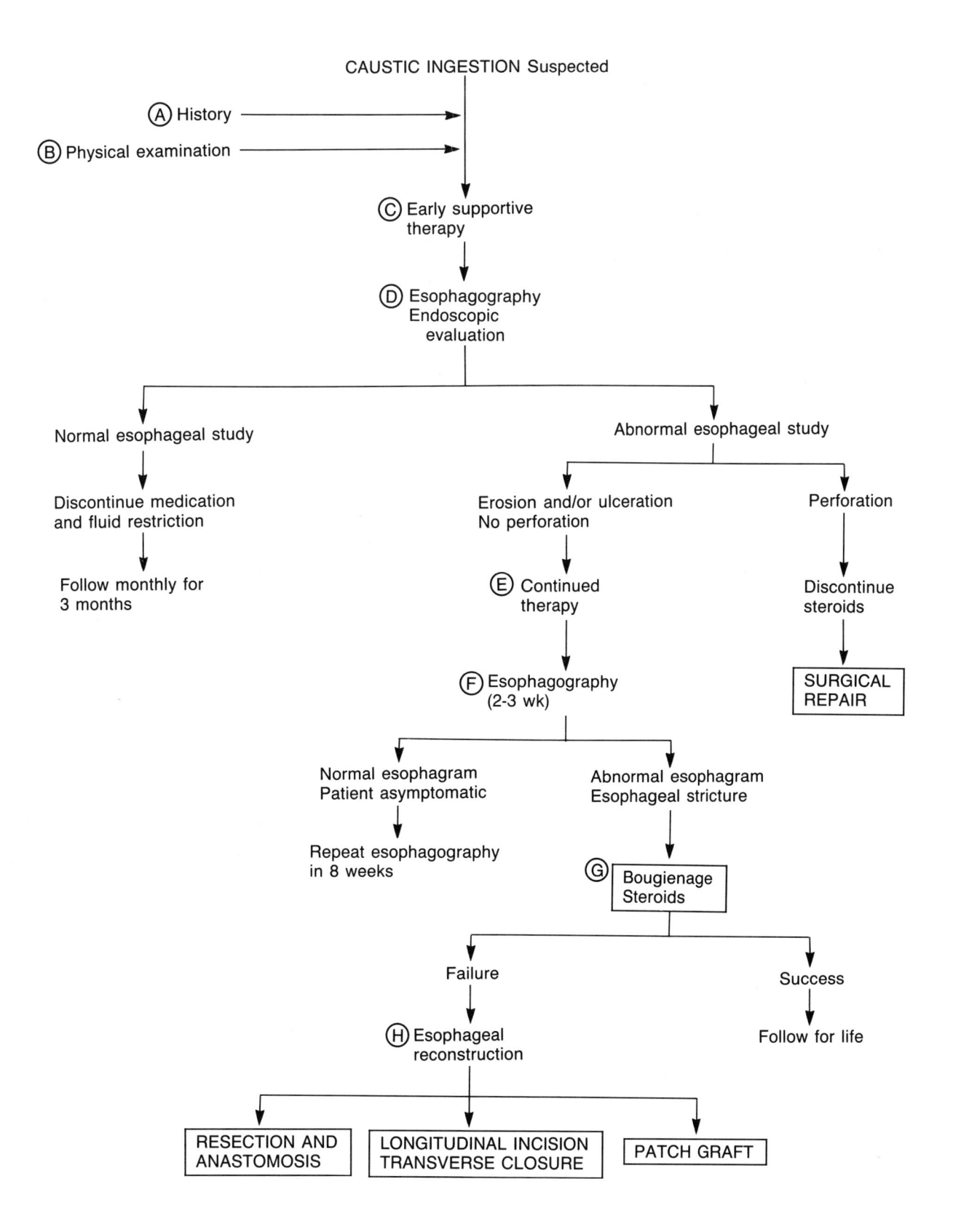

- (A) History
- (B) Physical examination
- (C) Early supportive therapy
- (D) Esophagography / Endoscopic evaluation

Normal esophageal study
- Discontinue medication and fluid restriction
- Follow monthly for 3 months

Abnormal esophageal study

Erosion and/or ulceration, No perforation
- (E) Continued therapy
- (F) Esophagography (2-3 wk)
  - Normal esophagram, Patient asymptomatic → Repeat esophagography in 8 weeks
  - Abnormal esophagram, Esophageal stricture → (G) Bougienage, Steroids
    - Success → Follow for life
    - Failure → (H) Esophageal reconstruction
      - RESECTION AND ANASTOMOSIS
      - LONGITUDINAL INCISION TRANSVERSE CLOSURE
      - PATCH GRAFT

Perforation
- Discontinue steroids
- SURGICAL REPAIR

CRICOPHARYNGEAL ACHALASIA

Howard B. Seim III

A. Patients affected with cricopharyngeal achalasia generally present with a history of persistent dysphagia that begins soon after weaning. Repeated attempts to swallow are followed by forceful regurgitation and violent episodes of coughing. Patients should be evaluated for respiratory disorders secondary to aspiration.

B. The asynchronous closure of the cricopharyngeal muscle in response to a bolus of food results in immediate regurgitation after feeding. Dogs fed a canned food diet can be expected to regurgitate within 30 seconds of feeding. Delayed regurgitation implies an esophageal disorder. It is important to distinguish between vomition and regurgitation. If the patient is truly vomiting, gastric or proximal small bowel disease is inferred.

C. Cinefluorography or videofluorography, in conjunction with barium administration, allows careful assessment of the entire swallowing mechanism. Asynchronous constriction of the cricopharyngeal muscle can be visualized as the barium bolus is delivered to the cricopharyngeal passageway; little or no contrast media is observed passing into the esophagus, but is instead retained in a markedly distended caudal pharynx.

D. A cricopharyngeal myotomy is performed to correct the achalasia (Fig. 1). A ventral midline incision is centered over the laryngeal region. The larynx is exposed and rotated 180 degrees to allow exposure of the cricopharyngeal muscle and dorsal esophagus. The cricopharyngeus is distinguished from the esophagus by its transverse muscle fibers. The muscle is then dissected free from the underlying mucosa and transected. Closure is routine. Improved swallowing is immediate.

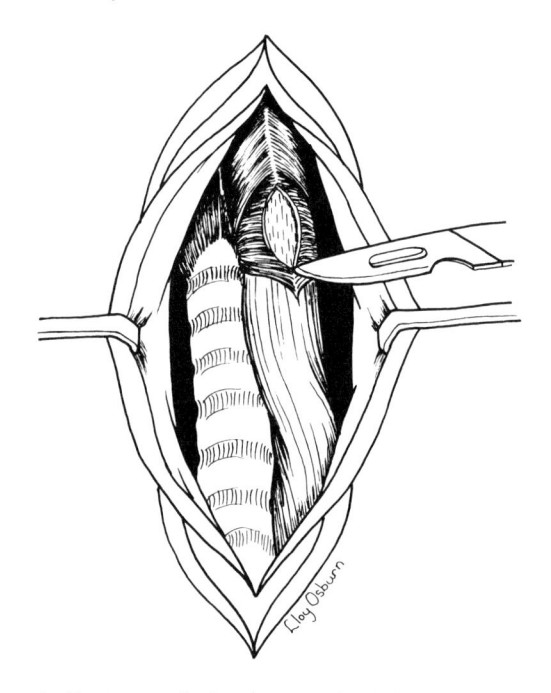

Figure 1 Treatment of cricopharyngeal achalasia by myotomy of cricopharyngeal muscle and associated cranial esophageal musculature allowing bulging of the intact esophageal mucosa.

References

Goring RL, Kagan KG. Cricopharyngeal achalasia in the dog: radiographic evaluation and surgical management. Comp Cont Ed 1982; 4(5):438.

Hoffer RE. Surgical esophageal diseases. In: Bojrab MJ, ed. Pathophysiology in small animal surgery. Philadelphia: Lea & Febiger, 1981: 90.

Shelton GD. Swallowing disorders in the dog. Comp Cont Ed 1982; 4:(7):608.

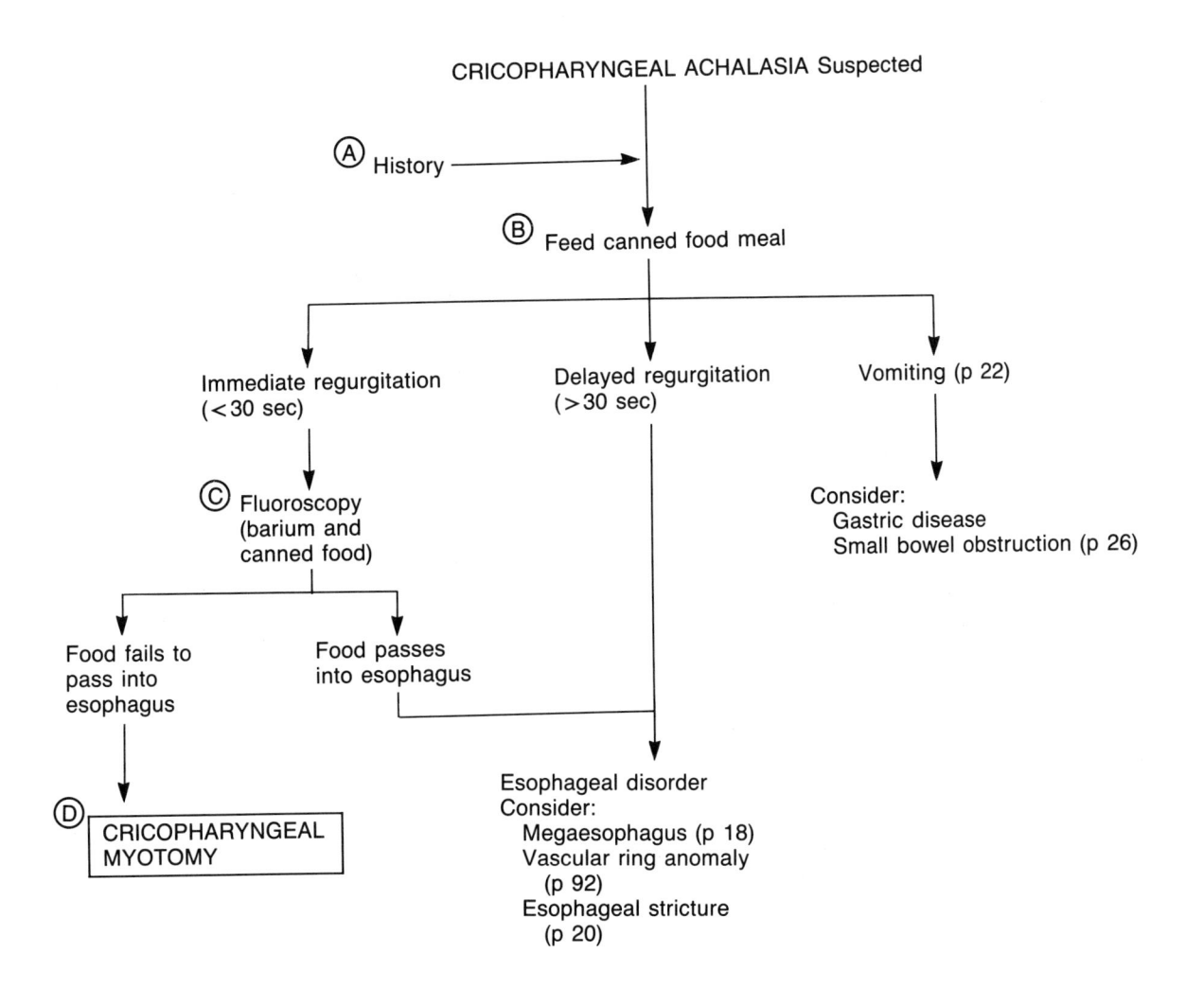

CRICOPHARYNGEAL ACHALASIA Suspected

- (A) History
- (B) Feed canned food meal

Immediate regurgitation (<30 sec)
- (C) Fluoroscopy (barium and canned food)
  - Food fails to pass into esophagus
    - (D) **CRICOPHARYNGEAL MYOTOMY**
  - Food passes into esophagus

Delayed regurgitation (>30 sec)
Esophageal disorder
Consider:
  Megaesophagus (p 18)
  Vascular ring anomaly (p 92)
  Esophageal stricture (p 20)

Vomiting (p 22)
Consider:
  Gastric disease
  Small bowel obstruction (p 26)

CERVICAL ESOPHAGEAL FOREIGN BODY

Howard B. Seim III

A. Patients with an esophageal foreign body may present with a variety of signs depending upon the duration of pathology. Initially, drooling, gagging, retching, and regurgitation are common signs. Some patients may exhibit dysphagia, distress, or slow continual swallowing. Later these signs may disappear, and the patient may exhibit nonspecific signs such as depression, anorexia, and weight loss.

B. The majority of esophageal foreign bodies are firm objects (bone, wood, cartilage), which are easily palpated if lodged in the cervical esophagus. In the case of nonpalpable foreign bodies, a cervical radiograph and/or barium swallow will reveal the foreign body.

C. Approximately 90 percent of esophageal foreign bodies may be removed without surgical intervention. Visualization and retrieval with rigid or flexible endoscopy is the method of choice. A technique utilizing two Foley catheters has been developed for removing soft, blunt, foreign bodies. The first Foley catheter is passed down the esophagus just beyond the foreign body. The second Foley catheter is passed just cranial to the foreign body. The bulbs of the Foley catheters are inflated, thus dilating the esophagus away from the foreign body. The catheters are gently pulled out, bringing the foreign body with them.

D. Cervical esophageal foreign bodies can be approached via a midline cervical incision. Attempts at gently milking and teasing the foreign body to encourage oral removal is done first. If unsuccessful, a longitudinal esophagotomy is performed in healthy tissue (generally aboral) and the foreign body removed. The incision is closed in two layers: the mucosal layer in a simple interrupted pattern with knots tied into the lumen and the muscular layer with interrupted horizontal mattress sutures.

E. After removal of the esophageal foreign body, an endoscope should be passed and the esophageal mucosa evaluated for evidence of esophagitis, erosion, ulceration, or perforation. Contrast radiography can also be used to evaluate the esophagus. Esophagitis should be treated aggressively to prevent post-removal stricture (p 10).

F. Cervical esophagotomy incisions that have a high potential for breakdown and leakage can be "patched" with the sternothyroideus muscle. The muscle is dissected from its attachment to surrounding tissue and mobilized to esophagotomy site. Simple interrupted sutures are used to secure the muscle to the esophagus. A gastrostomy tube should be placed to feed the patient for the first 7 to 10 days postoperatively. A large-bore Foley catheter (24 to 26 F) is placed into the fundus of the stomach through a left paracostal grid approach. Esophagography is performed prior to removal of the gastrostomy tube to assess esophageal closure.

References

Howard DR, Lammerding JJ, Dewevre PB. Esophageal reinforcement with sternothyroideus muscle in the dog. Canine Pract 1975; 2(4):30.

Ryan WW, Greene RW. The conservative management of esophageal foreign bodies and their complications: a review of 66 cases in dogs and cats. JAAHA 1975; 11:243.

Zimmer JF. Canine esophageal foreign bodies: endoscopic, surgical and medical management. JAAHA 1984; 20:669.

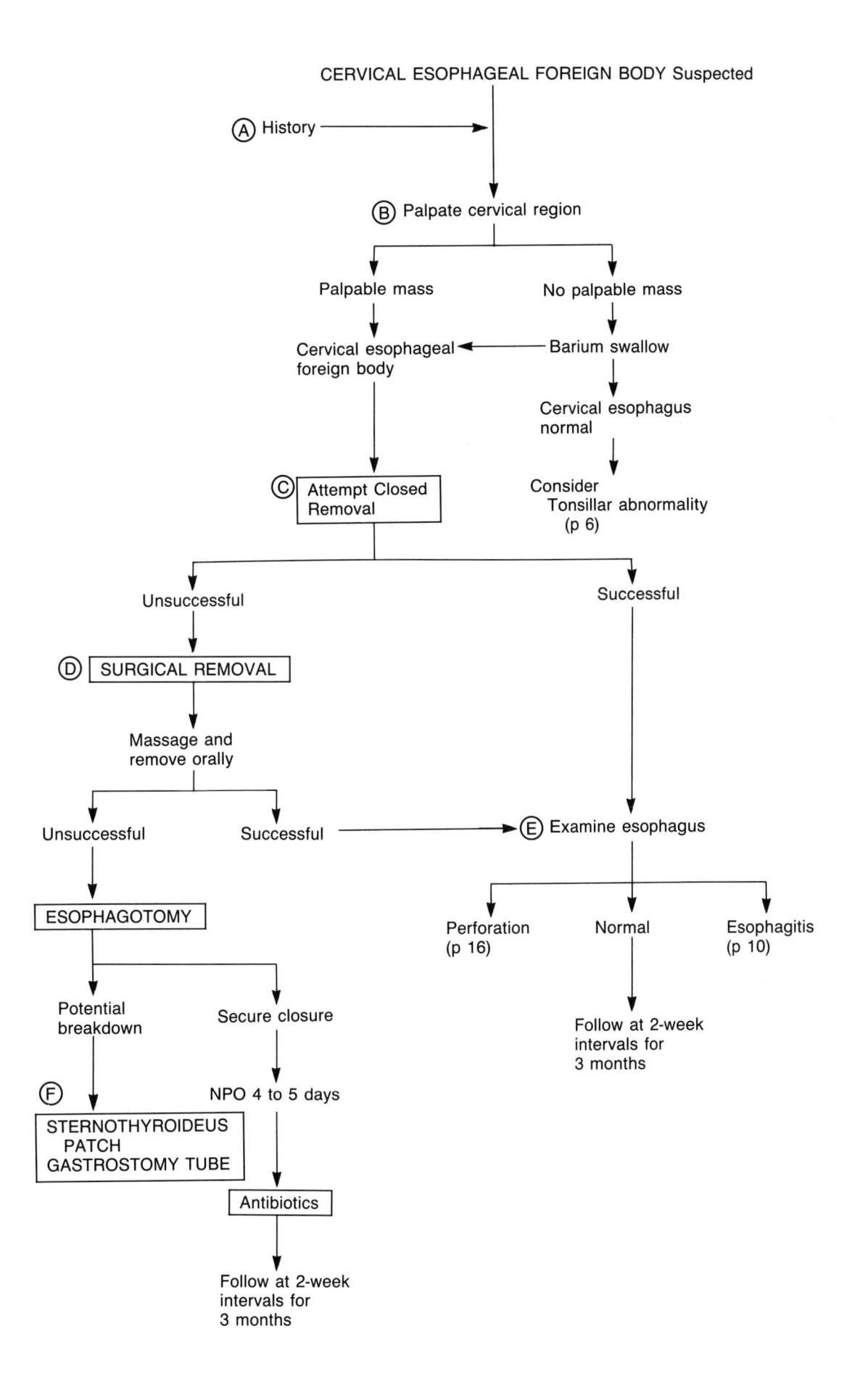

CERVICAL ESOPHAGEAL FOREIGN BODY Suspected

- (A) History
- (B) Palpate cervical region
  - Palpable mass → Cervical esophageal foreign body
  - No palpable mass → Barium swallow
    - Cervical esophageal foreign body (←)
    - Cervical esophagus normal → Consider Tonsillar abnormality (p 6)
- (C) Attempt Closed Removal
  - Successful → (E) Examine esophagus
    - Perforation (p 16)
    - Normal → Follow at 2-week intervals for 3 months
    - Esophagitis (p 10)
  - Unsuccessful → (D) SURGICAL REMOVAL
    - Massage and remove orally
      - Successful → (E) Examine esophagus
      - Unsuccessful → ESOPHAGOTOMY
        - Potential breakdown → (F) STERNOTHYROIDEUS PATCH GASTROSTOMY TUBE
        - Secure closure → NPO 4 to 5 days → Antibiotics → Follow at 2-week intervals for 3 months

THORACIC ESOPHAGEAL FOREIGN BODY

Howard B. Seim III

A. Patients with esophageal foreign bodies may present with a variety of signs depending upon the duration of pathology. Initially, drooling, gagging, retching, and regurgitation are common signs. Some patients may exhibit dysphagia, distress, or slow continual swallowing. Later these signs may disappear, and the patient may exhibit nonspecific signs such as depression, anorexia, and weight loss.

B. Physical examination may reveal a normal to slightly depressed patient with or without the classical signs of drooling and gagging. Careful palpation of the cervical esophagus rules out the presence of a cervical esophageal foreign body (p 14).

C. Definitive diagnosis and location of a thoracic esophageal foreign body is best done by initial chest radiographs. Approximately 50 percent of esophageal foreign bodies are radiopaque. Barium swallow or endoscopic examination of the esophagus confirms the presence of nonradiopaque foreign bodies.

D. Approximately 90 percent of esophageal foreign bodies may be removed without surgical intervention. Visualization and retrieval with rigid or flexible endoscopy are the methods of choice. A technique utilizing two Foley catheters has been developed for removing soft, blunt, foreign bodies. The first Foley catheter is passed down the esophagus just beyond the foreign body. The second Foley catheter is passed just cranial to the foreign body. The bulbs of the Foley catheters are inflated, thus dilating the esophagus away from the foreign body. The catheters are gently pulled out, bringing the foreign body with them.

E. Unsuccessful closed removal of an esophageal foreign body at the thoracic inlet requires a ventral cervical approach (p 14). If the esophagus cannot be adequately exposed, a median sternotomy is performed.

F. Unsuccessful closed removal of an esophageal foreign body at the heart base requires a left fifth or sixth intercostal thoracotomy. The exact interspace is dictated by the location of the foreign body on a lateral thoracic radiograph.

G. Unsuccessful closed removal of an esophageal foreign body at the esophageal hiatus requires a left eighth intercostal thoracotomy. If massage and removal is unsuccessful, a transdiaphragmatic approach may be used. An incision in the dome of the diaphragm is made, the stomach located, a gastrotomy performed, and the foreign body removed through the stomach. If this technique fails, an esophagotomy is performed (p 14). If the foreign body is distal to the esophageal hiatus, a ventral midline celiotomy and gastrotomy may be successful in removing the foreign body. The disadvantage of celiotomy and gastrotomy is the inability to visualize and massage the distal esophagus to encourage foreign body removal. Failure to remove the foreign body through this approach would subsequently require a left intercostal thoracotomy.

H. Successful closed removal of an esophageal foreign body that leaves the esophagus with perforations less than 2 mm in length may be treated conservatively with antibiotics, nothing by mouth, and frequent follow-up radiographs (daily for 3 to 5 days). Perforations greater than 2 mm in length must be surgically debrided and sutured primarily as described for esophagotomy closure (p 14).

I. Distal esophagotomy incisions that have a high potential for breakdown and leakage can be "patched" with a vascular muscle pedicle from the diaphragm. A vascular pedicle of diaphragm is developed and transferred to the esophagotomy incision. The patch is sutured to the esophagus with a simple continuous pattern using 4-0 or 5-0 PDS. Care is taken to preserve the vascular pedicle.

References

Lammerding J, Howard DR, Noser GA. Diaphragmatic pedicle flaps for repair of distal esophageal defects in dogs. JAAHA 1976; 12:588.

Ryan WW, Greene RW. The conservative management of esophageal foreign bodies and their complications: a review of 66 cases in dogs and cats. JAAHA 1975; 11:243.

Taylor RA. Transdiaphragmatic approach to distal esophageal foreign bodies. JAAHA 1982; 18:749.

Zimmer JF. Canine esophageal foreign bodies: endoscopic, surgical and medical management. JAAHA 1984; 20:669.

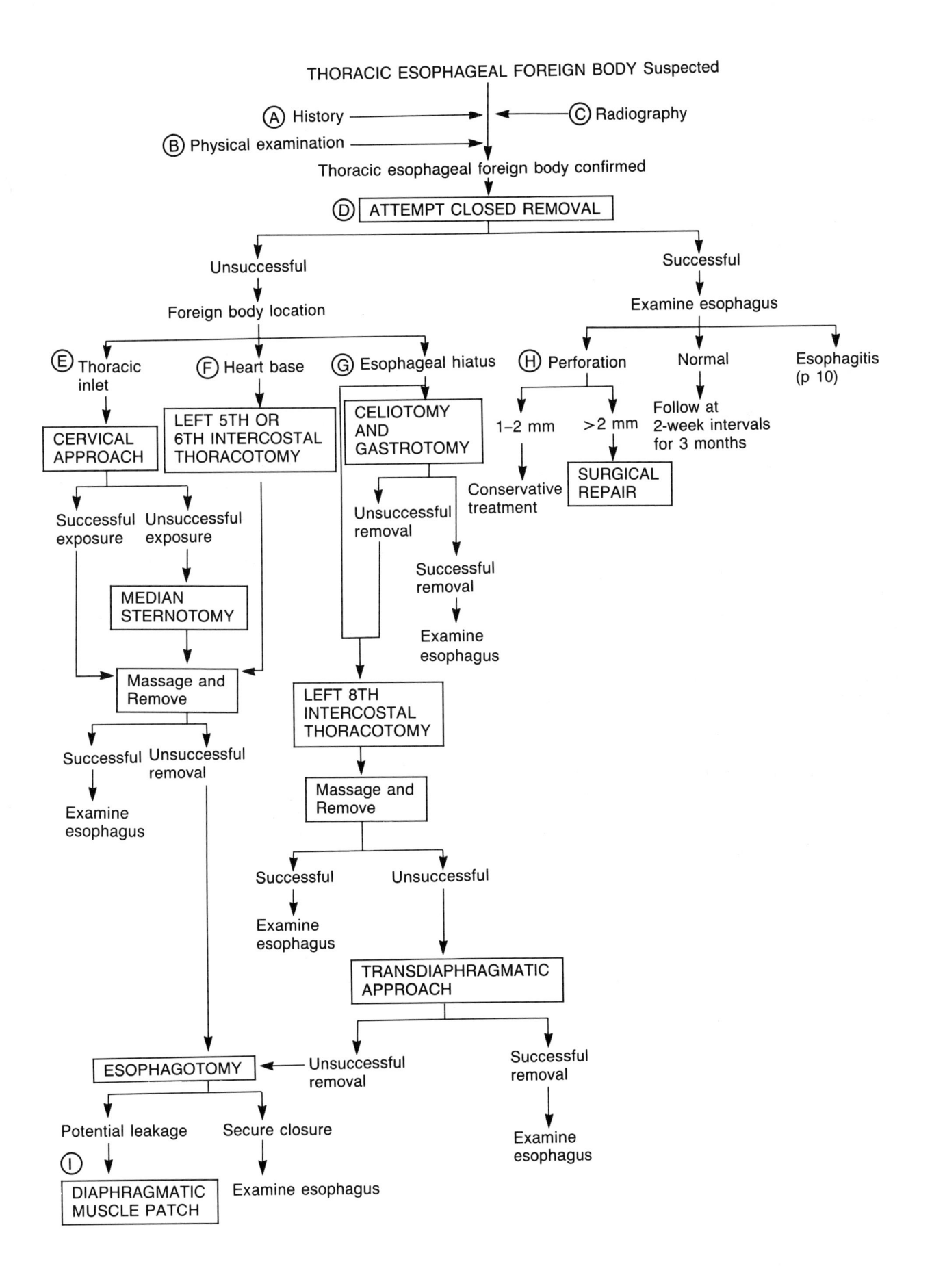

THORACIC ESOPHAGEAL FOREIGN BODY Suspected

- Ⓐ History
- Ⓑ Physical examination
- Ⓒ Radiography

→ Thoracic esophageal foreign body confirmed

Ⓓ **ATTEMPT CLOSED REMOVAL**

- Unsuccessful → Foreign body location:
  - Ⓔ Thoracic inlet → **CERVICAL APPROACH**
    - Successful exposure → Massage and Remove
    - Unsuccessful exposure → **MEDIAN STERNOTOMY** → Massage and Remove
      - Successful → Examine esophagus
      - Unsuccessful removal → ESOPHAGOTOMY
  - Ⓕ Heart base → **LEFT 5TH OR 6TH INTERCOSTAL THORACOTOMY** → (to Massage and Remove / ESOPHAGOTOMY)
  - Ⓖ Esophageal hiatus → **CELIOTOMY AND GASTROTOMY**
    - Successful removal → Examine esophagus
    - Unsuccessful removal → **LEFT 8TH INTERCOSTAL THORACOTOMY** → Massage and Remove
      - Successful → Examine esophagus
      - Unsuccessful → **TRANSDIAPHRAGMATIC APPROACH**
        - Successful removal → Examine esophagus
        - Unsuccessful removal → **ESOPHAGOTOMY**
          - Potential leakage → Ⓘ **DIAPHRAGMATIC MUSCLE PATCH**
          - Secure closure → Examine esophagus

- Successful → Examine esophagus
  - Ⓗ Perforation
    - 1–2 mm → Conservative treatment
    - >2 mm → **SURGICAL REPAIR**
  - Normal → Follow at 2-week intervals for 3 months
  - Esophagitis (p 10)

MEGAESOPHAGUS

Howard B. Seim III

A. Patients with megaesophagus present with a history of regurgitation of undigested food minutes to hours after eating. Clinical signs become apparent at weaning. It is imperative to differentiate regurgitation from vomiting and to determine the time interval between eating and regurgitation. Frequency of regurgitation varies from once every 2 to 3 days to 10 to 20 times per day.

B. Patients should be evaluated for respiratory disorders secondary to aspiration of food. Older patients may present with significant weight loss, regurgitation, and respiratory problems.

C. Plain and contrast radiography of the cervical and thoracic esophagus is helpful in evaluation of regurgitation. Feeding a canned food mixed with barium sulfate allows differential diagnosis of esophageal foreign body, esophageal stricture, vascular ring anomaly, and megaesophagus.

D. Cinefluorography, in conjunction with barium administration, allows careful assessment of primary and secondary esophageal peristalsis and the synchronous or asynchronous function of the lower esophageal sphincter (LES).

E. Patients that lack normal primary and secondary esophageal peristalsis, yet retain normal LES pressure as revealed by manometric studies, may have idiopathic or acquired megaesophagus. In idiopathic megaesophagus, the exact location of the defect has not been identified; however isolated studies have incriminated the nucleus ambiguous and/or local muscle abnormalities. These cases usually occur in young dogs; upright feeding with a diet of varying consistency has helped in the management of these cases. Acquired megaesophagus generally occurs in older dogs and can be caused by the following: lead poisoning, hypoadrenocorticism, myasthenia gravis, distemper, polymyositis, neoplasia, and systemic lupus erythematosus. These diseases must be ruled in, or out, in order to definitively diagnose acquired megaesophagus.

F. Patients with evidence of primary and secondary esophageal peristalsis, in which manometric studies reveal asynchronous closure (spasm) of the LES, are diagnosed as having achalasia. A modified Heller's procedure (LES myotomy) may be helpful in patients with true achalasia. A left eighth intercostal thoracotomy is performed, the esophagus is isolated and mobilized cranially, and a longitudinal incision is made through the diaphragm at the esophageal hiatus to expose the LES. An incision through the muscle fibers of the LES is made in the same direction as that in the diaphragm. The incision is carried through all layers of the esophagus except for the mucosal layer. The mucosa bulges through the myotomy incision when the appropriate depth is reached. The incision in the diaphragm is closed transversely, and the thoracotomy incision is closed routinely. The prognosis for cure is guarded. Many patients require continued upright feeding.

References

Hoffer RE, McCoy DM, Quick CB, Barclay SM, Rendaro VT. Management of acquired achalasia in dogs. JAVMA 1979; 175:814.

Leib MS, Hall RL. Megaesophagus in the dog. Part II. Clinical aspects. Comp Cont Ed 1984; 6(1):11.

Shelton GD. Swallowing disorders in the dog. Comp Cont Ed 1982; 4(7):607.

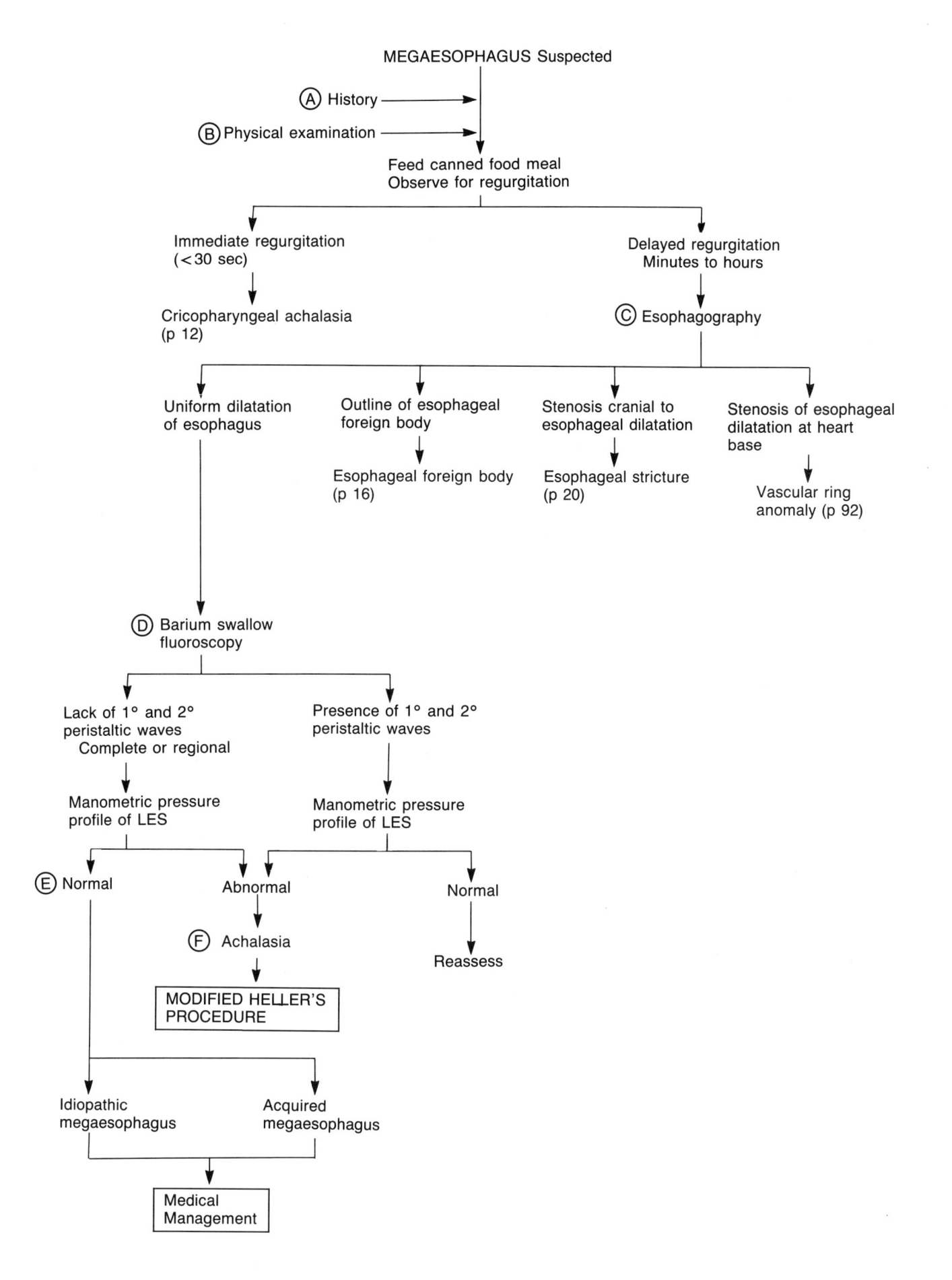

```
                    MEGAESOPHAGUS Suspected
                            │
              (A) History ──────────▶
                                     │
              (B) Physical examination ──▶
                            │
                    Feed canned food meal
                    Observe for regurgitation
                            │
           ┌────────────────┴────────────────┐
           ▼                                 ▼
   Immediate regurgitation            Delayed regurgitation
        (<30 sec)                       Minutes to hours
           │                                 │
           ▼                                 ▼
   Cricopharyngeal achalasia          (C) Esophagography
        (p 12)                               │
           │            ┌───────────┬────────┴────────┬─────────────────┐
           ▼            ▼           ▼                 ▼                 ▼
    Uniform dilatation  Outline of        Stenosis cranial to    Stenosis of esophageal
    of esophagus        esophageal        esophageal dilatation  dilatation at heart
                        foreign body                             base
                            │                 │                     │
                            ▼                 ▼                     ▼
                    Esophageal foreign body  Esophageal stricture  Vascular ring
                        (p 16)                (p 20)               anomaly (p 92)
           │
           ▼
    (D) Barium swallow
        fluoroscopy
           │
    ┌──────┴──────┐
    ▼             ▼
Lack of 1° and 2°    Presence of 1° and 2°
peristaltic waves    peristaltic waves
Complete or regional
    │                     │
    ▼                     ▼
Manometric pressure   Manometric pressure
profile of LES        profile of LES
    │                     │
 ┌──┴──┐              ┌───┴───┐
 ▼     ▼              ▼       ▼
(E) Normal  Abnormal  Normal
 │          │         │
 │          ▼         ▼
 │     (F) Achalasia  Reassess
 │          │
 │          ▼
 │    ┌──────────────┐
 │    │MODIFIED HELLER'S│
 │    │  PROCEDURE   │
 │    └──────────────┘
 │
 ┌────┴────┐
 ▼         ▼
Idiopathic  Acquired
megaesophagus  megaesophagus
      │
      ▼
  ┌──────────┐
  │ Medical  │
  │Management│
  └──────────┘
```

ESOPHAGEAL STRICTURE

Howard B. Seim III

A. Patients with acquired esophageal stricture present with frequent dysphagia and regurgitation, which are manifested by the decreased ability to eat solid food. A history of recent anesthesia, exposure to caustic chemicals, esophageal foreign body, or esophageal surgery are factors that may lead to diagnosis of esophageal stricture.

B. The physical examination is often unremarkable. It is helpful diagnostically to feed the patient a solid diet and to then observe for dysphagia and regurgitation.

C. Definitive diagnosis and localization of an esophageal stricture is made by positive-contrast esophageal radiography. A barium paste swallow demonstrates segmental narrowing of the esophageal lumen as well as indicating the length of the strictured area. Endoscopic examination allows diagnosis of the stricture and evaluation of the appearance and pliability of the esophageal wall.

D. Bougienage is accomplished by dilation of the esophagus at the strictured area. Esophageal dilators (bougies), either steel stem or mercury-filled rubber and ranging in gauge up to 60, are ideal for bougienage. The patient is anesthetized, the stricture is located with esophagoscopy, and the dilator is introduced. In cats and small dogs, a minimum bougie of 1 cm is recommended; medium-sized to large dogs should have a 1 to 1.5 cm diameter. Bougienage is repeated weekly or biweekly for up to 3 months. Administer prednisolone 0.5 mg per kilogram daily for 1 to 2 weeks, then reduce the dose to 0.2 mg per kilogram daily for an additional 2 to 4 weeks. Patients are kept on a permanent diet of slurried or soft food. Successful treatment can be expected in approximately 75 percent of patients treated with bougienage.

E. Use sternothyroideus or diaphragmatic patch grafts to facilitate closure in patients that undergo surgical correction of esophageal stricture in the cervical or the distal thoracic esophagus respectively.

F. Longitudinal esophagotomy through the stricture, with a transverse closure, may be effective in treating esophageal strictures less than 1 cm long. Close the esophagotomy incision in two layers by the use of simple interrupted sutures in the mucosa and submucosa, with knots tied into the lumen using 3-0 or 4-0 synthetic absorbable or nonabsorbable suture, and by the use of interrupted horizontal mattress sutures in the muscle, with a similar size and type of suture material (Fig. 1).

G. Locate the cranial and caudal limits of the stricture area and resect the appropriate amount of esophagus. The anastomosis is performed in a similar manner to the esophagotomy closure. Tension on the anastomosis is a major intraoperative danger that predisposes to significant postoperative complications. Perform tension-relieving techniques such as phrenic nerve blockage or sectioning, traction suturing from 1 cm caudal to the

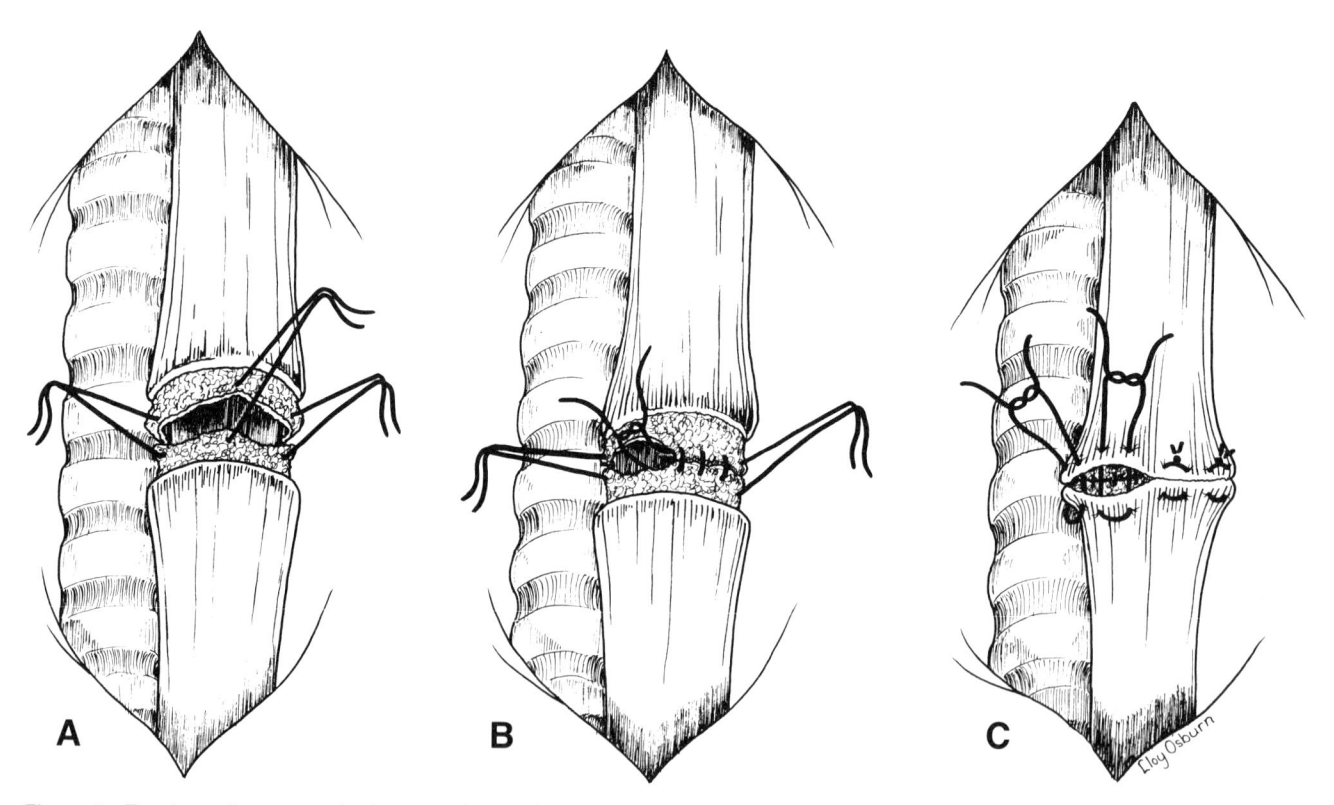

Figure 1 Esophageal anastomosis: *A*, mucosal approximation and alignment with stay sutures; *B*, mucosal closure with simple interrupted sutures, with knots within the lumen; and *C*, muscularis closed with horizontal mattress sutures.

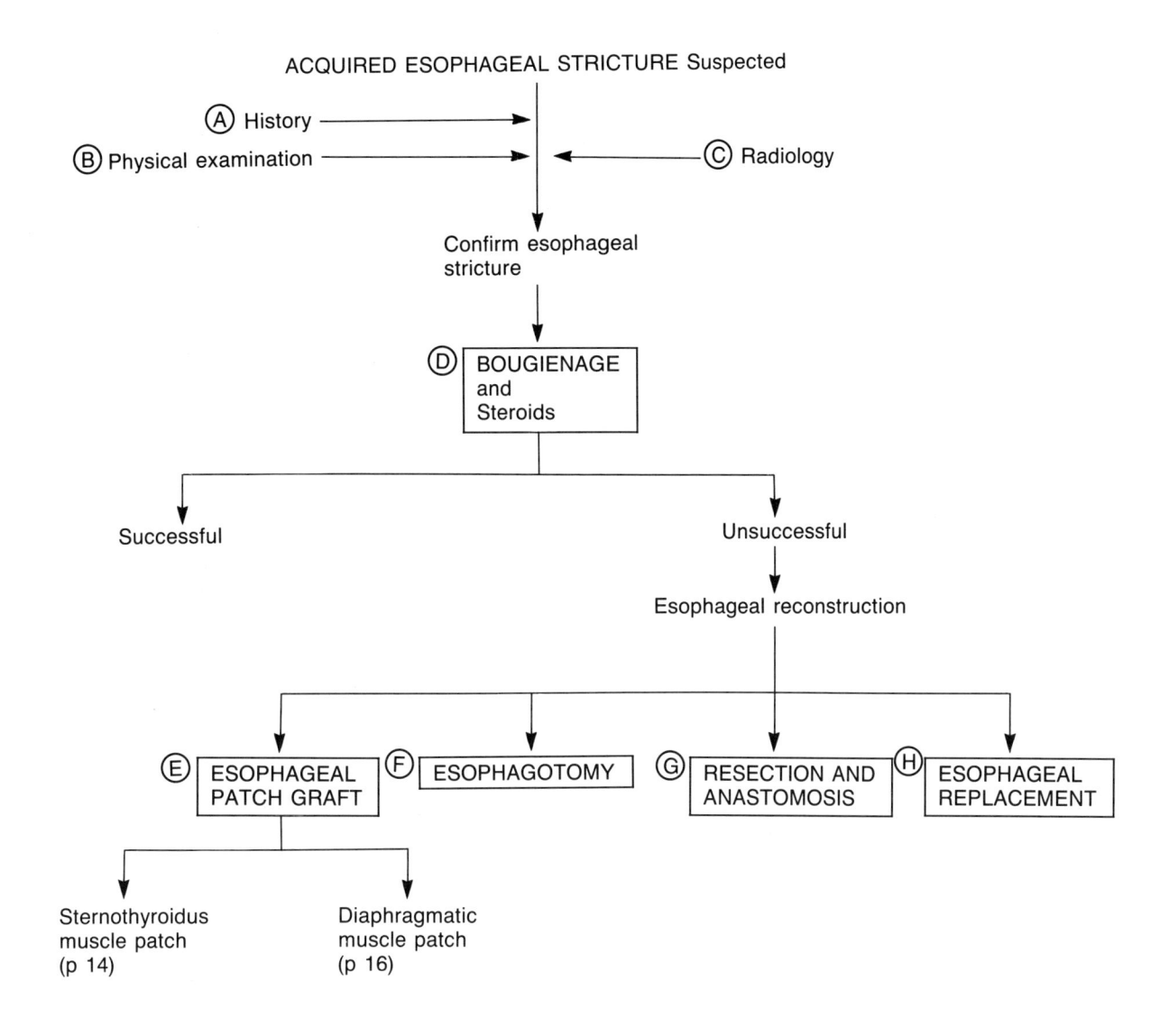

ACQUIRED ESOPHAGEAL STRICTURE Suspected

- (A) History
- (B) Physical examination
- (C) Radiology

↓ Confirm esophageal stricture

(D) **BOUGIENAGE and Steroids**

- Successful
- Unsuccessful → Esophageal reconstruction
  - (E) **ESOPHAGEAL PATCH GRAFT**
    - Sternothyroidus muscle patch (p 14)
    - Diaphragmatic muscle patch (p 16)
  - (F) **ESOPHAGOTOMY**
  - (G) **RESECTION AND ANASTOMOSIS**
  - (H) **ESOPHAGEAL REPLACEMENT**

anastomosis to the prevertebral fascia, circular myotomy of the outer longitudinal muscle layer, or patch grafting. Placement of a feeding gastrostomy tube is recommended for the first 1 to 2 postoperative weeks.

H. Elaborate techniques for esophageal replacement, utilizing pedicled GI segments (stomach, colon, jejunum), inverse tubed skin segments, and various patching and grafting techniques have been described. These procedures are technically difficult and have high morbidity and mortality rates; they are regarded as salvage procedures.

Reference

Harvey CE. Conservative treatment of acquired esophageal stricture. In: Slatter DH, ed. Textbook of small animal surgery. Philadelphia: WB Saunders, 1985:661.

VOMITING

Howard B. Seim III

A. The history of a patient that presents with vomiting may offer the most diagnostic information. It is important to differentiate between vomiting and regurgitation. The history should include general information such as environmental and vaccination history, previous medical problems, present medication, parasitic control program, dietary information, the nature of the illness as well as the onset, the duration, and the character of the vomitus.

B. A complete physical examination is performed with emphasis on palpation and auscultation of the cranial and midabdominal regions.

C. Depending upon the historical and physical findings, the minimum data base may include complete blood count, electrolyte analysis, acid-base evaluation, complete biochemical profile, and urinalysis.

D. The patient is stabilized as dictated by the physical examination and clinical pathologic findings. It is important to realize that vomiting is a clinical sign, not a disease; it can result from many mechanisms. The origin of the stimulus for vomiting must be determined. The history, clinical pathology, and the physical and neurologic examinations may point to one of the following pathogenic mechanisms.

E. Direct stimulation of the vomiting center results in the reflex act of emesis. This direct stimulation may be in the form of elevated CSF pressure, CNS neoplasia, or CNS inflammation. Diagnosis is generally confirmed on EEG, CSF evaluation, radiography, or CT scanning.

F. Indirect stimulation of the vomiting center may occur from cerebrocortical stimulation (higher centers), chemoreceptor trigger zone (CTZ) stimulation, or peripheral receptor stimulation.

G. Stimulation of the higher centers may originate from stressful situations, severe pain, or fear. Treatment is directed at controlling the signs and removing the cause.

H. Stimulation of the CTZ may occur due to drug toxicities (apomorphine, morphine, digitalis), radiation sickness, metabolic disorders (uremia, acidosis), bacterial endotoxins or motion sickness. Treatment is directed at controlling the signs and removing the cause.

I. Stimulation of various peripheral receptors may result in vomition. Sites of peripheral stimulation include the pharynx, gastrointestinal tract, pancreas, liver, mesentery, peritoneum, urinary tract and heart. The stimulus is generally mediated by the vagal and sympathetic nerves in the GI tract and abdominal viscera, and the glossopharyngeal nerve in the pharynx. Stimulus may come in the form of inflammation, irritation, distention or hyperosmolality.

J. Evaluation of the peripheral receptors includes radiography (routine films as well as contrast studies), endoscopy and biopsy procedures. Gastric fluid analysis and gastric secretory testing may also be used in complicated cases.

Reference

Twedt DC. Differential diagnosis and therapy of vomiting. Vet Clin North Am 1983; 13(3):503.

VOMITING Suspected

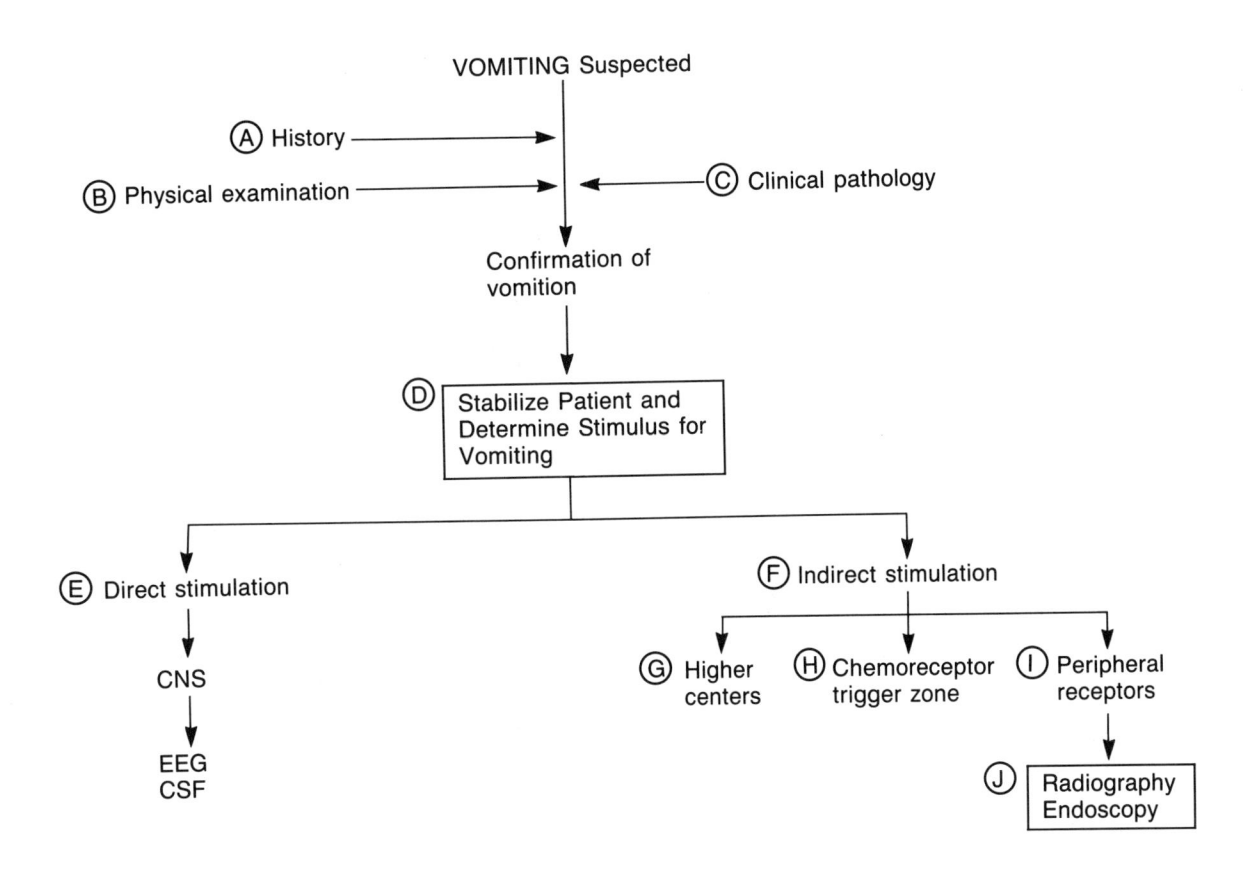

- (A) History
- (B) Physical examination
- (C) Clinical pathology

↓

Confirmation of vomition

↓

(D) Stabilize Patient and Determine Stimulus for Vomiting

- (E) Direct stimulation
  ↓
  CNS
  ↓
  EEG
  CSF

- (F) Indirect stimulation
  - (G) Higher centers
  - (H) Chemoreceptor trigger zone
  - (I) Peripheral receptors
    ↓
    (J) Radiography Endoscopy

GASTRIC DILATATION-VOLVULUS

Howard B. Seim III

A. The classic history for a dog with gastric dilatation-volvulus (GDV) is a large, deep-chested breed that has recently ingested a large quantity of food and/or water, has shortly thereafter been taken for a walk or run, and is beginning to show signs of sudden abdominal distention and nonproductive retching.

B. The immediate physical examination reveals abdominal distention, tympany in the cranial abdominal region, mental and respiratory depression, and shock.

C. Patients that present with the above history and physical findings require immediate stabilization. Simultaneous therapy for hypovolemic shock and gastric dilatation is mandatory and begins with volume replacement polyionic isotonic fluids, steroids, and antibiotics. Decompression can be accomplished by orogastric intubation or temporary gastrostomy. Orogastric intubation can be accomplished in 80 to 90 percent of GDV patients. This technique may be facilitated by prior gastric trocarization with two or three 16 to 18 gauge needles. If intubation is not successful, temporary gastrostomy may be necessary for patient stabilization prior to anesthesia induction. Careful cardiac monitoring is an essential part of the preoperative preparation.

D. Definitive surgical correction should not be considered until the gastric decompression and hypovolemic shock therapy have accomplished patient stabilization. Viability of the gastric wall is determined by evaluation of serosal color, the degree of active bleeding from the incised gastric wall, and palpation of the gastric wall. Viability determination dictates the initial surgical plan: gastrectomy or gastropexy. Patients with gastric wall necrosis may benefit from partial or total gastrectomy. Patients with a viable gastric wall should have a gastropexy performed (Fig. 1). Tube gastrostomy, circumcostal gastropexy, and incision- or scarified-type gastropexy have shown to be successful in both experimental and clinical cases. The use of concurrent pyloromyotomy or pyloroplasty is controversial. Splenectomy may be necessary (p 212).

E. Feeding of the postoperative GDV patient is dictated by stomach viability and surgical procedure performed. In complicated partial or total gastrectomy, the surgical site should be bypassed by placement of a needle catheter jejunostomy feeding tube. This can remain until feeding per os is tolerated by the patient. In gastropexy-treated patients with questionable gastric wall viability, oral feeding is postponed for 3 to 4 days. If the gastric wall is viable, feeding can commence within 24 to 48 hours postoperatively.

F. The occurrence of cardiac arrhythmias in patients with GDV has been reported to be as high as 42 percent. The majority are of ventricular origin and occur within 24 hours of hospitalization. The most common life-threatening arrhythmia is ventricular tachycardia.* In general, GDV arrhythmias are refractory and difficult to control. However, vigorous treatment, although not often reversing the arrhythmia, often improves cardiac output enough to maintain the animal's life. Ventricular tachycardia is initially treated with a bolus (2 to 4 mg per kilogram) of 2 percent lidocaine (without epinephrine). This can be repeated two to four times, then a constant infusion of 50 μg per kilogram per minute is used to keep the heart converted. Quinidine gluconate (6 to 22 mg per kilogram, two to three times a day) may be used for long-term conversion. If quinidine fails to resolve the arrhythmia, oral procainamide (125 to 500 mg, three to four times per day, not to exceed 33 to 50 mg per kilogram per day) can be attempted. Frequent ECG evaluations should be done to determine success of therapy. Most patients can be tapered off medication in 3 to 4 days, although some cases may require treatment for as long as 3 to 4 weeks. An ECG should be used to monitor success of withdrawal.

*Treatment of ventricular tachycardia is somewhat controversial; some authors feel that with more than 5 premature beats per minute, treatment should be instituted; others use 15 premature beats per minute as the critical level.

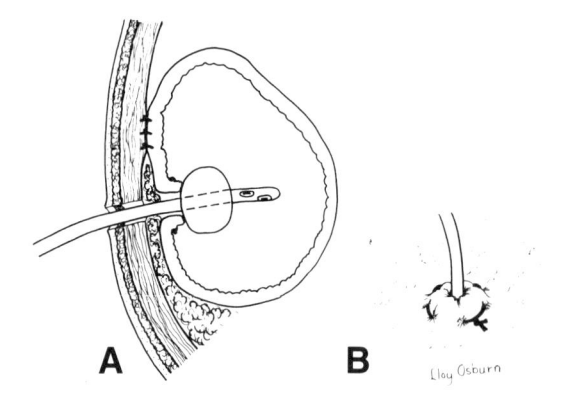

Figure 1 Tube gastropexy using a Foley catheter; *A*, the omentum is interpositioned between the gastric and abdominal walls to ensure a seal and the gastric and abdominal walls are approximated with sutures; *B*, the tube exits the gastric wall through a stab incision that is tightly closed with a pursestring suture.

References

Fallah AM, Lumb WV, Nelson AW, Frandson RD, Withrow SJ. Circumcostal gastropexy in the dog: a preliminary study. Vet Surg 1982; 11(1):9

Johnson RG, Barrus J, Greene RW. Gastric dilatation-volvulus: recurrence rate following tube gastrostomy. JAAHA 1984; 20:33.

Leib MS, Blass CE. Gastric dilatation-volvulus in dogs: an update. Comp Cont Ed 1984; 6(11):961.

MacCoy DM, Sykes GP, Hoffer RE, Harvey HJ. A gastropexy technique for permanent fixation of the pyloric antrum. JAAHA 1982; 18:763.

Matthiesen DT. Partial gastrectomy as treatment of gastric volvulus: results in 30 dogs. Vet Surg 1985; 14(3):185.

Muir WW, Bonagura JD. Treatment of cardiac arrhythmias in dogs with gastric distention-volvulus. JAVMA 1984; 184:(2):1366.

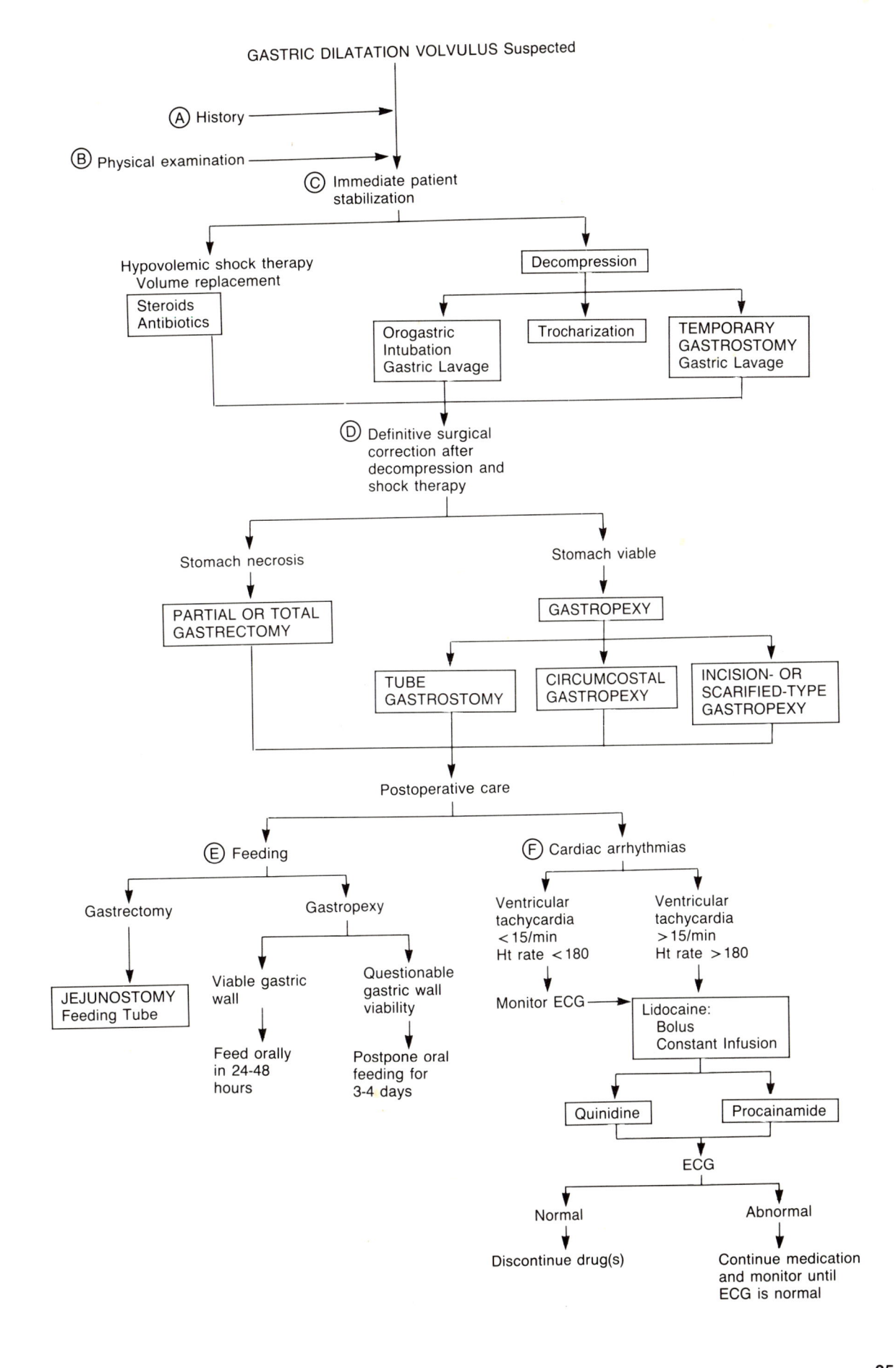

GASTRIC DILATATION VOLVULUS Suspected

- (A) History
- (B) Physical examination
- (C) Immediate patient stabilization
  - Hypovolemic shock therapy / Volume replacement
    - Steroids
    - Antibiotics
  - Decompression
    - Orogastric Intubation / Gastric Lavage
    - Trocharization
    - TEMPORARY GASTROSTOMY / Gastric Lavage
- (D) Definitive surgical correction after decompression and shock therapy
  - Stomach necrosis → PARTIAL OR TOTAL GASTRECTOMY
  - Stomach viable → GASTROPEXY
    - TUBE GASTROSTOMY
    - CIRCUMCOSTAL GASTROPEXY
    - INCISION- OR SCARIFIED-TYPE GASTROPEXY

Postoperative care

- (E) Feeding
  - Gastrectomy → JEJUNOSTOMY Feeding Tube
  - Gastropexy
    - Viable gastric wall → Feed orally in 24-48 hours
    - Questionable gastric wall viability → Postpone oral feeding for 3-4 days
- (F) Cardiac arrhythmias
  - Ventricular tachycardia <15/min, Ht rate <180 → Monitor ECG
  - Ventricular tachycardia >15/min, Ht rate >180 → Lidocaine: Bolus, Constant Infusion
    - Quinidine
    - Procainamide
  - ECG
    - Normal → Discontinue drug(s)
    - Abnormal → Continue medication and monitor until ECG is normal

OBSTRUCTION OF THE SMALL INTESTINE

Howard B. Seim III

A. One of the greatest pitfalls of intestinal obstruction is a delay in establishing the diagnosis. Whenever a patient presents with gastrointestinal signs such as acute or chronic vomiting, diarrhea, abdominal tenderness, dehydration, anorexia, and depression, intestinal obstruction should be included on the list of differential diagnoses. Careful historical examination may help in determining the location of the obstruction (e.g., proximal versus distal).

B. A thorough physical examination of the vomiting patient must be performed with particular attention to abdominal palpation. Careful palpation with positional changes (e.g., front legs off the ground) may allow diagnosis of suspected intestinal obstruction, particularly in cases of intussusception (p 28) and foreign bodies (p 30). Examination of hydration and mucous membrane perfusion and color may help determine preoperative therapy.

C. The minimum data base should include complete blood count (CBC), electrolytes, BUN, glucose, and acid-base status. The CBC may reveal sepsis and gives a baseline for comparison in the event of postoperative complications. Electrolyte evaluation, particularly sodium, potassium, and chloride, allows proper selection of fluid for volume replacement. Renal function should be assessed in order to select appropriate fluid volume. Glucose is measured to assess the presence or absence of sepsis. Blood gas evaluation ensures accurate assessment of the patient's acid-base status and dictates appropriate therapy.

D. Plain abdominal x-rays should be evaluated for signs of gastrointestinal obstruction including ileus, loss of detail of abdominal structures, and free gas in the abdominal cavity. Contrast radiography (upper GI series) should be performed in patients that have inconclusive radiographic findings, yet have a history of gastrointestinal signs consistent with obstructive disease.

E. Preoperative stabilization depends on the patient's preoperative status and the minimum data base results. In general, volume replacement with polyionic, isotonic fluids is required, and broad-spectrum antibiotics should be administered. Patients suspected of being septic should have steroids, glucose, and banamine (1 mg per kilogram) added to the preoperative treatment regimen before performing exploratory celiotomy.

F. Another potential pitfall in cases of intestinal obstruction is the ability to accurately evaluate viable versus nonviable bowel. Standard criteria include bowel colors, peristalsis, pulsation of arteries to the suspect segment, and blood flow from a cut bowel surface. Bowel viability can best be evaluated by intravenous injection of fluorescein dye. The characteristic fluorescent pattern of viability versus nonviability provides an accurate evaluation of the bowel intraoperatively.

G. If an enterotomy is indicated (e.g., intraluminal foreign body) the incision is best placed on the healthy side of the foreign body (generally aboral). The closure may be accomplished by simple interrupted apposing, simple interrupted crushing, or simple continuous apposing suture patterns, using 4-0 or 5-0 monofilament nonabsorbable or synthetic absorbable suture material on a reverse cutting or taper-cut needle.

H. Resection and anastomosis may be performed by any of the techniques previously described for enterotomy closure. Generally, the remaining small intestine can compensate for a 50 to 60 percent resection. However, if 70 to 80 percent of the small bowel is resected, a hyperacidic environment occurs and significantly decreases the compensatory ability of the remaining small bowel, as well as inhibiting the action of digestive enzymes, particularly lipase. The majority of these patients can be managed with cimetidine therapy (44 mg per kilogram three times a day).

I. In situations of potential leakage or existing peritonitis, the enterotomy or anastomosis can be protected by suturing a healthy piece of bowel (generally jejunum) to the incision site in order to form a serosal patch. Polypropylene (4-0 or 5-0) in a simple interrupted pattern is used to suture the patch in place.

J. Delay in postoperative feeding is based on the preoperative status of the patient, intraoperative status of the bowel, procedures performed, and the postoperative status of the patient.

References

Crowe DT Jr. The serosal patch: clinical use in 12 animals. Vet Surg 1984; 13(1):29.

Ellison GW, Jokinen MP, Park RD. End-to-end approximating intestinal anastamosis in the dog: a comparative fluorescein dye, angiographic and histopathologic evaluation. JAAHA 1982; 18:729.

Lantz GC. The pathophysiology of acute mechanical small bowel obstruction. Comp Cont Ed 1981; 3(10):910.

Wheaton LG, Strandberg JD, Hamiliton SR, Bulkley GB. A comparison of three techniques for intraoperative prediction of small intestinal injury. JAAHA 1983; 19:897.

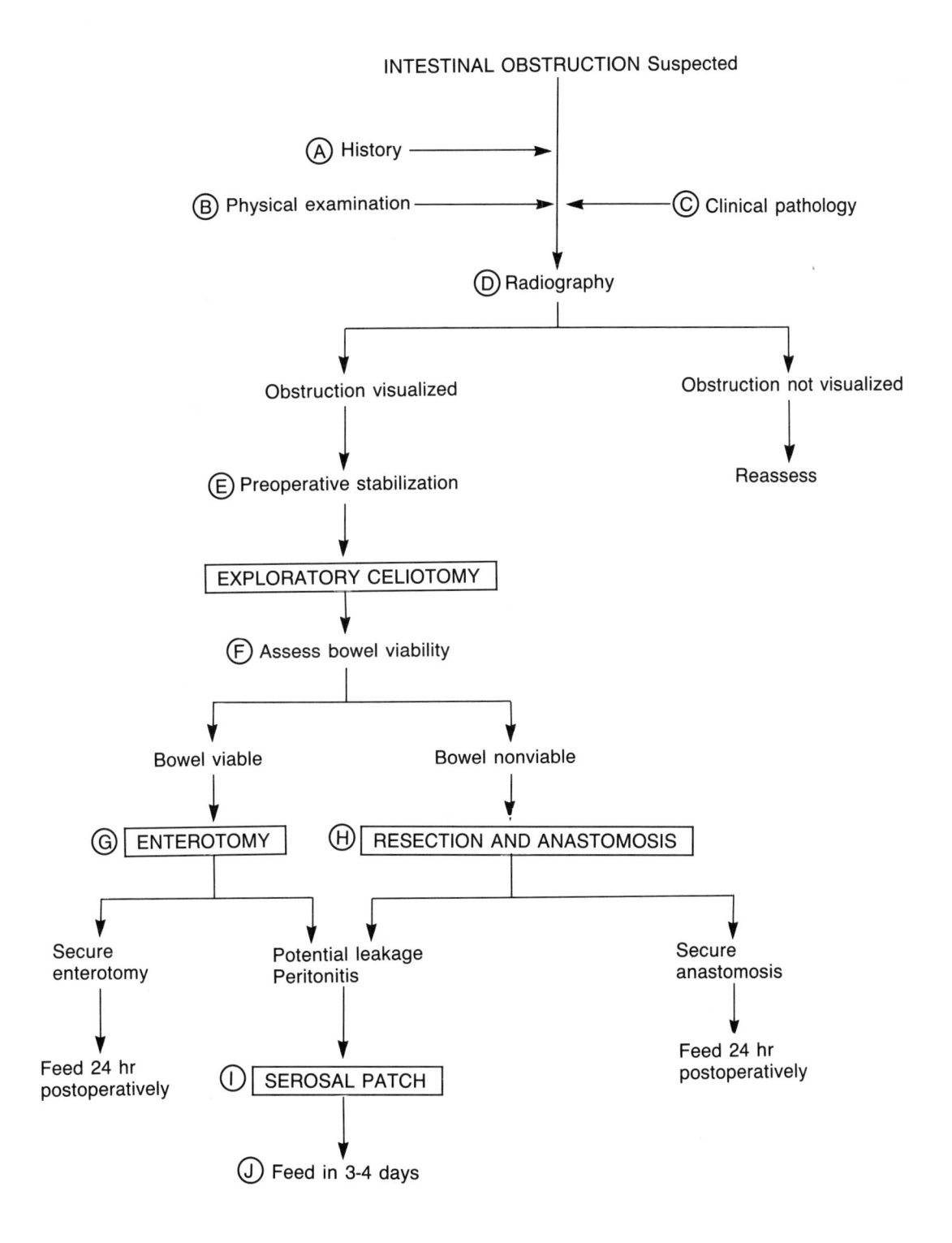

```
                    INTESTINAL OBSTRUCTION Suspected
                                  │
         Ⓐ History ───────────────▶│
                                  │
    Ⓑ Physical examination ──────▶│◀────── Ⓒ Clinical pathology
                                  ▼
                           Ⓓ Radiography
                          ┌───────┴────────┐
                          ▼                ▼
                 Obstruction visualized   Obstruction not visualized
                          │                │
                          ▼                ▼
              Ⓔ Preoperative stabilization  Reassess
                          │
                          ▼
                ┌─────────────────────┐
                │ EXPLORATORY CELIOTOMY│
                └─────────────────────┘
                          │
                          ▼
                 Ⓕ Assess bowel viability
                    ┌─────┴─────┐
                    ▼           ▼
               Bowel viable  Bowel nonviable
                    │           │
                    ▼           ▼
            Ⓖ┌───────────┐  Ⓗ┌──────────────────────────┐
              │ENTEROTOMY │    │ RESECTION AND ANASTOMOSIS│
              └───────────┘    └──────────────────────────┘
                ┌──────┴────────┬──────────┬──────────┐
                ▼               ▼          ▼          ▼
             Secure        Potential leakage      Secure
           enterotomy        Peritonitis        anastomosis
                │               │                   │
                ▼               ▼                   ▼
            Feed 24 hr    Ⓘ┌──────────────┐    Feed 24 hr
          postoperatively   │SEROSAL PATCH │   postoperatively
                            └──────────────┘
                                  │
                                  ▼
                          Ⓙ Feed in 3-4 days
```

INTUSSUSCEPTION

Howard B. Seim III

A. Intussusception should be suspected in any young dog or cat that presents with a history consistent with intestinal obstruction (p 26). Abdominal palpation may result in discomfort and often reveals a sausage-like mass. The mass may come and go if the patient has a sliding intussusception. Older patients rarely present with spontaneous intussusception.

B. Plain radiographs may reveal an obstructive pattern. A barium enema and/or an upper GI series are generally successful in outlining the intussusception.

C. Prior to surgical intervention, the patient should be stabilized with polyionic, isotonic fluids (volume replacement), systemic antibiotics, and treatment for sepsis if indicated by the physical examination, and the minimum data base results.

D. Patients with a "sliding" intussusception may present with periodic signs of intestinal obstruction and a palpable abdominal mass that comes and goes. These patients should be reassessed by frequent careful palpation for 2 to 3 days to document the presence or absence of an intussusception. If the intussusception does not recur, the patient is discharged with careful instructions to watch for signs of intestinal obstruction. If the intussusception recurs, a celiotomy should be performed, the intussusception reduced or resected, and the bowel plicated.

E. A celiotomy is performed and the affected bowel gently exteriorized. When attempting to reduce the intussusception, *push* distally and gently pull proximally (do not pull hard) on the bowel. Most intussesceptions can be reduced in this manner without significant serosal tears or disruption of the mesenteric blood supply.

F. If the intussusception is reducible and viable, plication may be necessary to prevent recurrence, if no initiating cause is found. The bowel is gently plicated from the distal duodenum to the distal ileum. The seromuscular layers of adjoining bowel loops are sutured with 4-0 absorbable suture in a simple interrupted pattern. Strong serosal adhesions will prevent reintussusception of the hypermotile bowel.

G. An irreducible intussusception or a reducible intussusception with nonviable bowel should be resected. The anastomosis is accomplished as described on p 26. If a foreign body, tumor, or other obvious cause of intussusception is present, plication is not necessary. However, if the cause cannot be determined, plication should be performed in order to prevent recurrence (Fig. 1).

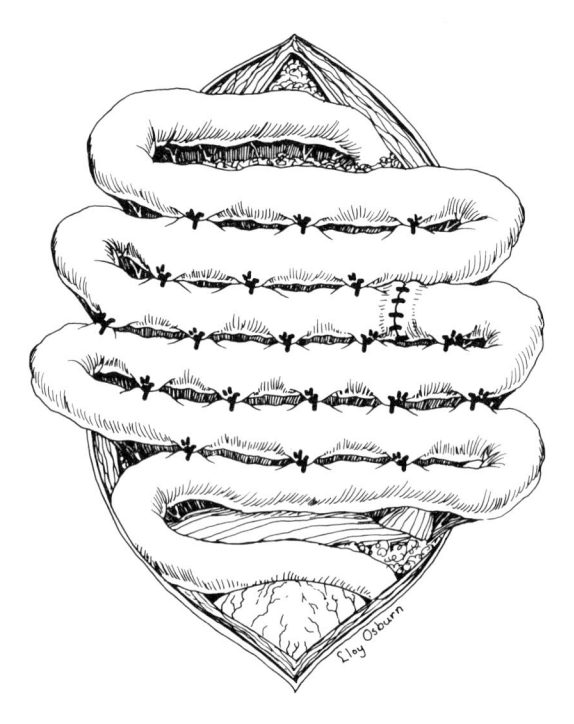

Figure 1 Reoccurrence of intussusception prevented by bowel plication.

References

Ragins H, Freeman L, Coomaraswamy R, et al. Clinical and experimental comparison of the Noble and Childs-Phillips plication of small bowel. Am J Surg 1966; 111:555.

Wilson GP, Burt JK. Intussusception in the dog and cat: a review of 45 cases. JAVMA 1974; 164(5):515.

Wolfe DA. Recurrent intestinal intussusception in the dog. JAVMA 1977; 171(6):553.

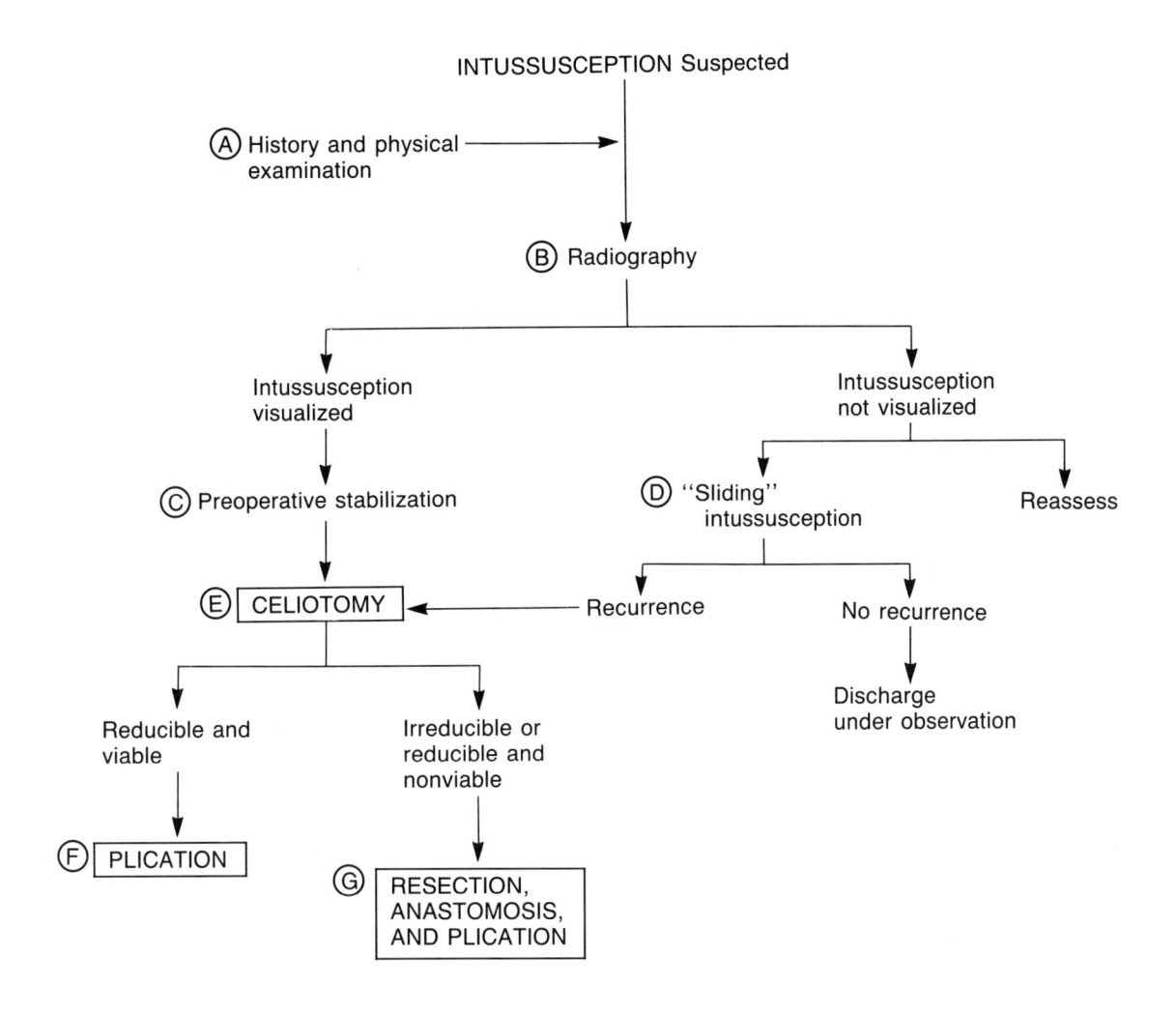

INTUSSUSCEPTION Suspected

- (A) History and physical examination
- (B) Radiography
  - Intussusception visualized
    - (C) Preoperative stabilization
    - (E) CELIOTOMY
      - Reducible and viable
        - (F) PLICATION
      - Irreducible or reducible and nonviable
        - (G) RESECTION, ANASTOMOSIS, AND PLICATION
  - Intussusception not visualized
    - (D) "Sliding" intussusception
      - Recurrence → (E) CELIOTOMY
      - No recurrence → Discharge under observation
    - Reassess

LINEAR INTESTINAL FOREIGN BODY

Howard B. Seim III

A. Patients with a linear foreign body (string, tinsel, yarn, plastic bags) generally present with an acute history of persistent vomiting, anorexia, and depression. These signs are common with many gastrointestinal disturbances, and linear foreign body should be included in the differential diagnosis. Occasionally, patients are presented late in the course of the disease and may have a history of occasional vomiting with anorexia, depression, and weight loss as the major presenting signs.

B. A thorough physical examination should be performed with emphasis on oral examination and abdominal palpation. Oral examination often finds the linear foreign body around the base of the tongue or an area of inflammation at the junction of the base of the tongue and frenulum. Abdominal palpation may reveal "bunched up" small intestine due to bowel plication. When this finding is made, the clinician must be very gentle with abdominal manipulations.

C. Definitive diagnosis is based on characteristic findings on plain and contrast radiography. Plain radiographs may reveal plicated bowel bunched up in the midabdominal region. Because of the plicated nature of the bowel, air accumulation forms a characteristic "tapered enteric gas bubble." Three or more tapered gas bubbles are diagnostic for linear foreign body. Patients with inconclusive plain radiographs should have an upper GI contrast study performed. This will reveal the typical plicated appearance of the bowel if there is a linear foreign body.

D. After appropriate preoperative preparation a celiotomy is performed. The most orad portion of the foreign body is located and dislodged (tongue, stomach, pylorus, or small intestine). The extent of the linear foreign body is determined, and two or three enterotomies are performed to allow its atraumatic removal. Care is taken to remove the linear foreign body in segments short enough that further cutting of the intestine does not occur during removal, yet long enough to perform a minimum number of enterotomies. Colotomies are generally *not* indicated because once the string is in the colon, it can be passed with little danger of causing obstruction.

E. After the foreign body has been removed, a close examination of the mesenteric border is made for evidence of nonviable segments or perforation. All perforations should be debrided and sutured.

F. If multiple perforations occur, a resection and anastomosis may be necessary. Generally, the remaining small intestine can compensate for a 50 to 60 percent resection. However, if 70 to 80 percent of the small bowel is resected, a hyperacidic environment occurs and significantly decreases the compensatory ability of the remaining small bowel as well as inhibiting the action of digestive enzymes, particularly lipase. The majority of these patients can be managed with cimetidine therapy (44 mg per kilogram twice a day).

References

Felts JF, Fox PR, Burk RL. Thread and sewing needles as gastrointestinal foreign bodies in the cat: a review of 64 cases. JAVMA 1984; 184(1):56.

Root CR, Lord PF. Linear radiolucent gastrointestinal foreign bodies in, cats and dogs: their radiographic appearance. J Am Vet Radiol Soc 1971; 12:45.

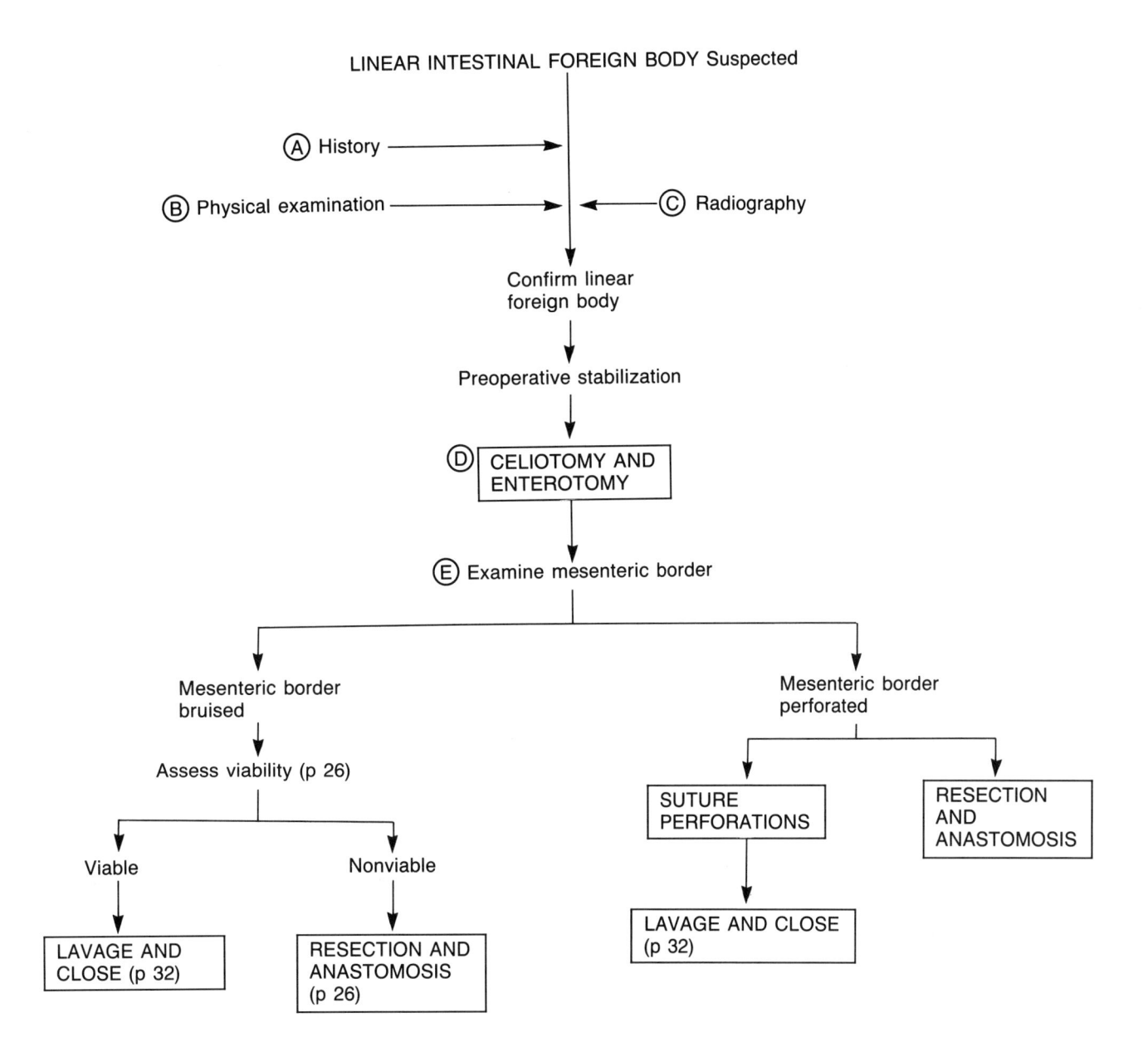

LINEAR INTESTINAL FOREIGN BODY Suspected

- (A) History
- (B) Physical examination
- (C) Radiography

Confirm linear foreign body

Preoperative stabilization

(D) **CELIOTOMY AND ENTEROTOMY**

(E) Examine mesenteric border

- Mesenteric border bruised
  - Assess viability (p 26)
    - Viable → **LAVAGE AND CLOSE (p 32)**
    - Nonviable → **RESECTION AND ANASTOMOSIS (p 26)**
- Mesenteric border perforated
  - **SUTURE PERFORATIONS** → **LAVAGE AND CLOSE (p 32)**
  - **RESECTION AND ANASTOMOSIS**

31

INTESTINAL PERFORATION

Howard B. Seim III

A. Patients presenting with acute, severe abdominal pain (acute abdomen), vomiting, depression, anorexia, and particularly those patients with a recent history of intestinal surgery or a penetrating abdominal wound, should be suspected of having an intestinal perforation.

B. The physical findings are nonspecific and may include abdominal tenderness, abdominal distention, fever, severe depression, and purple or muddy-colored mucous membranes. The minimum data base results may reveal early signs of sepsis.

C. Confirmation of intestinal perforation may be accomplished by a combination of radiography and paracentesis. Plain abdominal radiographs may reveal an obstructive pattern and/or free gas in the peritoneal cavity. An upper GI series may be performed in suspected cases that do not show characteristic plain film findings. Due to the severe peritoneal irritation caused by barium, organic iodides are the contrast agent of choice. Cytology evaluated from a four quadrant peritoneal tap or diagnostic peritoneal lavage may reveal characteristic findings associated with intestinal perforation that include the following: toxic neutrophils, phagocytized bacteria, free bacteria, and free particles of ingesta. A degenerative left shift and decreased glucose level may imply sepsis.

D. Preoperative management includes a shock dose of polyionic isotonic fluids (80 ml per kilogram), corticosteroids, broad-spectrum antibiotics (aerobic and anaerobic spectrum), glucose, and banamine (1 mg per kilogram). During the administration of fluids, paracentesis and removal of abdominal fluid is performed.

E. An exploratory celiotomy is performed. Fluid that has accumulated in the peritoneal cavity is evacuated by suction to facilitate visualization of abdominal structures. A systematic approach is used when evaluating abdominal viscera in order to locate all injured or perforated viscera. Bowel perforations are debrided and sutured as described for enterotomy (p 26). All questionably secure enterotomies and anastomoses are examined and either resutured or secured with a serosal patch (Fig. 1).

F. After evaluation and repair of the perforated segment(s) of bowel, the peritoneal cavity should be irrigated with copious amounts (5 to 6 liters) of warm, sterile, physiologic saline solution. The lavage helps float away debris, dilutes organism numbers and endotoxin load, and distributes intraperitoneal antibiotics. Penicillin or cephalosporin may be added to the lavage solution.

G. Minor contamination of the peritoneal cavity can be managed by intraoperative peritoneal lavage and primary closure. No postoperative lavage management is needed in these cases.

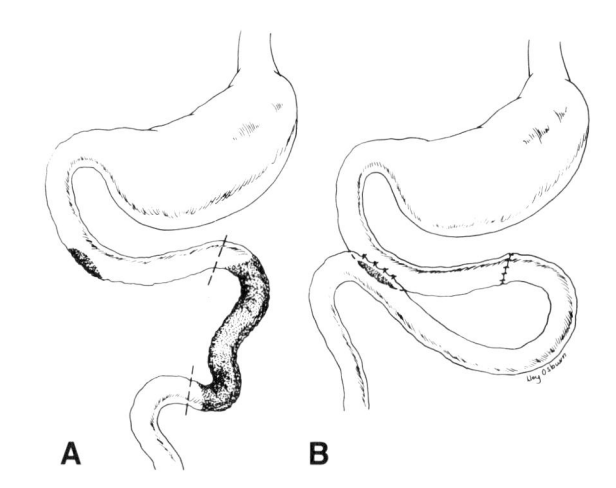

Figure 1 *A*, Resection of perforated bowel; and *B*, use of a loop of jejunum as a serosal patch to cover a perforation in the descending duodenum.

H. Patients with existing peritonitis may require active peritoneal lavage. An ingress-egress lavage system is placed. An appropriate lavage solution is infused two to three times per day until the cytology of the fluid removed reveals the presence of healthy neutrophils and no bacteria. Peritoneal dialysis catheters may be used to facilitate closed lavage efficiency.

I. Patients with severe intra-abdominal sepsis may be treated by open peritoneal drainage. The abdominal incision is left open and packed with sterile nonadhering pads, then covered with gauze sponges, and held in place with an abdominal bandage. The bandage is changed daily until the cytology of the drainage fluid appears healthy (generally 3 to 5 days). The abdomen is then closed routinely.

References

Botte RJ, Rosin E. Cytology of peritoneal effusion following intestinal anastomosis and experimental peritonitis. Vet Surg 1983; 12(1):20.

Crowe DT Jr. Diagnostic abdominal paracentesis techniques: clinical evaluation in 129 dogs and cats. JAAHA 1984; 20:223.

Orsher RJ, Rosin E. Open peritoneal drainage in experimental peritonitis in dogs. Vet Surg 1984; 13(4):222.

Vercoutere AL, Humphrey R. Improved method for intra-abdominal drainage. Surg Gynecol Obstet 1984; 158:587.

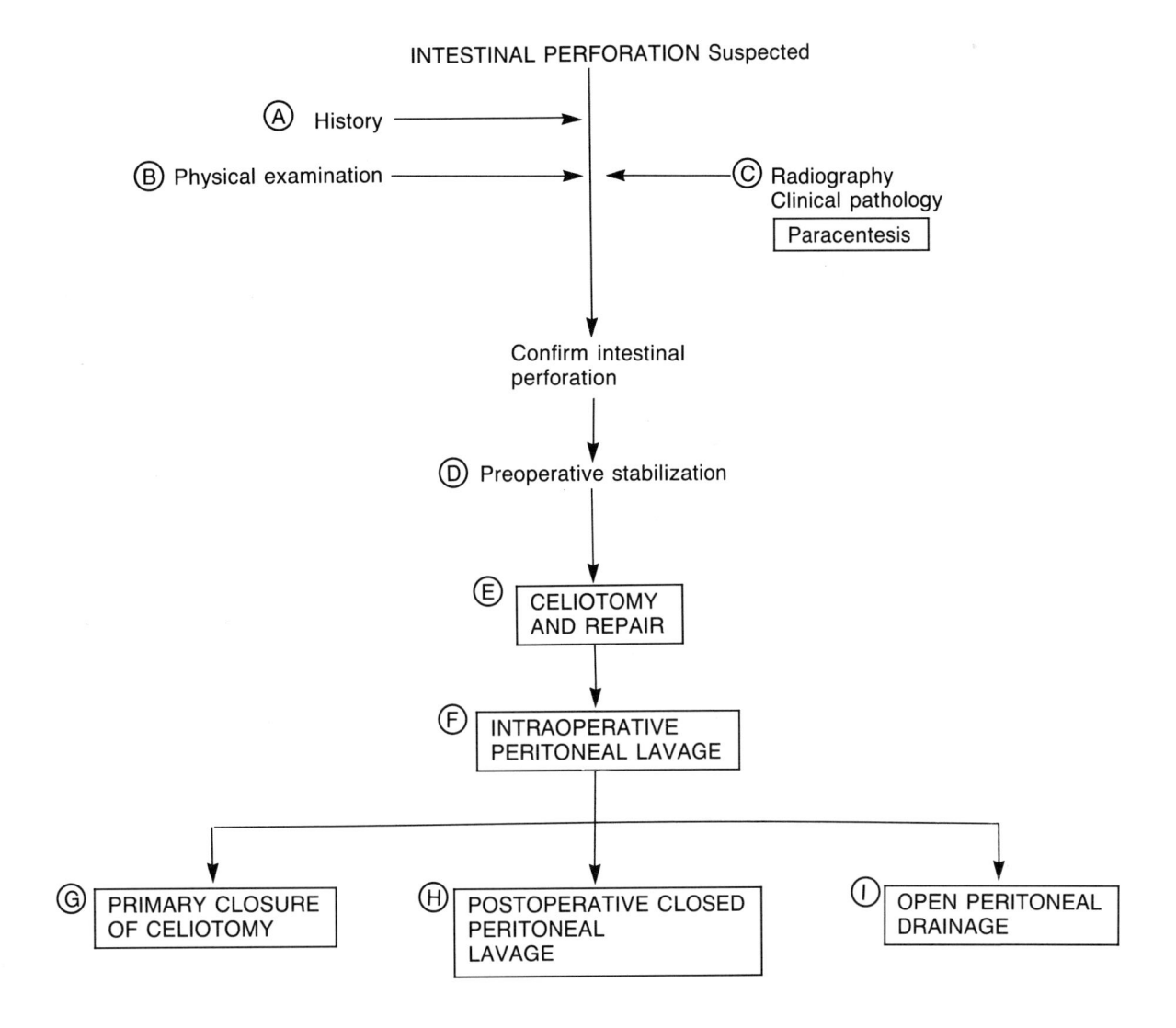

INTESTINAL PERFORATION Suspected

- (A) History
- (B) Physical examination
- (C) Radiography / Clinical pathology
  - Paracentesis

↓

Confirm intestinal perforation

↓

(D) Preoperative stabilization

↓

(E) **CELIOTOMY AND REPAIR**

↓

(F) **INTRAOPERATIVE PERITONEAL LAVAGE**

↓

- (G) **PRIMARY CLOSURE OF CELIOTOMY**
- (H) **POSTOPERATIVE CLOSED PERITONEAL LAVAGE**
- (I) **OPEN PERITONEAL DRAINAGE**

COLONIC OBSTRUCTION

Howard B. Seim III

A. Patients with colonic obstruction often present with a nonspecific history of occasional vomiting (once a day or every other day), depression, anorexia, variable degrees of debilitation, and cachexia. Stools are often scanty, may be blood tinged, and are occasionally associated with straining.

B. Physical examination may reveal moderate to severe debilitation and depression. Careful abdominal palpation, particularly of the caudal abdomen, may reveal the presence of an abdominal mass.

C. Confirmation of the presence and location of the obstruction is accomplished by administration of a barium enema. Proctoscopic examination is helpful in identifying the obstructive mass and acquiring biopsy specimens if necessary. The major limitation of proctoscopic examination is the distance that can be adequately examined.

D. Colonic obstructions are not often life-threatening unless they are associated with perforation. Patients are generally presented with severe protein-calorie malnutrition and may be helped by preoperative nutrient supplementation of low residue diets via nasogastric, pharyngostomy, or gastrostomy tube. During this time, gut sterilization can commence by multiple betadine enemas, enteric antibiotics (neomycin, kanamycin, and metronidazole), and systemic antibiotics (cephalosporins or ampicillin).*

E. After appropriate patient preparation, a ventral midline exploratory celiotomy is performed from 2 to 3 cm cranial to the umbilicus to the pubis. Careful examination of the ascending, transverse, and descending colon is performed. Evaluation of the obstruction as to its location extramural, mural, or luminal) is determined. Colonic and sublumbar lymph nodes are carefully palpated and biopsied if enlarged.

F. Resection and anastomosis may be necessary in cases of mural masses, or luminal masses associated with nonviable bowel. Careful surgical manipulation is critical because of the colon's high bacterial content, the surgical stimulation of increased collagenase activity at 5 to 7 days postoperatively, its high pressure conduit nature, and the lack of a richly vascular mesenteric pedicle. Colonic anastomosis is accomplished by a single-layer, interrupted, inverting end-to-end closure using a Cushing, Lembert, or Connell suture pattern or simple interrupted sutures; 3-0 or 4-0 synthetic absorbable or monofilament nonabsorbable suture with a reverse-cutting or taper-cut needle are the suture materials of choice. In cases in which potential leakage may be a postoperative complication, the placement of a serosal patch is indicated. A low-residue diet should be started 24 to 48 hours postoperatively and continued for 2 weeks. If question arises as to the integrity of the colonic closure, a low pressure organic iodide enema can confirm this.

G. A colotomy incision may be necessary for the removal of a luminal mass that cannot be gently massaged out through the anus. The incision is centered over the most viable bowel (generally aboral), and the mass is gently removed. The colotomy is closed using the same suture patterns and materials as described for anastomosis. The use of a serosal patch and the postoperative feeding management is as described for resection and anastomosis patients.

* Editor's Note.
The use of nonabsorbable antibiotics for "gut sterilization" prior to surgery may alter the animal's colonization resistance and lead to superinfections with resistant strains. It may be more advantageous to create an effective serum level of the appropriate antibiotics during the surgical period.

References

Leveen HH, Wapnick S, Falk G, et al. Effects of prophylactic antibiotics on colonic healing . Am J Surg 1976; 131:47.
Richardson DC, Krahwinkel DJ Jr. Surgery of the colon. In: Bojrab MJ, ed. Current techniques in small animal surgery. 2nd ed. Philadelphia: Lea & Febiger, 1983: 187.
Stoloff D, Snider TG, Crawford MP, et al. End-to-end colonic anastamosis: a comparison of techniques in normal dogs. Vet Surg 1984; 13(2):76.

COLONIC OBSTRUCTION Suspected

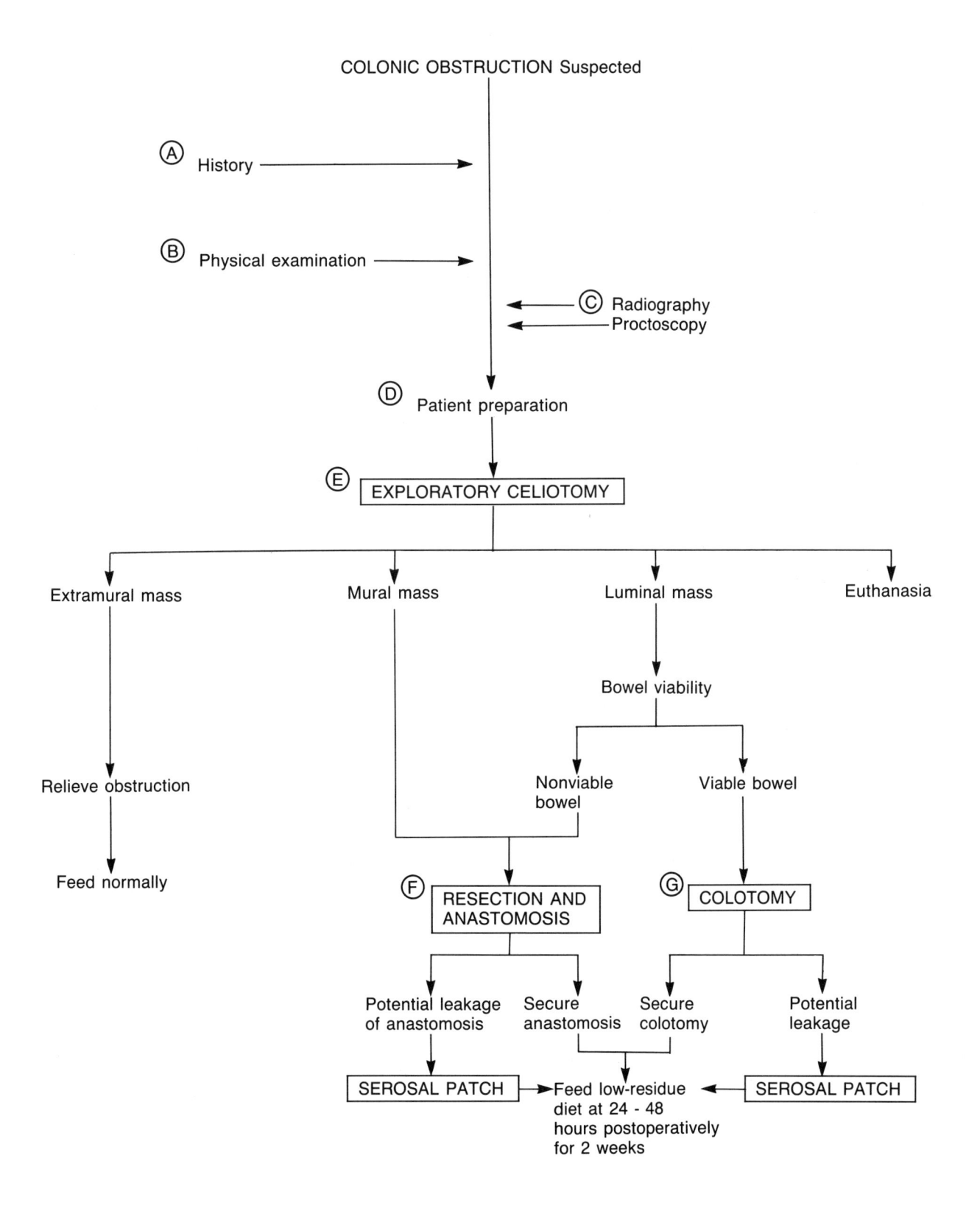

Ⓐ History

Ⓑ Physical examination

Ⓒ Radiography
Proctoscopy

Ⓓ Patient preparation

Ⓔ EXPLORATORY CELIOTOMY

- Extramural mass
- Mural mass
- Luminal mass
- Euthanasia

Extramural mass → Relieve obstruction → Feed normally

Luminal mass → Bowel viability → Nonviable bowel / Viable bowel

Ⓕ RESECTION AND ANASTOMOSIS (from Mural mass and Nonviable bowel)

Ⓖ COLOTOMY (from Viable bowel)

RESECTION AND ANASTOMOSIS → Potential leakage of anastomosis / Secure anastomosis

COLOTOMY → Secure colotomy / Potential leakage

Potential leakage of anastomosis → SEROSAL PATCH

Potential leakage → SEROSAL PATCH

SEROSAL PATCH, Secure anastomosis, Secure colotomy, SEROSAL PATCH → Feed low-residue diet at 24 - 48 hours postoperatively for 2 weeks

35

RECTAL PROLAPSE

Howard B. Seim III

A. Any disorder that causes severe prolonged tenesmus, particularly in young, unthrifty, or heavily parasitized animals can predispose to rectal prolapse. Diseases that have commonly been associated with rectal prolapse include severe enteritis, dystocia, urolithiasis, perineal hernia, rectal polyps, prostatic disease, and chronic constipation. Diagnosis is based on visual examination of a tube-like mass protruding from the anus.

B. Rectal prolapse must be differentiated from a prolapsed intussusception. Both conditions have a similar appearance on presentation; however, with an intussusception, a finger or long blunt probe can be passed between the rectal wall and the prolapsed mass. If this condition is present, an exploratory celiotomy and simple reduction or resection and anastomosis based on bowel viability is performed (p 26).

C. If a finger or probe does not pass between the prolapsed mucosa and anocutaneous junction, the patient has a prolapsed rectum (Fig.1). Treatment is based on rectal viability and reducibility.

D. If the prolapsed rectum is viable and reducible, a pursestring suture of 2-0 nylon should be placed. Reduction can be accomplished by first applying a hypertonic solution (50% glucose) to help relieve edema. After reduction and placement of the pursestring suture, topical application of a local anesthetic ointment (1% dibucaine) may help relieve post-reduction tenesmus. The pursestring suture is removed in 4 to 5 days.

E. If the prolapsed rectum is viable but nonreducible, or if the prolapse recurs after the pursestring suture is removed, a celiotomy and colopexy procedure is performed. A ventral midline abdominal incision is made in the posterior abdomen. The colon is located and the prolapse reduced by gentle cranial traction combined with digital anal reduction by an assistant. The colon is pulled cranially until slight tension is transmitted to the rectum. The seromuscular layer of the colon is scarified, and the peritoneum, 2 to 3 cm away from the abdominal incision, is also scarified. The two surfaces are sutured together with two rows of simple interrupted sutures using 2-0 or 3-0 absorbable suture material. Care is taken not to penetrate the bowel lumen.

F. If the prolapsed rectum is nonviable or nonreducible by celiotomy, amputation of the prolapsed portion is required. The index finger is placed into the lumen of the bowel. Three stay sutures (2-0 or 3-0 suture material) are placed through the full thickness of the prolapsed bowel. The prolapse is then amputated, and the anastomosis is performed using a single-layer closure with simple interrupted sutures (synthetic absorbable). The sutures are placed through the full thickness of the rectal wall to ensure penetration of the submucosal layer. The stay sutures are then removed, and the rectum is reduced manually inside the anus. Topical anesthetic is instilled postoperatively to prevent further tenesmus. Patients are placed on a stool softener and low-residue diet for 10 to 14 days postoperatively.

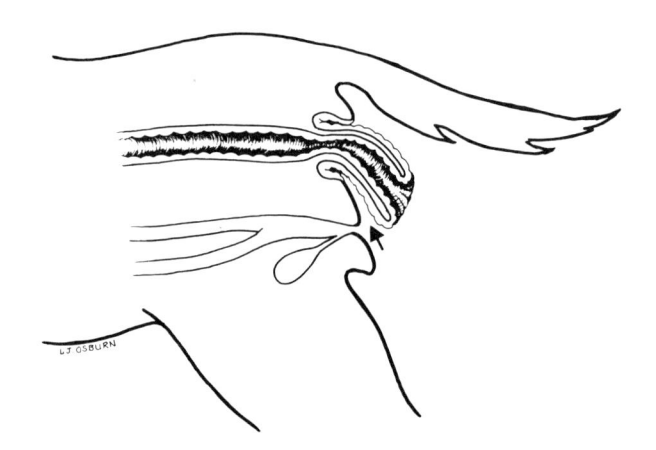

Figure 1 Rectal prolapse: Note that a probe cannot be advanced between the prolapsed mucosa and the anocutaneous junction.

Reference

Engen MH. Management of rectal prolapse. In: Bojrab MJ ed. Current techniques in small animal surgery. 2nd ed. Philadelphia: Lea & Febiger, 1983: 184.

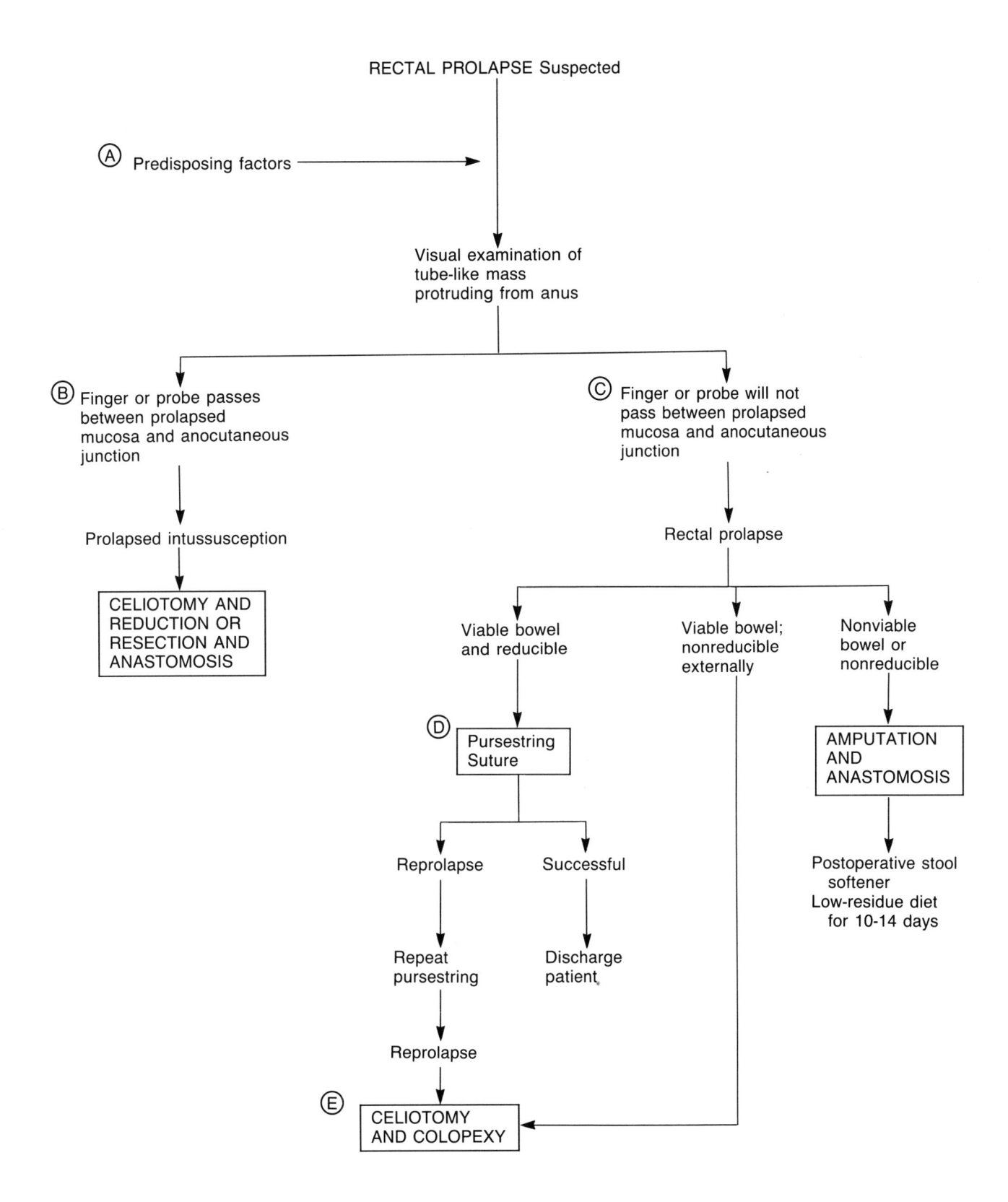

RECTAL PROLAPSE Suspected

(A) Predisposing factors →

Visual examination of tube-like mass protruding from anus

(B) Finger or probe passes between prolapsed mucosa and anocutaneous junction
→ Prolapsed intussusception
→ **CELIOTOMY AND REDUCTION OR RESECTION AND ANASTOMOSIS**

(C) Finger or probe will not pass between prolapsed mucosa and anocutaneous junction
→ Rectal prolapse

- Viable bowel and reducible → (D) **Pursestring Suture**
  - Reprolapse → Repeat pursestring → Reprolapse → (E) **CELIOTOMY AND COLOPEXY**
  - Successful → Discharge patient
- Viable bowel; nonreducible externally → (E) **CELIOTOMY AND COLOPEXY**
- Nonviable bowel or nonreducible → **AMPUTATION AND ANASTOMOSIS** → Postoperative stool softener; Low-residue diet for 10-14 days

RECTAL POLYP

Howard B. Seim III

A. Patients with rectal polyps generally present with a history of dyschezia and hematochezia. Occasionally, visualization of the polyp as it prolapses through the anus during defecation may be included as part of the presenting history.

B. Physical examination may reveal a prolapsed portion of the polyp. This generally appears as a red to reddish-purple fold of rectal mucosa. Diagnosis may be confirmed by careful digital rectal palpation, if the polyp is not beyond the level of the pelvic canal.

C. It is important to rule out the presence of multiple polyps as well as to definitively diagnose the presence of polyps beyond the reach of digital rectal palpation. The use of a barium enema may be helpful to evaluate the ascending, transverse, and descending colon. Proctoscopic examination is useful in evaluating the rectum and descending colon. A biopsy should be performed to rule out inflammatory disease and confirm the diagnosis of rectal polyp.

D. Multiple polyps occur rarely in dogs and cats. If two or three polyps are located in the distal colon and rectum, removal per rectum is possible. If the polyps are located further orad in the colon (ascending and transverse colon), a celiotomy for colotomy is the treatment of choice.

E. Treatment of a single rectal polyp is determined by its location from the anal orifice.

F. Rectal polyps located 1 to 3 cm from the anal orifice can be treated by digitally everting the polyp and excising it. If the polyp has a sessile base, cautery or cryosurgical excision is preferred. If the polyp is pedunculated, scalpel, cautery or cryosurgical excision can be easily performed.

G. Rectal polyps located 3 to 8 cm from the anal orifice require iatrogenic rectal prolapse for adequate exposure. Epidural anesthesia, an excellent muscle relaxant, is the anesthetic regimen of choice. The anus is digitally dilated to expose the folds of rectal mucosa. Three to four stay sutures are placed in the mucosal folds equidistant around the rectum. Gentle traction on the stay sutures allows prolapse of the rectal mucosa until the polyp comes into view. Excision of the polyp is performed as previously described. When excision is complete, the prolapse is reduced, a tampon is inserted for hemostasis, and a pursestring suture is placed in the anus to keep the tampon in place and to prevent recurrence of the prolapse. The pursestring suture is removed within 12 to 24 hours, and the patient is allowed to pass the tampon.

H. The prognosis for rectal polyp removal is generally favorable. Polyps that possess a pedunculated base are easier to remove completely, and recurrence of the polyp is rare. Polyps with a sessile base are more difficult to remove completely; recurrence is more common, often requiring several procedures to effect a cure. Rectal polyps may be premalignant in nature and may transform into rectal adenocarcinoma. Histologic evaluation of each excised polyp should be performed.

References

Holt PE, Lucke VM. Rectal neoplasia in the dog: a clinicopathological review of 31 cases. Vet Rec 1985; 116:400.

Nelson D, Gourley IM. Rectal neoplasia in the dog. Mod Vet Pract 1977; 58(6): 525.

Seiler RJ. Colorectal polyps of the dog: a clinicopathologic study of 17 cases. JAVMA 1979; 174(1):72.

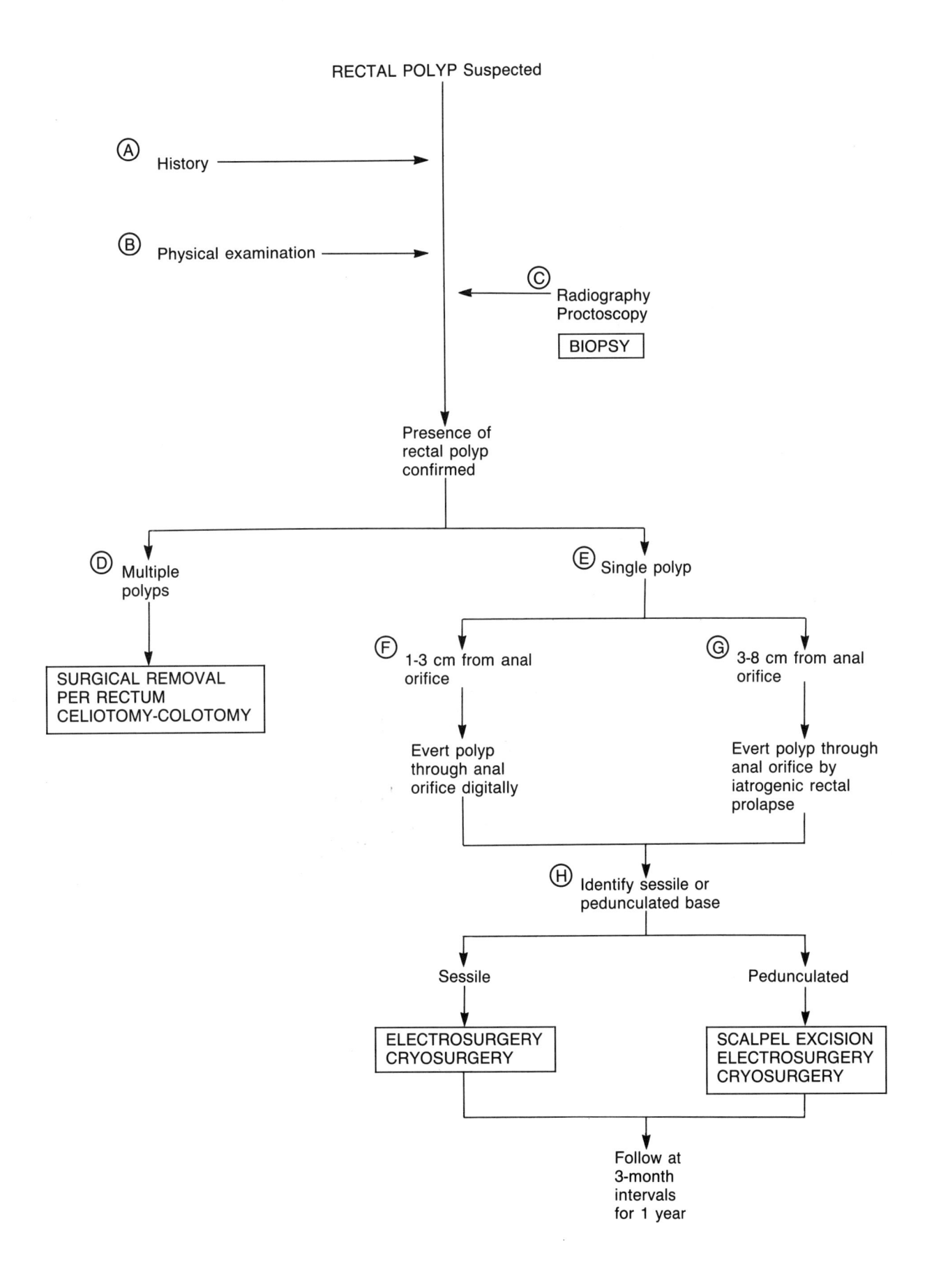

RECTAL POLYP Suspected

- (A) History
- (B) Physical examination
- (C) Radiography / Proctoscopy — **BIOPSY**

Presence of rectal polyp confirmed

- (D) Multiple polyps → **SURGICAL REMOVAL PER RECTUM CELIOTOMY-COLOTOMY**
- (E) Single polyp
  - (F) 1-3 cm from anal orifice → Evert polyp through anal orifice digitally
  - (G) 3-8 cm from anal orifice → Evert polyp through anal orifice by iatrogenic rectal prolapse

(H) Identify sessile or pedunculated base

- Sessile → **ELECTROSURGERY CRYOSURGERY**
- Pedunculated → **SCALPEL EXCISION ELECTROSURGERY CRYOSURGERY**

Follow at 3-month intervals for 1 year

PERIANAL NEOPLASIA

Howard B. Seim III

A. Patients with perianal neoplasia generally present with signs that include scooting, anal licking, and hematochezia with single or multiple masses in the perianal region. These neoplasms occur in both males and females and generally occur in middle- to older-aged dogs.

B. Physical examination of the perianal region verifies the presence of ulcerated and raised lesions. Digital rectal examination of the perianal skin may reveal smaller masses (2 to 3 mm diameter) that might otherwise go unnoticed.

C. Included in the patient's minimum data base should be serum calcium levels. Hypercalcemia may be seen, particularly in spayed females with anal sac involvement.

D. Perianal gland adenomas generally occur in middle-aged and older intact male dogs. Females are seldom affected. The adenoma is testosterone-dependent. The most effective form of therapy is castration and excision (cold-knife, cryosurgery, or electroscalpel). Definitive diagnosis must be established by histopathologic examination of excised tissue. The prognosis is favorable.

E. Perianal gland adenocarcinoma generally occurs in middle-aged and older dogs. Males are more commonly affected than females. These neoplasms must be differentiated from perianal gland adenomas by histopathologic examination. Complete excision is often difficult because of the invasive nature of the tumor. Metastasis is generally to iliac and lumbar aortic lymph nodes and may be present at the time of diagnosis. Preoperative chest and abdominal radiographs are taken to help assess the presence or absence of metastasis. Therapy is directed at cytoreduction (debulking) of the primary and metastatic lesions by surgical excision followed by local radiation therapy. Castration does not affect the prognosis since the neoplasm does not seem to be hormonally dependent. Long-term prognosis is unfavorable owing to local recurrence and abdominal and thoracic metastasis.

F. Anal sac apocrine adenocarcinoma is a malignant tumor of the apocrine glands lining the walls of the anal sacs. It most commonly occurs in older spayed females. The tumor secretes a parathyroid hormone-like substance that results in hypercalcemia. Careful rectal palpation is necessary as some tumors are only 2 to 3 mm in diameter. Metastasis to the lumbar aortic lymph nodes often is present at the time of diagnosis. Treatment includes controlling the hypercalcemia, removing the tumor load (primary tumor as well as any metastatic involvement), and controlling recurrence. A guarded prognosis must be given for dogs with this neoplasm.

G. Perianal gland adenomas occur rarely in females. They resemble perianal gland adenomas in males, and must be differentiated from anal sac apocrine adenocarcinomas. The treatment of choice is local excision as for the male.

References

Hause WR, Stevenson S, Meuten DJ, Capen CC. Pseudohyperparathyroidism associated with adenocarcinomas of anal sac origin in four dogs. JAAHA 1981; 17:373.

Liska WD, Withrow SJ. Cryosurgical treatment of perianal gland adenomas in the dog. JAAHA 1978; 14:457.

Wilson GP, Hayes HM Jr. Castration for the treatment of perianal gland neoplasms in the dog. JAVMA 1979; 174(12):1301

```
                    PERIANAL NEOPLASIA Suspected
    Ⓐ History ─────────→    ←───── Ⓒ Clinical pathology
    Ⓑ Physical examination ──→
                              ↓
                         Sex of animal
                    ┌─────────┴─────────┐
                  Male                Female
                    ↓                   ↓
            EXCISIONAL OR       EXCISIONAL OR
            INCISIONAL          INCISIONAL
            BIOPSY              BIOPSY
```

Ⓓ Perianal gland adenoma → CASTRATION AND EXCISION → Follow at 4-month intervals for 1 year

Ⓔ Perianal gland adenocarcinoma → Chest and abdominal radiography → LOCAL EXCISION and Radiation → Follow for local recurrence and metastasis

Ⓕ Anal sac apocrine adenocarcinoma → Biochemical profile: Hypercalcemia → Chest and abdominal radiography → EXCISION OF PRIMARY AND METASTATIC TUMORS → Postoperative Chemotherapy

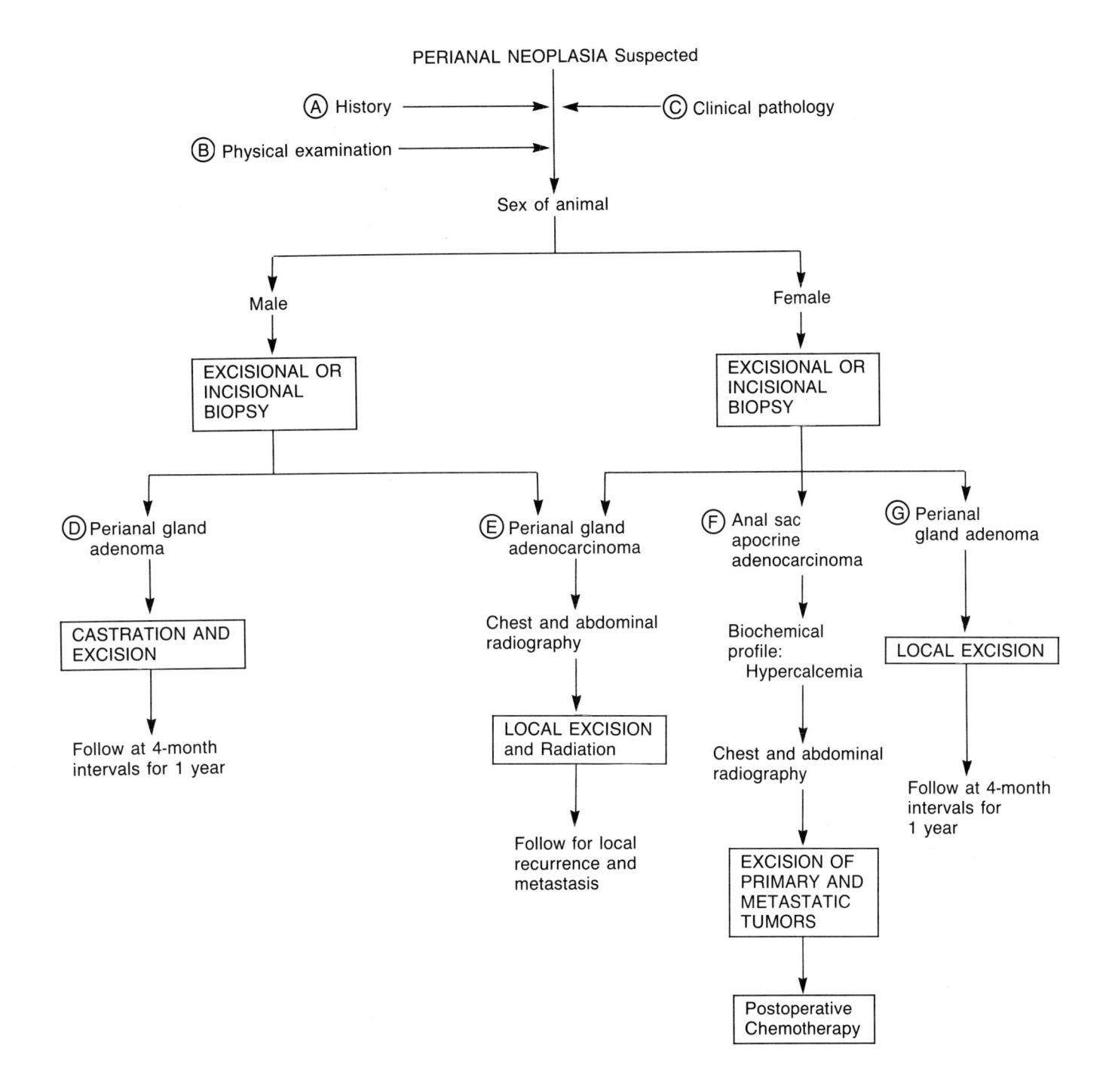

Ⓖ Perianal gland adenoma → LOCAL EXCISION → Follow at 4-month intervals for 1 year

IMPERFORATE ANUS

Howard B. Seim III

A. Patients with imperforate anus generally present with a history of not defecating since birth. Abdominal distension may be recognized grossly, particularly in chronic cases.

B. Diagnosis of imperforate anus is made by visual examination of a membrane covering the anal opening. At this time, a sharp probe or needle should be used to stimulate the anal sphincter reflex. This determines the presence or absence of a functioning anal sphincter. Also, a blunt instrument (thermometer, hemostat) should be used to gently attempt penetration of the anal membrane.

C. If the blunt instrument easily penetrates the anal membrane (imperforate anus type I) and a normal anal reflex is present, the patient is released and followed at weekly intervals for 3 weeks to assess patency and function.

D. If the membrane is not easily penetrated, a lateral abdominal radiograph with the hind end slightly elevated allows visualization of gas in the terminal rectum. If the membrane covering the anus is 5 to 10 mm thick (imperforate anus type II), a perineal approach can be used to remove the membrane. If the air density only reaches the pubic brim (imperforate anus type III), an abdominoperineal approach is necessary.

E. Treatment of imperforate anus type II is directed at locating the anal dimple, dissecting the membrane to the level of the rectal mucosa, and suturing the mucosa to the subcutaneous tissue and perianal skin. The prognosis is favorable if the anal sphincter muscle is intact and functional.

F. Treatment for imperforate anus type III requires exposure of the distal rectum or colon abdominally to allow delivery through the pelvic canal to an opening made in the anal dimple. Rectal mucosa is then sutured to the subcutaneous tissue and skin in the perianal region. The prognosis is guarded. Patients may remain incontinent postoperatively.

References

Horney FD, Archibald J. Colon, rectum and anus. In: Archibald J, ed. Canine surgery. 2nd ed. Santa Barbara: American Veterinary Publications 1974: 603.

Kiesewetter WB, Bill AH, Nixon HH. Imperforate anus. Arch Surg 1976; 3:518.

Smith EI, Tunell WP, Rainey WG. A clinical evaluation of the surgical treatment of anorectal malformations (imperforate anus). Ann Surg 1978; 187(6):583.

IMPERFORATE ANUS Suspected

- (A) History
- (B) Physical examination

Imperforate anus confirmed

- (C) Imperforate anus type I
  → Follow weekly for 3 weeks
  Keep anus open

- (D) Abdominal radiography
  - (E) Imperforate anus type II
    → **SURGICAL REPAIR: PERINEAL APPROACH**
  - (F) Imperforate anus type III
    → **SURGICAL REPAIR: ABDOMINOPERINEAL APPROACH**

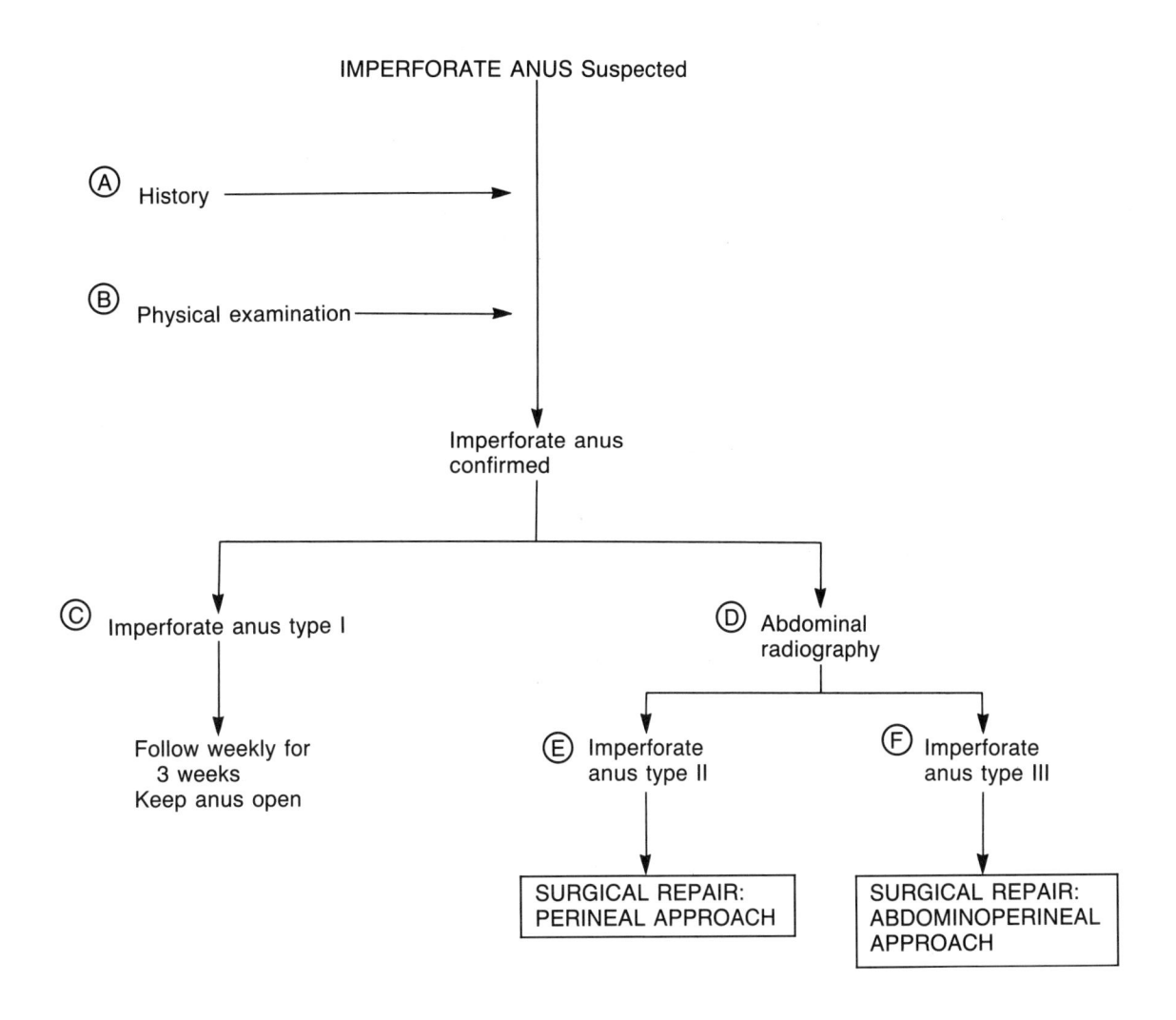

ANAL SAC ABSCESS

Howard B. Seim III

A. Patients with anal sac abscess or chronic, recurrent anal sacculitis generally present with a history of scooting, anal licking, discharge in the anal sac region, perianal bleeding, and pain during defecation. Small breeds of dogs (Toy Poodle, Shih Tzu, Pomeranian) are the most commonly affected.

B. Diagnosis is based on visual examination of the perianal region and digital rectal palpation. The area of the anal sac may look inflamed, swollen, and, in cases of ruptured abscess, a serosanguineous to purulent discharge may be present. Digital rectal palpation is often painful, and palpation of the anal sacs may reveal swollen, impacted sacs with thick, often inspissated material. Expression of the material may cause rupture of the sac.

C. Initial treatment for patients that present with one episode of anal sacculitis is appropriate drainage of the anal sac, flushing of the perianal region with antiseptic solution, and instillation of an antibiotic ointment. If the patient presents with recurrent episodes, medical management should be attempted one or two more times. If the problem does not resolve, bilateral anal sacculectomy should be recommended.

D. Anal sacculectomy is the treatment of choice for chronic, recurrent (two to three episodes in less than 3 months), anal sacculitis or abscessation. Prior to surgery, the patient should be treated with local therapy until the acute exacerbation is under control (1 to 2 weeks). This presurgical treatment makes identification of the anal sac and external anal sphincter muscle much easier and uncomplicated wound healing more predictable. The patient is readmitted and scheduled for elective anal sacculectomy. The patient is placed in a perineal position, the anal sacs expressed, a tampon placed in the rectum, and the perineal skin routinely prepared for aseptic surgery (Fig. 1). A probe is placed in the anal sac orifice and gently pushed to the end of the sac. The sac is then incised to expose the interior epithelial surface. The edge of the sac is grasped and adhering structures (subcutaneous tissue, scar tissue and external anal sphincter muscle) are carefully scraped off the sac wall. After complete removal of the anal sac, the incised portion of the external anal sphincter muscle is sutured. The subcutaneous tissues and skin are closed routinely. Alternately, following exposure of the inner epithelial surface of the anal sac, it may be destroyed using a double freeze-thaw cryosurgery procedure. The wound is left to heal by second intention.

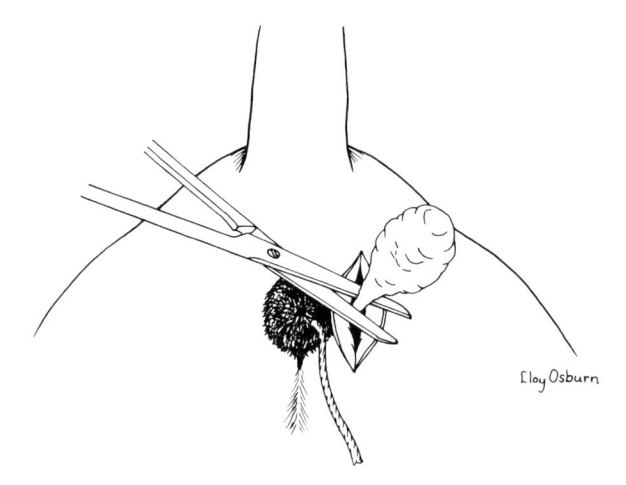

Figure 1 Anal sac resection following packing with string or other material (plaster of paris, agar gel, latex rubber).

References

Harvey CE. Incidence and distribution of anal sac disease in the dog. JAAHA 1974; 10:573.

Horney FD, Archibald J. Colon, rectum and anus. In: Archibald J, ed. Canine surgery. 2nd ed. Santa Barbara: American Veterinary Publications, 1974:622.

Johnston DE. Surgical diseases of the rectum and anus. In: Slatter DH, ed. Textbook of small animal surgery. Philadelphia: WB Saunders, 1985:775.

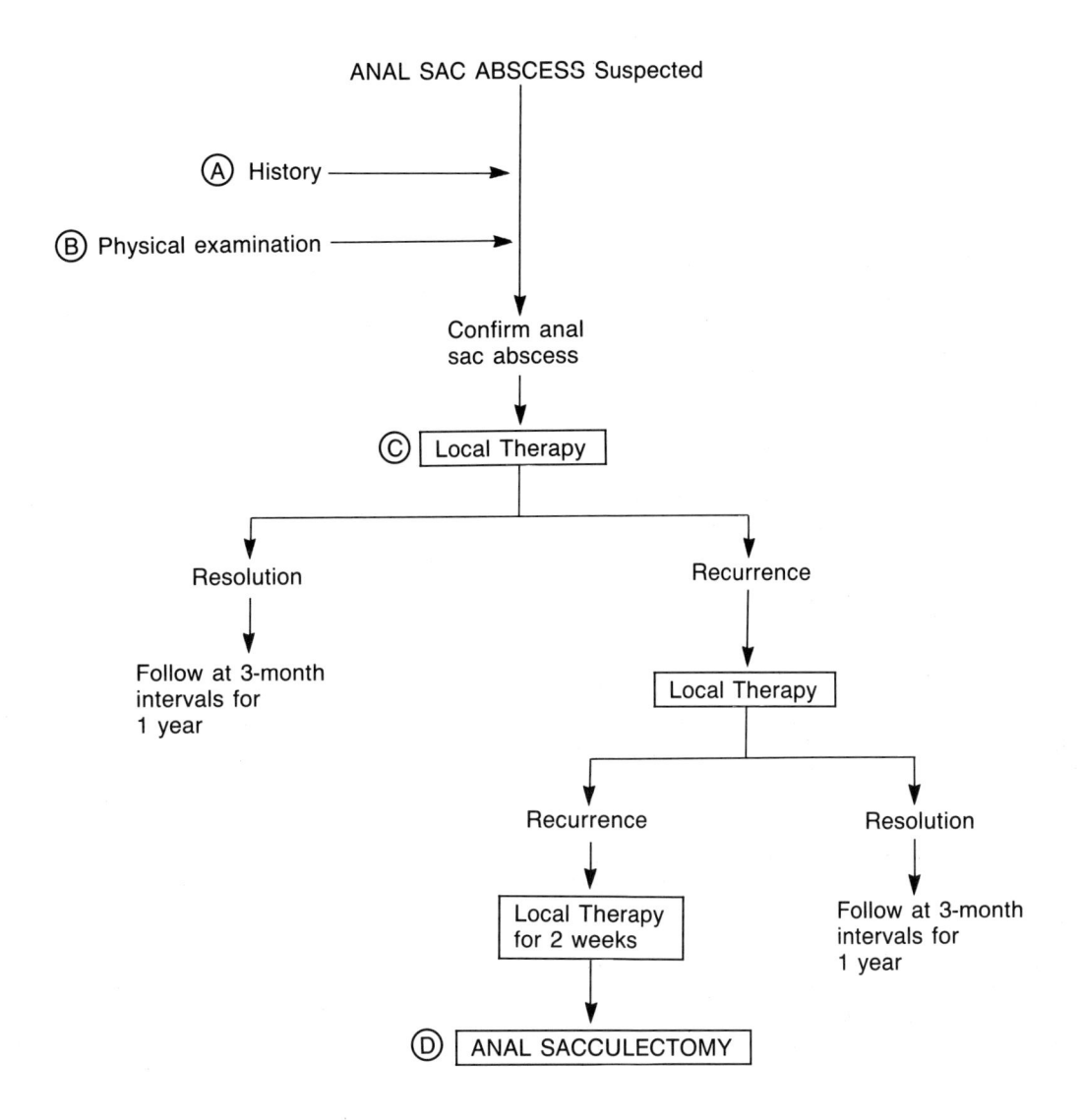

```
                    ANAL SAC ABSCESS Suspected
                                │
        (A) History ────────────▶│
                                │
        (B) Physical examination ▶│
                                │
                                ▼
                         Confirm anal
                         sac abscess
                                │
                                ▼
                        (C) │ Local Therapy │
                    ┌───────────┴───────────┐
                    ▼                       ▼
                Resolution              Recurrence
                    │                       │
                    ▼                       ▼
            Follow at 3-month       │ Local Therapy │
            intervals for           ┌───────┴───────┐
            1 year                  ▼               ▼
                                Recurrence      Resolution
                                    │               │
                                    ▼               ▼
                            │ Local Therapy │   Follow at 3-month
                            │ for 2 weeks   │   intervals for
                                    │           1 year
                                    ▼
                        (D) │ ANAL SACCULECTOMY │
```

45

PERIANAL FISTULA

Howard B. Seim III

A. Patients with perianal fistula most commonly present with a history of tenesmus, hematochezia, diarrhea, and anal licking. The most common breeds affected include German Shepherds, Irish Setters, and Labrador Retrievers, although other large breeds are also affected. The male to female ratio is approximately 2 to 1.

B. The diagnosis is based on clinical signs and visual examination of the perianal region. Visual examination reveals multiple fistulous tracts opening in the perianal skin. The severity ranges from one single tract to extensive 360 degree anal involvement.

C. Treatment of perianal fistulas is based on the degree of involvement of the perianal tissues. Involvement may be divided into the following categories: less than 90 degrees, 90 to 180 degrees, and 180 to 360 degrees.

D. If 90 degrees or less of the perianal skin is involved, the options for treatment include medical management or various forms of surgical management. Medical management includes the use of systemic and topical antibiotics, chemical cauterization of fistulous tracts, antiseptic flush, and elevation or amputation of the tail. This treatment may resolve the early single tract or mildly affected cases, but resolution is often only temporary. It is generally accepted that some form of surgery is necessary to treat perianal fistulas successfully. Patients with up to 90 degree involvement can be successfully treated by anoplasty, cryosurgery, or electrosurgical debridement and fulguration. A second procedure may be required at 4 to 6 weeks if recurrence or stricture occurs postoperatively. The prognosis for return to normal function is favorable.

E. If 90 to 180 degrees of the perianal skin is involved, anoplasty or electrosurgical debridement and fulguration are the procedures of choice. Bilateral anal sacculectomy is also performed. Cases that recur are generally managed by cryosurgery or a second debridement and fulguration. Postoperative strictures may be handled by anoplasty. The prognosis for return to normal function is guarded.

F. If 180 to 360 degrees of the perianal skin is involved, a two-stage electrosurgical debridement and fulguration procedure is performed. The first stage includes debridement and fulguration of 180 degrees of involved tissue. Bilateral anal sacculectomy is performed during the first stage. Four to 6 weeks later, the second 180 degrees of involved tissue is treated by electrosurgical debridement and fulguration. If there is recurrence of tracts on the previously operated side, excision, cautery, or cryosurgery can be used at this time for treatment. Stricture or recurrence of fistulas are treated as previously described. The prognosis for return to normal function is guarded. Postoperative fecal incontinence may result from excessive muscle damage or nerve injury.

References

Elkins AD, Hobson HP. Management of perianal fistulae: a retrospective study of 23 cases. Vet Surg 1982; 11:110.

Liska WD, Greiner TP, Withrow SJ. Cryosurgery in the treatment of perianal fistulae. Vet Clin North Am 1975; 5(3):449.

Vasseur PB. Perianal fistulae in dogs: a restrospective analysis of surgical techniques. JAAHA 1981; 17:177.

Vasseur PB. Results of surgical excision of perianal fistulas in dogs. JAVMA 1984; 185:60.

Walshaw R. Perianal fistula in the dog. In: Bojrab MJ, ed. Current techniques in small animal surgery. 2nd ed. Philadelphia: Lea & Febiger, 1983:191.

PERIANAL FISTULA Suspected

- (A) History
- (B) Physical examination
- (C) Assess degree of involvement

(D) < 90° involvement

Medical management
- Antibiotics
- Perianal Lavage
- Chemical Cautery
- Tail Elevation

→ Resolution → Follow at 3-month intervals for 1 year

→ Recurrence → SURGICAL MANAGEMENT

Surgical management
- ANOPLASTY
- CRYOSURGERY
- ELECTROSURGICAL DEBRIDEMENT
- ANAL SACCULECTOMY

→ Recurrence → SURGICAL MANAGEMENT

(E) 90°–180° involvement

ANOPLASTY OR ELECTROSURGICAL DEBRIDEMENT ANAL SACCULECTOMY

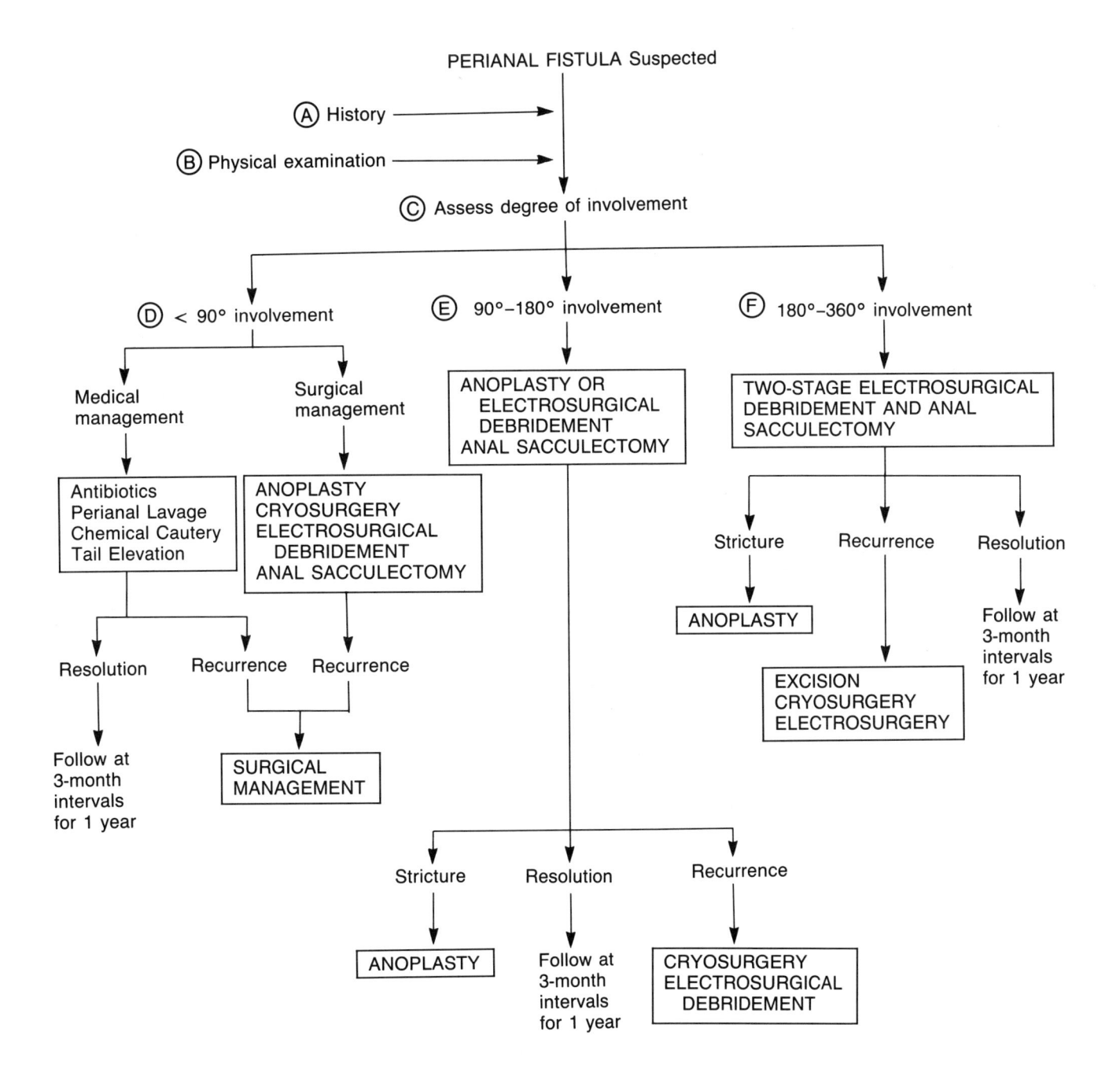

- Stricture → ANOPLASTY
- Resolution → Follow at 3-month intervals for 1 year
- Recurrence → CRYOSURGERY ELECTROSURGICAL DEBRIDEMENT

(F) 180°–360° involvement

TWO-STAGE ELECTROSURGICAL DEBRIDEMENT AND ANAL SACCULECTOMY

- Stricture → ANOPLASTY
- Recurrence → EXCISION CRYOSURGERY ELECTROSURGERY
- Resolution → Follow at 3-month intervals for 1 year

47

ACUTE DIARRHEA

David C. Twedt

A. The onset, duration, and character of the stool should classify the disease as acute diarrhea. The vaccination status and any history concerning deworming or other drug therapy should be determined. Investigate any history of dietary indiscretions or exposure to environmental toxins. Note symptoms that may be related to systemic disease. There may be a history of exposure to other animals that also have diarrhea. Record the type and amount of food and water intake.

B. Assess the animal's general condition and hydration status through skin turgor, mucous membranes, and capillary refill. Perform careful palpation of the abdomen in the case of abnormalities such as fluid-distended loops of bowel, foreign bodies, or pain. Perform a rectal examination, assess the character of the stool. Note any extraintestinal manifestations of systemic disease.

C. Obtain basic laboratory tests, including hematocrit, total protein, and fecal flotation, and perform microscopic examination of direct and stained fecal smears.

D. Based on the history, physical examination, and limited laboratory findings, the patient should be categorized as to the degree of severity. Animals with mild, self-limiting disease appear well hydrated and are alert and active. Generally, these patients are treated on an outpatient basis with symptomatic management. Moderately sick animals have mild dehydration and may be lethargic. Severely affected patients have significant fluid loss, dehydration, and electrolyte alterations. The diarrhea may be bloody. Such life-threatening diarrheas require in-depth diagnostic evaluation and an aggressive therapeutic approach.

E. The moderately-to-severely-ill patient should have an expanded laboratory investigation. A complete blood count (CBC), biochemical profile, and urinalysis are generally indicated to exclude the possibility of systemic disorders causing the diarrhea and to detect the presence of azotemia, acidosis, or electrolyte abnormalities. With such information, a therapeutic plan is instituted.

F. The goal of symptomatic therapy is first to rest the bowel by withholding food for 24 to 48 hours. For mild dehydration, oral replacement using water or electrolyte solutions is recommended. Short-term therapy with motility modifiers (anticholinergics or narcotic analgesic agents) may be considered, but frequently is not required. Proctectants may be used. Antibiotics are not indicated for simple nonspecific diarrhea. With resolution of the diarrhea, a bland diet such as boiled rice and meat or a prescription intestinal diet should be given in small, frequent feedings. The original diet is reintroduced over a 2 to 3 day period.

G. Calculate and replace the fluid and electrolyte deficits with intravenous rehydration (p 190). Fluid replacement should include daily maintenance needs and replacement of any continued loss from diarrhea.

H. An attempt is made to identify the underlying etiology by means of specific diagnostic tests. A leukopenia in an unvaccinated dog suggests a viral etiology and tests for viral detection are indicated. A leukocytosis with an inflammatory fecal cytology suggests a bacterial component and indicates the need for a stool culture. Other specific tests such as fecal flotations or radiology may aid in the diagnosis.

I. A poor response to symptomatic treatment over a reasonable period of time requires further diagnostic evaluations or dietary or empirical anthelmintic or protozoal therapy.

References

DeNovo RC. Therapeutics of gastrointestinal disease. In: Kirk RW, ed. Current veterinary therapy IX. Philadelphia: WB Saunders, 1986:862.

Dillon R. Bacterial enteritis. In: Kirk RW, ed. Current veterinary therapy IX. Philadelphia: WB Saunders, 1986:872.

Hendrix CM, Blagburn BL. Common gastrointestinal parasites. Vet Clin North Am 1983; 13(3):627.

Pollock RVH, Carmichael LE. Canine viral enteritis. Vet Clin North Am 1983; 13(3):551.

Sherding RG. Diseases of the small bowel. In: Ettinger SJ, ed. Textbook of veterinary internal medicine. Philadelphia: WB Saunders, 1983:1278.

Strombeck DR. Acute diarrhea, hemorrhagic enteritis, and gastroenteritis. In: Strombeck DR, ed. Small animal gastroenterology. Davis, CA: Stonegate Publishing, 1979:179.

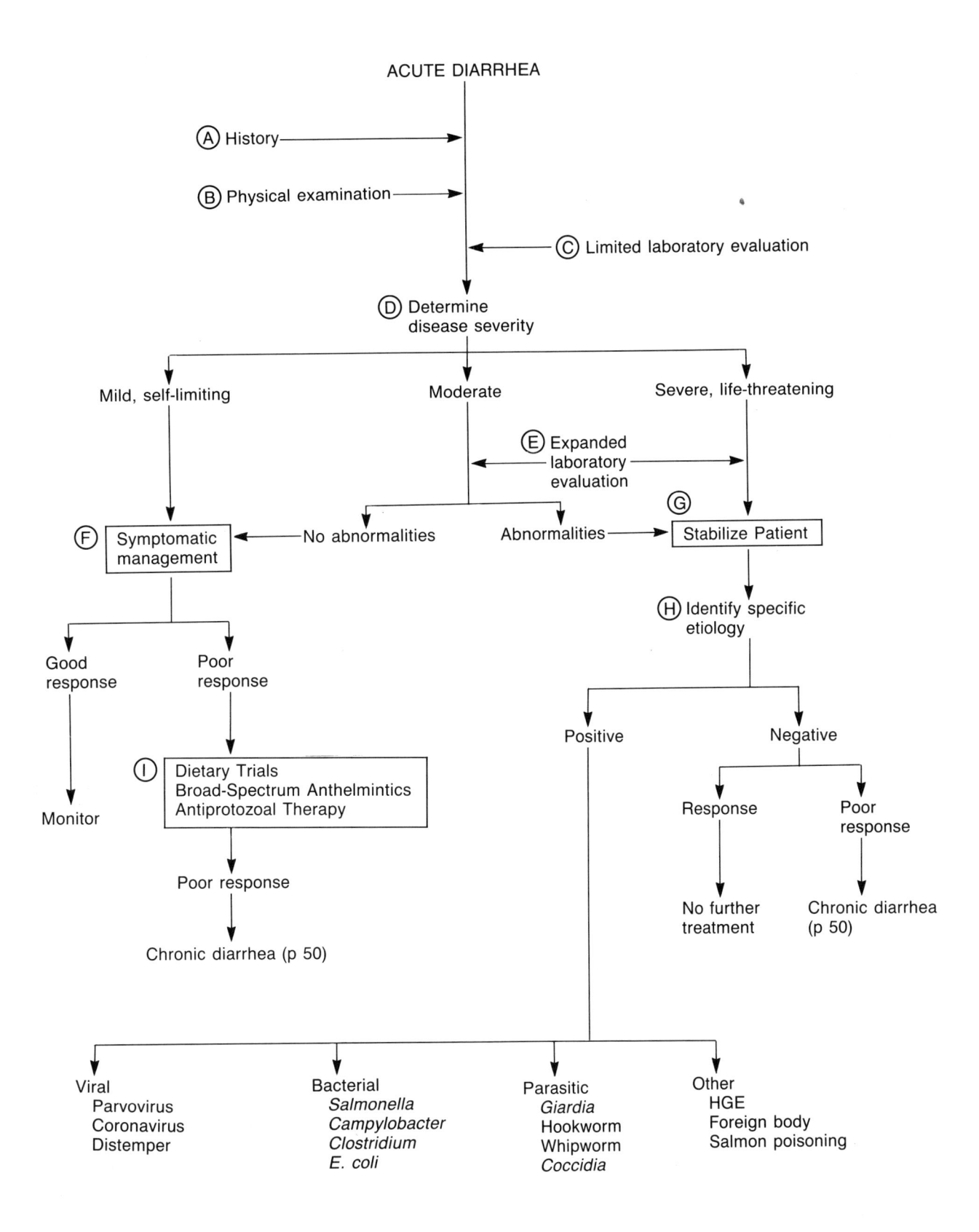

ACUTE DIARRHEA

- Ⓐ History
- Ⓑ Physical examination
- Ⓒ Limited laboratory evaluation
- Ⓓ Determine disease severity
  - Mild, self-limiting
  - Moderate
    - Ⓔ Expanded laboratory evaluation
      - No abnormalities
      - Abnormalities
  - Severe, life-threatening
    - Ⓖ Stabilize Patient
      - Ⓗ Identify specific etiology
        - Positive
          - Response → No further treatment
        - Negative
          - Poor response → Chronic diarrhea (p 50)

- Ⓕ Symptomatic management
  - Good response → Monitor
  - Poor response
    - Ⓘ Dietary Trials
      Broad-Spectrum Anthelmintics
      Antiprotozoal Therapy
      - Poor response → Chronic diarrhea (p 50)

Viral
Parvovirus
Coronavirus
Distemper

Bacterial
Salmonella
Campylobacter
Clostridium
E. coli

Parasitic
Giardia
Hookworm
Whipworm
Coccidia

Other
HGE
Foreign body
Salmon poisoning

49

CHRONIC DIARRHEA

David C. Twedt

A. Chronic diarrhea is diarrhea that (1) has persisted for a considerable length of time (usually greater than 2 weeks) or (2) has failed to respond to symptomatic therapy. Questions should be asked in order to investigate the duration, character, and frequency of the diarrhea. Further information should be gathered as to the diet, appetite, and possible environmental aspects. Determine the degree of weight loss as well as signs that are associated with systemic or primary extraintestinal disorders.

B. A complete examination with a review of all systems is required. Careful palpation of the intestinal tract and a rectal examination should be part of the physical examination.

C. Comprehensive laboratory evaluation, which is required in order to rule out systemic disease, may give a clue to the etiology of the diarrhea. A neutrophilia suggests inflammatory disease. A lymphopenia is frequently observed with lymphangiectasia, and an eosinophilia occurs with both endoparasites and eosinophilic gastroenteritis. Hypoproteinemia is associated with conditions that cause a protein-losing enteropathy. A comprehensive fecal examination, which includes evaluation for parasites as well as fecal cytology techniques, is required.

D. Based on the initial evaluation, the lesion should be localized anatomically to either large bowel or small bowel diarrhea. Small bowel diarrhea is characterized by a slight increase in frequency, large volume, and often watery nature. Melena, steatorrhea, and weight loss may be present. Large bowel diarrhea is one of increased frequency, urgency, tenesmus, and small volume, often with fresh blood and mucus. Weight loss is rare and steatorrhea absent.

E. With signs of large bowel diarrhea, proceed directly to evaluation of the colon with fecal cytology, proctoscopic examination, and mucosal biopsy. If it is not possible to examine the entire length of the colon, a barium enema should be performed.

F. Reasonably healthy animals with minimal disease may be treated symptomatically if signs are not severe and a delay in diagnosis would not be detrimental. Dietary trials and therapy for metazoan parasites (such as fenbendazole) and *Giardia* (quinacrine or metronidazole) are acceptable before embarking on an in-depth, diagnostic work-up. Response to such therapy supports the diagnosis.

G. When weight loss and debilitation result from chronic diarrhea, a maldigestion or malabsorption disorder should be suspected. Documentation of steatorrhea, either through positive fecal-staining with Sudan or quantitation of abnormal fecal fat excretion, supports a diagnosis, and should be the first step in evaluating a suspected case. With Sudan fecal-staining techniques, the steatorrhea can often be further separated into split and unsplit fats.

H. Unsplit or undigested fats in the feces stain as orange droplets and indicate maldigestion. Maldigested starch stains blue-black with iodine. Other screening tests include plasma turbidity, x-ray film, gelatin digestion, PABA digestion, and the trypsin-like immunoreactivity assay. Positive tests support the diagnosis of exocrine pancreatic insufficiency.

I. Digested fat in the feces stains with Sudan after first being mixed with acetic acid. A diagnosis of malabsorption is supported by an abnormal oral D-xylose or glucose tolerance test. In most cases, definitive diagnosis of malabsorptive conditions requires an intestinal mucosal biopsy. Full-thickness biopsy of the duodenum, jejunum, and ileum is indicated. Obtain a small amount of proximal intestinal fluid, and perform a direct smear examination for *Giardia*. Bacterial culture and quantitation of bacterial numbers for bacterial overgrowth should be considered.

J. A barium series is performed when other tests fail to determine the cause. Barium studies may demonstrate mucosal lesions, regional lesions, tumors, or strictures.

K. When no organic lesion is identified, irritable bowel syndrome, a functional diarrhea due to a motility disorder, should be considered and treated with diet, tranquilization, and/or motility modifiers. Dietary intolerance, which may show no mucosal lesions, should be considered and dietary trials initiated. Bacterial overgrowth and gastrointestinal parasites should be approached with a trial therapy as indicated.

L. The following intestinal lesions cause malabsorption: plasmacytic lymphocytic enteritis, eosinophilic enteritis, gluten enteropathy (villus atrophy), neutrophilic enteritis, lymphangiectasia, lymphosarcoma, histoplasmosis, granulomatous enteritis.

References

Burrows CF. Chronic diarrhea in the dog. Vet Clin North Am 1983; 13(3):521.

Chiapella A. Diagnosis and management of chronic colitis in the dog and cat. In: Kirk RW, ed. Current veterinary therapy IX. Philadelphia: WB Saunders, 1986:896.

Franklin RT, Jones BD, Feldman BF. Medical diseases of the small intestine. In: Jones BD, ed. Canine and feline gastroenterology. Philadelphia: WB Saunders, 1986:161.

Sherding RG. Diseases of the small bowel. In: Ettinger SJ, ed. Textbook of veterinary internal medicine. Philadelphia: WB Saunders, 1983:1278.

Strombeck DR. Maldigestion and Malabsorption. In: Small animal gastroenterology. Davis, CA: Stonegate Publishing, 1979:201.

Tams TR, Twedt DC. Canine protein losing gastroenteropathy syndrome. Comp Cont Ed 1981:105.

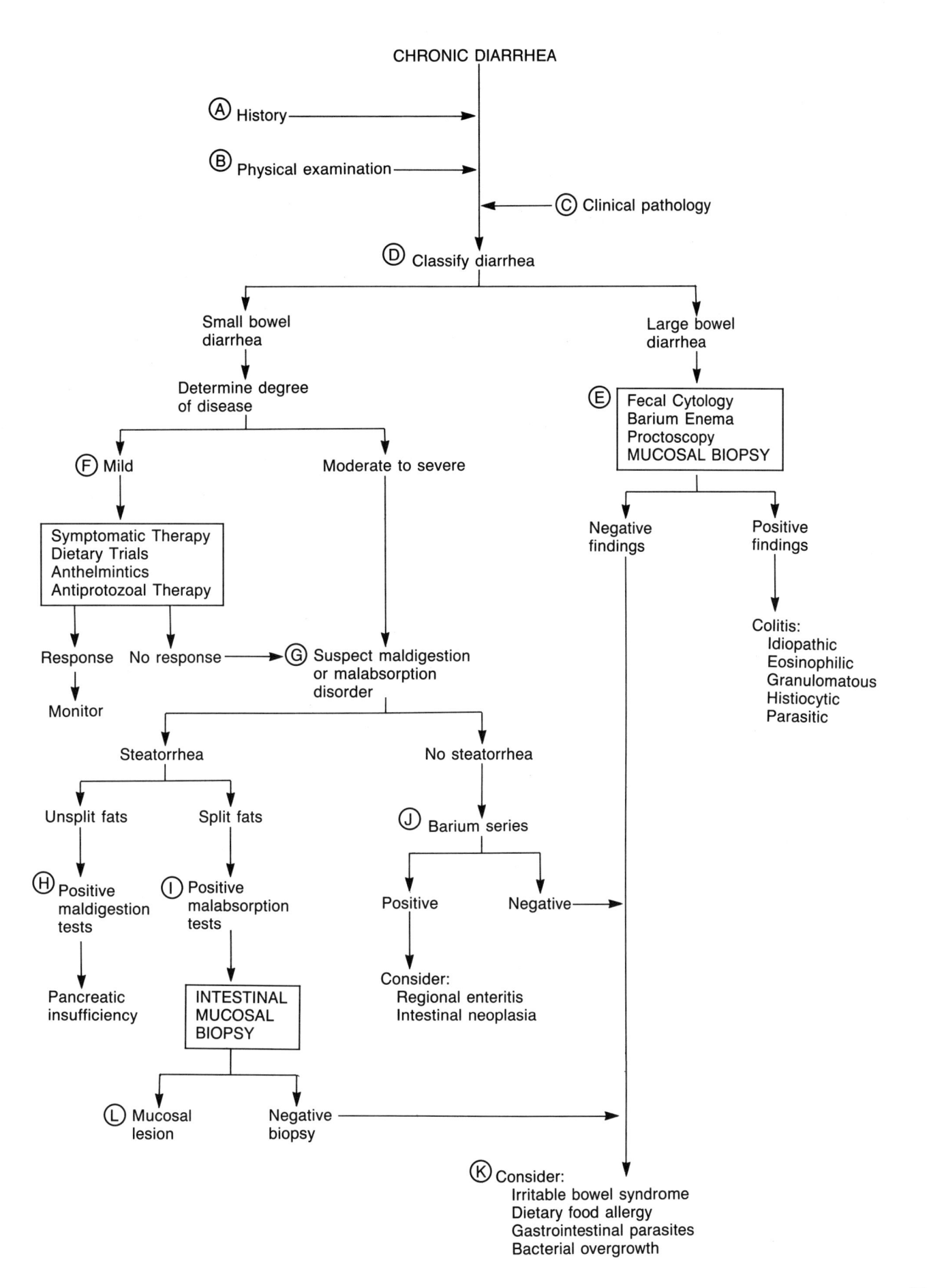

CHRONIC DIARRHEA

- Ⓐ History
- Ⓑ Physical examination
- Ⓒ Clinical pathology
- Ⓓ Classify diarrhea
  - Small bowel diarrhea
    - Determine degree of disease
      - Ⓕ Mild
        - Symptomatic Therapy
        - Dietary Trials
        - Anthelmintics
        - Antiprotozoal Therapy
          - Response → Monitor
          - No response → Ⓖ Suspect maldigestion or malabsorption disorder
      - Moderate to severe → Ⓖ Suspect maldigestion or malabsorption disorder
        - Steatorrhea
          - Unsplit fats → Ⓗ Positive maldigestion tests → Pancreatic insufficiency
          - Split fats → Ⓘ Positive malabsorption tests → INTESTINAL MUCOSAL BIOPSY
            - Ⓛ Mucosal lesion
            - Negative biopsy → Ⓚ
        - No steatorrhea
          - Ⓙ Barium series
            - Positive → Consider: Regional enteritis, Intestinal neoplasia
            - Negative → Ⓚ
  - Large bowel diarrhea
    - Ⓔ Fecal Cytology, Barium Enema, Proctoscopy, MUCOSAL BIOPSY
      - Negative findings → Ⓚ
      - Positive findings → Colitis: Idiopathic, Eosinophilic, Granulomatous, Histiocytic, Parasitic

Ⓚ Consider:
- Irritable bowel syndrome
- Dietary food allergy
- Gastrointestinal parasites
- Bacterial overgrowth

ACUTE LIVER TRAUMA

Karol A. Mathews

A. Liver injuries frequently occur as a result of motor vehicle accidents, but penetrating objects such as bullets, wooden sticks, and fractured ribs may also injure the liver. Small lacerations of the liver usually cause minimal bleeding and resolve spontaneously; however, large lacerations result in severe hemorrhage and shock. Isolated liver injury is rare; concurrent injuries to other organs must be considered.

B. The animal may be presented in hypovolemic shock. There may be anterior abdominal pain and fluid in the abdomen.

C. Obtain blood for packed cell volume (PCV), total protein (TP), and urea analysis prior to institution of shock therapy. Although the acute peripheral hematocrit is not a reliable indicator of blood loss, it does provide a baseline value for future assessment. The use of broad-spectrum antibiotics is recommended as liver trauma may result in tissue ischemia and proliferation of resident bacteria.

D. If the hematocrit of the abdominal fluid is less than 5 percent, hemorrhage is not the primary problem, and the fluid should be evaluated further (p 204). If there is a free flow of nonclotting blood that has a PCV and white blood cell count similar to peripheral blood, or if a PCV >5 percent is obtained upon peritoneal lavage, significant hemorrhage has occurred.

E. Obtain radiographs of the chest and abdomen in order to rule out thoracic injuries or a diaphragmatic hernia.

F. If a diaphragmatic injury is suspected, carry out exploratory laparotomy as soon as possible.

G. If there is no evidence or suspicion of a diaphragmatic hernia, conservative management should be instituted initially. Hemorrhage can frequently be managed by maintaining normovolemia with intravenous fluid therapy or whole blood (p 190). Use a compressive abdominal wrap to control the abdominal bleeding. Care must be taken not to compromise respiration, and compressive bandages must not be used if diaphragmatic injury is suspected. Assess vital signs hourly, and adjust fluid or whole blood requirements accordingly. Assessment of abdominal bleeding, as well as PCV and TP of the abdominal fluid, should be carried out hourly. A steady rise in abdominal fluid hematocrit indicates continued intra-abdominal bleeding, and exploratory laparotomy should be considered. If the patient continues to deteriorate although hemorrhaging is judged to be controlled, assess other organ systems.

H. When bleeding has been identified as coming from an injured liver, attempt hemostasis by direct pressure. Ligate individual bleeders. Deep lacerations may be enlarged in order to provide adequate exposure so as to facilitate vessel ligation, but exposure of tracts that have been caused by penetrating wounds is not necessary and may lead to uncontrollable hemorrhage. If hemorrhage continues or recurs, digital compression of the portal and hepatic veins (Pringle maneuvre) may control hemorrhage sufficiently to allow identification of the bleeding vessel. The Pringle maneuvre should last no longer than 15 minutes. Control persistent arterial bleeding by selected dearterialization. Control persistent oozing by suturing omentum over the wound or by applying a hemostatic agent. Absorbable gelatin or cellulose sponge should not be used as these have been associated with abscess formation. All devitalized and markedly traumatized tissue should be removed in order to avoid subsequent abscess formation, but contained hematomas should not be disturbed. To minimize the risk of abscessation, defects in healthy liver should not be closed, and the use of full-thickness, overlapping mattress sutures should be avoided. If injury is extensive, a lobectomy or partial lobectomy of the liver may be required.

References

Crowe DT, Bjorling DE. Peritoneum and peritoneal cavity. In: Slatter DH, ed. Textbook of small animal surgery. Philadelphia: WB Saunders, 1985:571.

Walshaw R. Surgical diseases of the liver and biliary system. In: Slatter DH, ed. Textbook of small animal surgery. Philadelphia: WB Saunders, 1985:798.

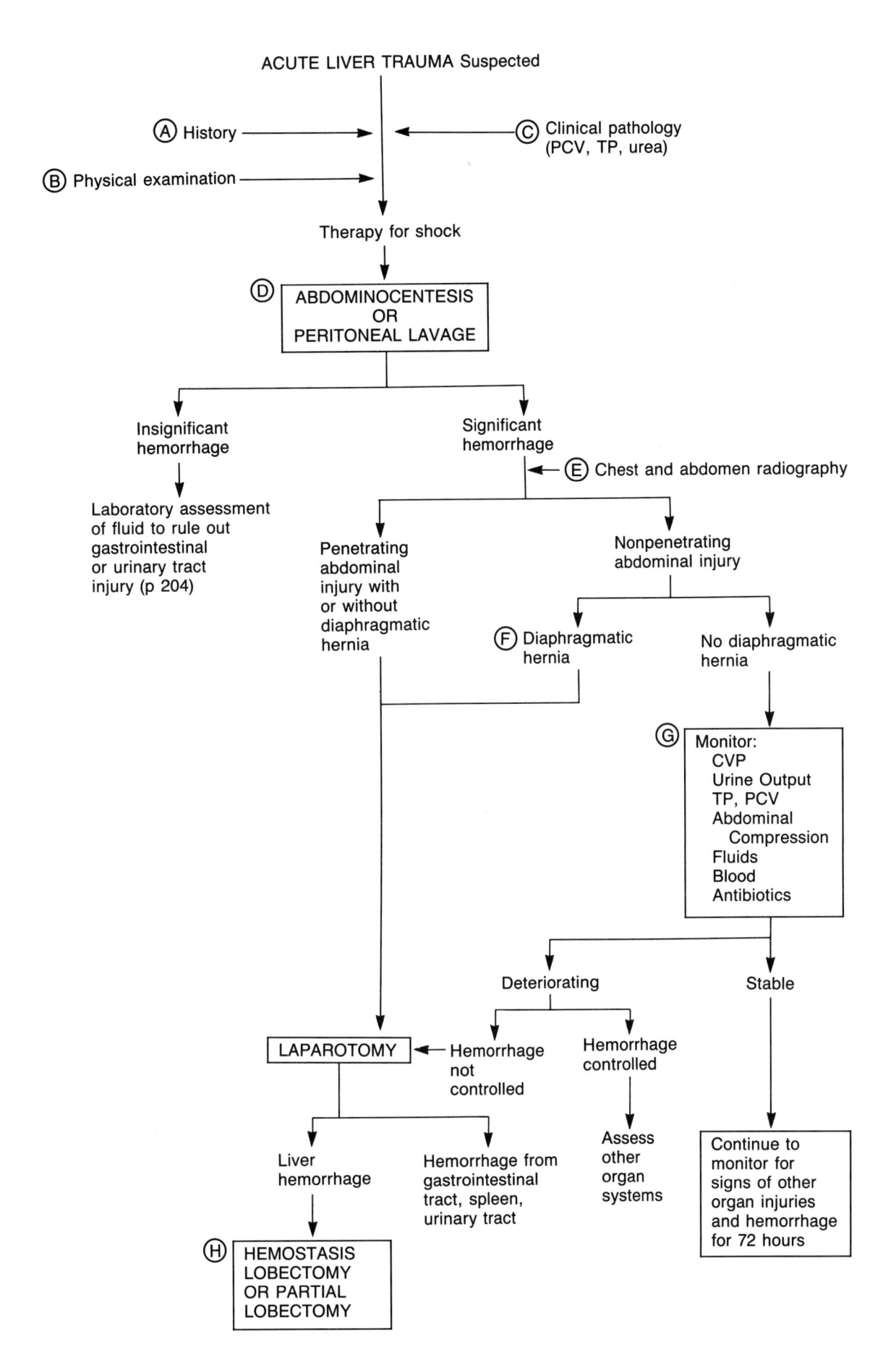

```
                    ACUTE LIVER TRAUMA Suspected
                                │
     Ⓐ History ──────────→      │      ←────── Ⓒ Clinical pathology
                                │                 (PCV, TP, urea)
     Ⓑ Physical examination ──→ │
                                ▼
                          Therapy for shock
                                │
                                ▼
                    ┌───────────────────────┐
                 Ⓓ │   ABDOMINOCENTESIS    │
                    │          OR           │
                    │   PERITONEAL LAVAGE   │
                    └───────────────────────┘
                         │              │
              Insignificant          Significant
              hemorrhage            hemorrhage    ←── Ⓔ Chest and abdomen radiography
                   │                     │
                   ▼                ┌────┴─────┐
         Laboratory assessment      │          │
         of fluid to rule out    Penetrating   Nonpenetrating
         gastrointestinal        abdominal     abdominal injury
         or urinary tract        injury with        │
         injury (p 204)          or without    ┌────┴────┐
                                 diaphragmatic │         │
                                 hernia     Ⓕ Diaphragmatic   No diaphragmatic
                                              hernia          hernia
                                                │                │
                                                │                ▼
                                                │        ┌─────────────────┐
                                                │      Ⓖ │ Monitor:         │
                                                │        │   CVP            │
                                                │        │   Urine Output   │
                                                │        │   TP, PCV        │
                                                │        │   Abdominal      │
                                                │        │    Compression   │
                                                │        │   Fluids         │
                                                │        │   Blood          │
                                                │        │   Antibiotics    │
                                                │        └─────────────────┘
                                                │             │         │
                                                │        Deteriorating  Stable
                                                │          │      │       │
                                                ▼          │      │       │
                                    ┌──────────────┐       │      │       │
                                    │  LAPAROTOMY  │←── Hemorrhage  Hemorrhage
                                    └──────────────┘   not          controlled
                                       │      │       controlled       │
                                       ▼      ▼                        ▼
                                   Liver   Hemorrhage from         Assess
                                   hemorrhage  gastrointestinal    other
                                       │    tract, spleen,         organ
                                       ▼    urinary tract          systems
                               ┌─────────────┐
                            Ⓗ │ HEMOSTASIS  │                  ┌──────────────┐
                               │  LOBECTOMY  │                  │ Continue to  │
                               │ OR PARTIAL  │                  │ monitor for  │
                               │  LOBECTOMY  │                  │ signs of other│
                               └─────────────┘                  │ organ injuries│
                                                                │ and hemorrhage│
                                                                │ for 72 hours  │
                                                                └──────────────┘
```

HEPATIC MASS

Karol A Mathews

A. The history of a patient with a hepatic tumor or abscess is often one of gradual weight loss, lethargy, and depression. The presenting signs may include abdominal pain, vomiting, abdominal distention, or acute collapse. A previous episode of acute collapse may be reported. A history of abdominal trauma or liver surgery may be suggestive of an abscess.

B. On physical examination, pain may be elicited on palpation of the anterior abdomen. A fever may be present. The degree of wasting varies with the duration of the clinical course. Icterus rarely occurs. Occasionally an abdominal mass may be detected on routine physical examination although there is no related clinical history.

C. Serum alanine aminotransferase (SALT), serum alkaline phosphatase (SAP), and bilirubin concentration are rarely elevated with focal hepatic lesions. Increased SALT, SAP, and possibly bilirubin levels may be evidence of a more extensive lesion. An animal with a hepatic abscess or necrotic tumor often has a neutrophilic leukocytosis with a left shift. White blood cell counts of 10,000 to 30,000 per μl are common but may exceed 50,000 per μl. The animal may be anemic from blood loss, chronic infection, or malignancy. Evaluate blood urea, electrolytes, and blood gases in critical cases.

D. Hepatic tumors may rupture, which results in abdominal hemorrhage and collapse. Hepatic abscesses that rupture may also lead to collapse as a result of hypodynamic septic shock.

E. Liver masses may be identified on survey abdominal radiographs or by ultrasonography. Gas pockets within the liver are highly suggestive of hepatic abscessation. Free fluid within the abdomen may obscure the hepatic shadow.

F. Diagnosis of septic peritonitis, or of abdominal hemorrhage, is based on analysis of the abdominal fluid (p 204).

G. If a tumor is suspected, thoracic radiographs should be taken prior to exploratory laparotomy in order to rule out pulmonary metastases.

H. The most common primary liver neoplasms are hepatocellular adenoma (hepatoma), hepatocellular carcinoma, hepatic carcinoid (tumor of biliary epithelium), and bile duct carcinoma. Less common primary tumors include fibroma, fibrosarcoma, hemangioma, and leiomyosarcoma. Hepatocellular adenomas are usually focal, well circumscribed, and highly vascular. They are friable and therefore commonly rupture. Hepatocellular carcinomas and bile duct carcinomas can be nodular, diffuse, or massive (large mass from a single liver lobe, frequently associated with smaller nodules in other lobes). Metastasis to the liver from other organs is common. These lesions are commonly diffuse, but may occasionally be single.

I. If possible, a large vascular tumor (especially if ruptured) should be excised by partial or total lobectomy, even if there is diffuse hepatic involvement. If a single tumor is nonresectable, selective hepatic artery ligation may reduce tumor growth. Hepatic artery ligation or embolization combined with infusion chemotherapy is currently being used in humans.

References

Hardy RM. Diseases of the liver. In: Ettinger SJ, ed. Textbook of veterinary internal medicine. Philadelphia: WB Saunders, 1983: 1372.

Magne ML, Withrow SJ. Hepatic neoplasia. Vet Clin North Am 1985; 15:243.

Walshaw R. Surgical diseases of the liver and biliary system. In: Slatter DH, ed. Textbook of small animal surgery. Philadelphia: WB Saunders, 1985: 798.

HEPATIC MASS Suspected

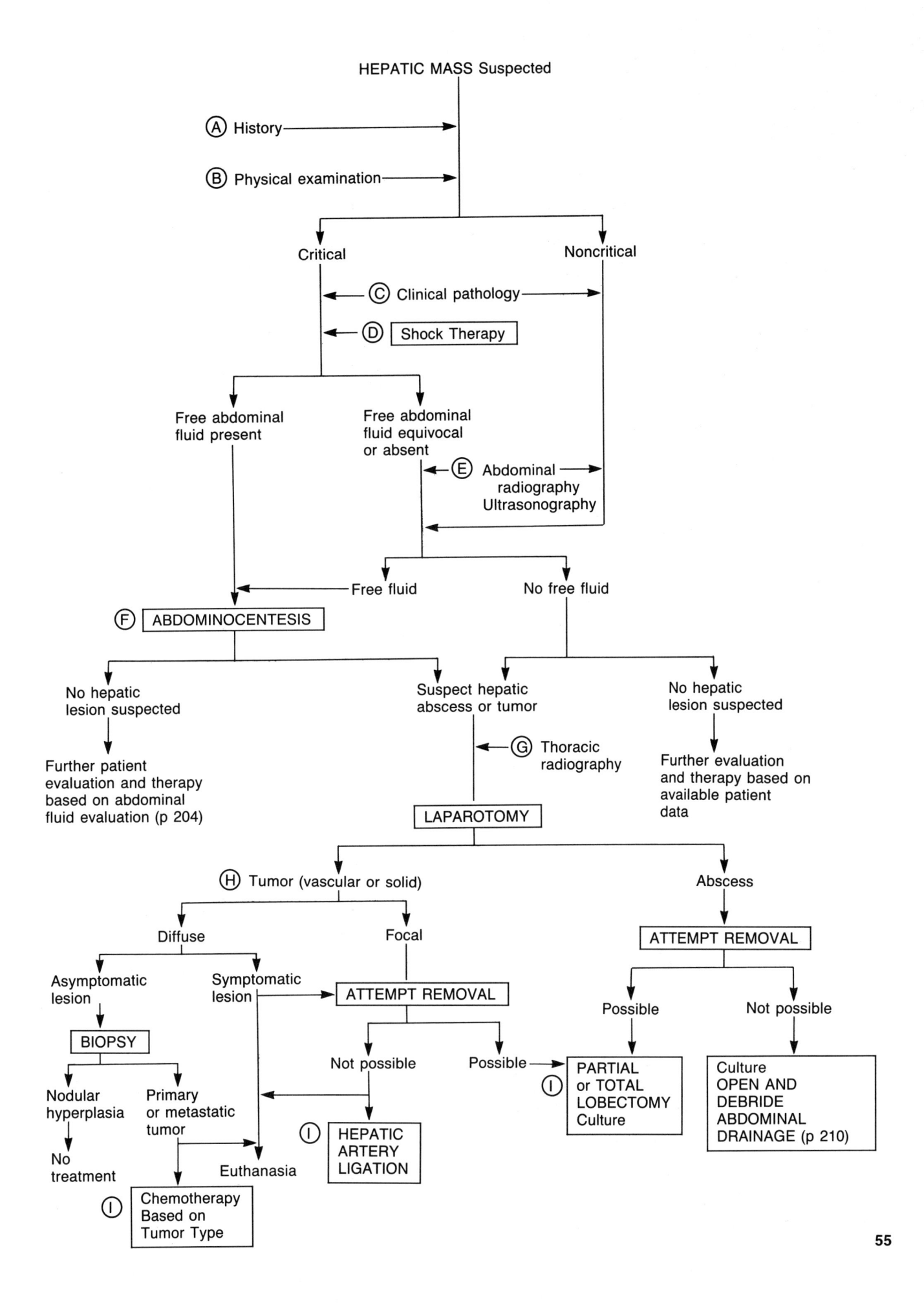

- Ⓐ History
- Ⓑ Physical examination

→ Critical / Noncritical

- Ⓒ Clinical pathology
- Ⓓ Shock Therapy

Critical → Free abdominal fluid present / Free abdominal fluid equivocal or absent

- Ⓔ Abdominal radiography / Ultrasonography

→ Free fluid / No free fluid

- Ⓕ **ABDOMINOCENTESIS**

From ABDOMINOCENTESIS:
- No hepatic lesion suspected → Further patient evaluation and therapy based on abdominal fluid evaluation (p 204)
- Suspect hepatic abscess or tumor
- No hepatic lesion suspected → Further evaluation and therapy based on available patient data

- Ⓖ Thoracic radiography

LAPAROTOMY

- Ⓗ Tumor (vascular or solid) / Abscess

Tumor:
- Diffuse
  - Asymptomatic lesion → **BIOPSY**
    - Nodular hyperplasia → No treatment
    - Primary or metastatic tumor → Ⓘ Chemotherapy Based on Tumor Type
  - Symptomatic lesion → **ATTEMPT REMOVAL**
- Focal → **ATTEMPT REMOVAL**
  - Not possible → Euthanasia / Ⓘ **HEPATIC ARTERY LIGATION**
  - Possible → Ⓘ **PARTIAL or TOTAL LOBECTOMY** Culture

Abscess → **ATTEMPT REMOVAL**
- Possible → Ⓘ **PARTIAL or TOTAL LOBECTOMY** Culture
- Not possible → Culture **OPEN AND DEBRIDE ABDOMINAL DRAINAGE** (p 210)

55

BILIARY TRACT TRAUMA

Karol A. Mathews

A. Biliary tract injury usually does not become apparent until several days after the traumatic incident. During this time, the patient becomes progressively depressed and anorexic. Vomiting, abdominal pain, icterus, rust-colored urine, acholic feces, and an enlarging abdomen are frequently reported. If there is an extension of bile into the thorax, the resulting bile pleuritis may cause progressive dyspnea. Physical findings usually consist of icterus, dehydration, poor body condition, a fluid-distended abdomen, abdominal pain, fever, and tachycardia. If bile pleuritis is present, abnormalities can be detected on thoracic auscultation.

B. Turbid, green-to-dark-brown fluid may be obtained upon abdominocentesis (p 204). Although bile is sterile, bacterial contamination may occur if there is concurrent gastrointestinal injury; therefore, a culture and sensitivity should be performed.

C. Serum biochemical profile values may include conjugated and nonconjugated hyperbilirubinemia and an elevation in serum alkaline phosphatase, serum alanine aminotransferase, and serum aspartate aminotransferase. Hypoproteinemia, electrolyte imbalance, neutrophilia, and anemia are usually present.

D. After abdominal drainage, take abdominal and thoracic radiographs in order to assess the integrity of the diaphragm and to identify other injuries. Survey radiographs rarely provide information with regard to the biliary tract. Cholecystography is usually unrewarding because of the poor concentrating ability of the biliary system.

E. Repair simple tears by use of an inverting suture technique. Extensive injuries may require cholecystectomy.

F. Reimplant the bile duct by tunneling it between the mucosal and muscular layers of the duodenum. Alternatively, depending on the degree of duct dilation, an end-to-side or side-to-side choledochoenterostomy may be performed. If a choledochoeneteral anastomasis is not possible, a cholecystoenterostomy may be performed. An elliptical enterotomy, is made with removal of everting mucosa, in order to create a stoma that is a minimum of 2.5 cm in width.

G. Suturing the hepatic wound may repair the biliary leak. However, as this may lead to abscess formation, ligation of the ruptured duct is preferred.

H. Bile duct perforations may be amenable to a primary repair with or without a T-tube or straight tube stent (Fig. 1). Large perforations may require cholecystoenterostomy. A transected bile duct may be repaired by end-to-end anastomosis. If there is severe damage to the proximal stump of the bile duct, the gallbladder may be anastomosed to the distal part of the common bile duct or cholecystoenterostomy may be performed.

I. An avulsed hepatic duct may be ligated, and the associated bile duct defect may be closed. If hepatic duct avulsion results in a major bile duct defect, an attempt should be made to anastomose the hepatic duct to the bile duct. A simple interrupted-suture technique should be used and a T-tube placed.

J. Uncomplicated bile peritonitis is nonseptic and, therefore, does not require postoperative drainage. However, should the abdomen become contaminated prior to or during surgery, drainage is indicated. Carry out saline lavage at laparotomy.

K. The T-tube should have a minimal drainage to the exterior. If drainage is excessive, the duct or the tube, or both, may be obstructed. To avoid an ascending cholangitis, tube management should be aseptic. Bile cultures can be obtained from the tube and cholangiographic studies can be performed through the tube. In dogs, T-tubes have remained in place from 9 to 42 days. Stricture at the anastomotic site of any biliary procedure may occur whether or not a T-tube is used. Serum alkaline phosphatase levels should be measured periodically for several months in order to monitor for cholangitis secondary to obstruction or infection.

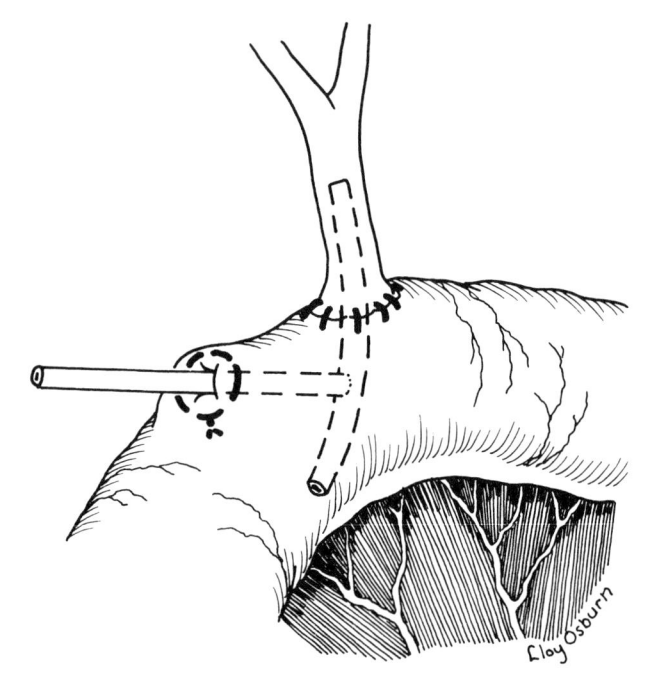

Figure 1 Use of a T-tube as a stent in choledochoduodenal anastomosis. The tube exits the intestine through a pursestring suture below the anastomosis.

References

Blass CE. Surgery of the biliary tract. Comp Cont Ed 1983; 5(10):801.

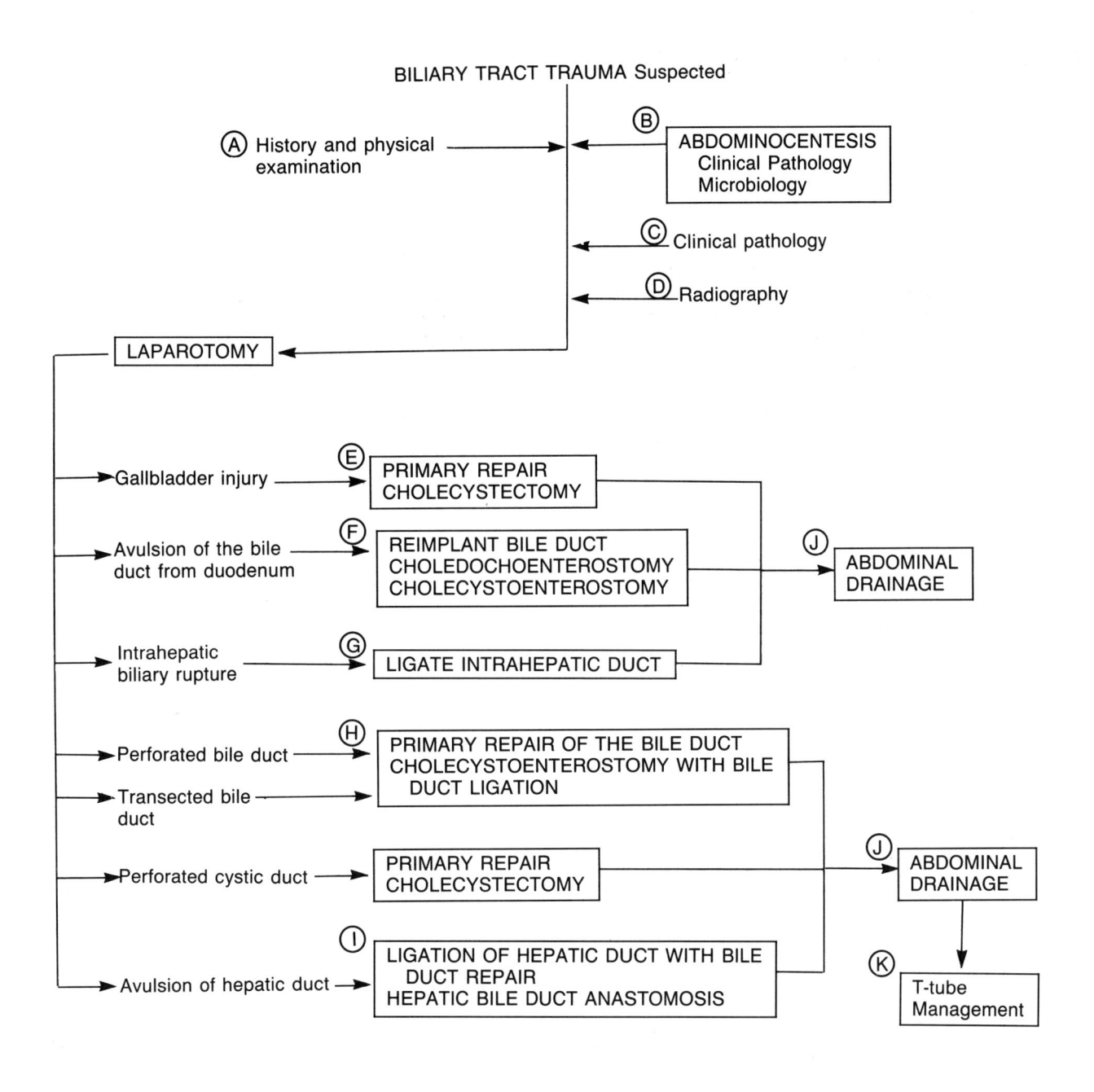

```
                            BILIARY TRACT TRAUMA Suspected
                                         │
         Ⓐ History and physical ─────────▶│◀──── Ⓑ  ABDOMINOCENTESIS
            examination                   │         Clinical Pathology
                                          │         Microbiology
                                          │
                                          │◀──── Ⓒ Clinical pathology
                                          │
                                          │◀──── Ⓓ Radiography
                                          ▼
                                    ┌──────────┐
                            ┌───────│LAPAROTOMY│
                            │       └──────────┘
```

- Gallbladder injury → **Ⓔ PRIMARY REPAIR / CHOLECYSTECTOMY**
- Avulsion of the bile duct from duodenum → **Ⓕ REIMPLANT BILE DUCT / CHOLEDOCHOENTEROSTOMY / CHOLECYSTOENTEROSTOMY** → **Ⓙ ABDOMINAL DRAINAGE**
- Intrahepatic biliary rupture → **Ⓖ LIGATE INTRAHEPATIC DUCT**
- Perforated bile duct / Transected bile duct → **Ⓗ PRIMARY REPAIR OF THE BILE DUCT / CHOLECYSTOENTEROSTOMY WITH BILE DUCT LIGATION**
- Perforated cystic duct → **PRIMARY REPAIR / CHOLECYSTECTOMY** → **Ⓙ ABDOMINAL DRAINAGE** → **Ⓚ T-tube Management**
- Avulsion of hepatic duct → **Ⓘ LIGATION OF HEPATIC DUCT WITH BILE DUCT REPAIR / HEPATIC BILE DUCT ANASTOMOSIS**

Dingwall JS. The liver and biliary system. In: Bojrab MJ, ed. Current techniques in small animal surgery. Philadelphia: Lea & Febiger, 1975:142.

Hertzer DR, Gray HW, Hoerr SO, Hermann RE. The use of T-tube splints in bile duct repairs. Surg Gynecol Obstet 1973; 137:414.

Hunt CA, Gofton N. Primary repairs of a transected bile duct. JAAMA 1984; 20:57.

Tangner CH. Cholecystoduodenostomy in the dog—comparison of two techniques. Vet Surg 1984; 13(3):126.

BILE DUCT OBSTRUCTION

Howard B. Seim III

A. Patients with bile duct obstruction generally present with depression, anorexia, vomiting, progressive weight loss, and persistent icterus. Cranial abdominal pain may be present depending upon the specific etiology. The most dramatic physical finding is icteric mucous membranes.

B. Survey radiographic studies are often unrewarding, as biliary calculi are infrequent and often radiolucent in dogs and cats. Cholecystography in icteric patients is often difficult to assess owing to the poor concentrating ability of the biliary system. Ultrasonography is helpful in detecting dilation of bile ducts in larger breed dogs. Laparoscopic placement of a catheter in the gallbladder and injection of radiopaque dye is helpful in assessing the biliary tree.

C. The biochemical profile may vary depending upon the duration of obstruction, the completeness of obstruction, and the amount of liver damage secondary to cholestasis-induced periportal inflammation. Generally, serum bilirubin is variably elevated with increases in both conjugated and unconjugated fractions. Acholic feces and negative urine urobilinogen are seen in cases of complete bile duct obstruction. Positive urobilinogen and normal-colored stools may suggest a partial obstruction. The alkaline phosphatase (ALP) is usually markedly elevated due to cholestatic induction of alkaline phosphatase synthesis. Alanine aminotransferase (ALT) and aspartate aminotransferase (AST) may show variable degrees of elevation, depending on the degree and duration of cholestasis. Coagulopathy may be present in patients with severe liver disease.

D. Cholecystotomy can be performed for removal of choleliths. After entering the gallbladder, a sample of bile is taken for aerobic and anaerobic culture and sensitivity testing, the choleliths are removed for analysis, and the common bile duct is irrigated. Closure of the cholecystotomy incision is performed using one or two continuous, inverting layers of synthetic absorbable suture material.

E. In cases of extramural or mural bile duct obstruction, the treatments of choice include cholecystoduodenostomy or cholecystojejunostomy using a Roux-en-Y loop. The choice of technique lies mainly in the surgeon's preference. Cholecystoduodenostomy involves freeing the gallbladder from its attachment to the liver; positioning the duodenum next to the gallbladder; making two parallel incisions 2.5 cm in length (one in the gallbladder and one in the duodenum); and anastomosing the two using a double-layer, simple, continuous pattern with absorbable suture material.

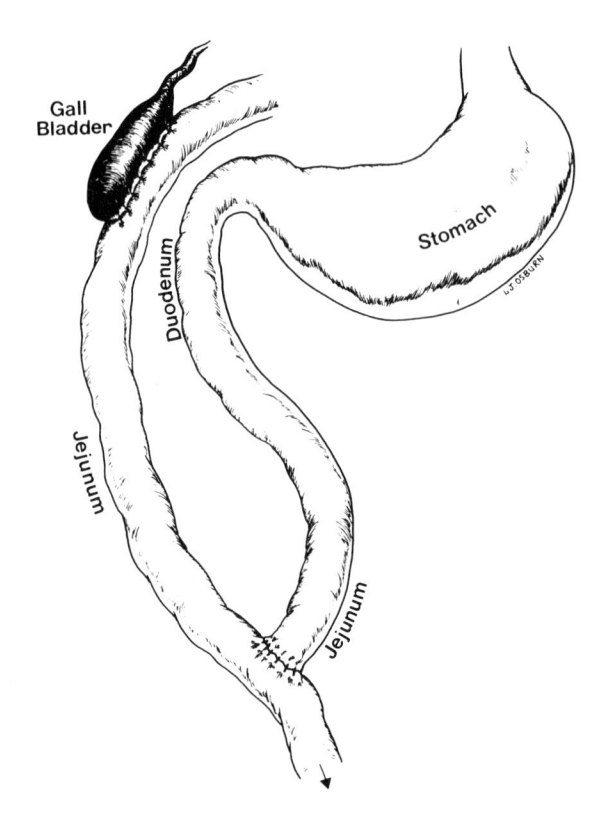

Figure 1 Cholecystojejunostomy: Gallbladder segment is approximately 40 cm in length.

F. Cholecystojejunostomy using a Roux-en-Y loop involves the advancement of a segment of jejunum (about 40 cm in length) to the gallbladder (Fig. 1). A cholecystojejunostomy is performed as described for cholecystoduodenostomy. And end-to-side jejunostomy is performed to restore intestinal continuity. The defunctioned limb of jejunum serves as a conduit for biliary secretions and helps to prevent enterobiliary reflux.

References

Blass CE, Seim HB,III. Surgical techniques for the liver and biliary tract. Vet Clin North Am 1985; 15(1):257.

Magne ML, Wrigley RH, Twedt DC. Cholecystography and cholecystoduodenostomy in the diagnosis and treatment of bile duct obstruction in a dog. JAVMA 1985; 187(5):509.

Tangner CH. Cholecystoduodenostomy in the dog: comparison of two techniques. Vet Surg 1984; 13(3):126.

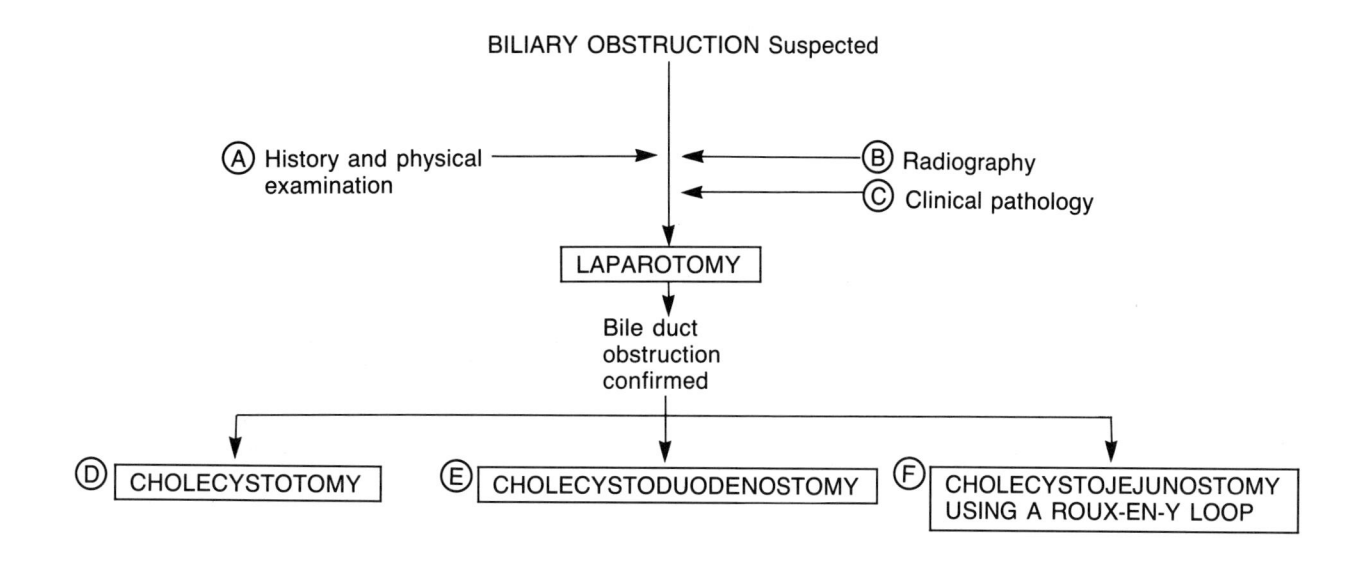

BILIARY OBSTRUCTION Suspected

- (A) History and physical examination
- (B) Radiography
- (C) Clinical pathology

↓

LAPAROTOMY

Bile duct obstruction confirmed

- (D) **CHOLECYSTOTOMY**
- (E) **CHOLECYSTODUODENOSTOMY**
- (F) **CHOLECYSTOJEJUNOSTOMY USING A ROUX-EN-Y LOOP**

PANCREATITIS

Howard B. Seim III

A. Pancreatitis can be a very serious clinical syndrome with potentially devastating consequences. The nonspecific presentation of sudden vomiting, diarrhea, depression, and anorexia in a middle- to older-aged and often obese patient may be misleading.

B. Tenderness on palpation of the right cranial abdominal quadrant may be a helpful physical finding. Other findings may include mild fever, dehydration, and cardiac arrhythmia.

C. The most common radiographic findings in patients with acute pancreatitis include increased density, diminished contrast and granularity of the right cranial abdominal quadrant, displacement of the stomach toward the left side of the abdomen, truncated pyloric antral border, presence of a fluid density medial to the proximal descending duodenum, and duodenal displacement toward the right flank. Any one or a combination of these findings is highly suggestive of pancreatitis.

D. Common abnormalities in the serum biochemistries are an increase in BUN, ALT, AST, alkaline phosphatase, glucose, amylase, and lipase. Any one or a combination of these abnormalities, along with the above historic, physical, and radiographic findings are strongly suggestive of pancreatitis.

E. Initial therapy should include replacement of fluid and electrolyte losses from dehydration and vomiting, then maintenance fluid replacement using polyionic isotonic fluid. Antibiotics are instituted to decrease the incidence of pancreatic and parapancreatic abscess formation and septicemia. Food is withheld for 3 to 5 days.

F. Patients that fail to respond favorably to medical management may benefit from closed peritoneal lavage. An ingress catheter is placed in the upper right abdominal quadrant (flank), and an egress sump drain is placed in the ventral abdomen. Inflow and outflow peritoneal lavage is carried out two to three times per day. Another technique that may increase the efficacy of peritoneal lavage is the use of a peritoneal dialysis catheter. The catheter is placed in the ventral abdominal region. Fluid at body temperature is infused into the peritoneal cavity, allowed to remain for 20 to 30 minutes, then removed. Lavage is continued until the fluid cytology reveals a nonsuppurative inflammation and the clinical signs begin to resolve.

G. If 3 to 5 days of closed peritoneal lavage is unsuccessful, exploratory celiotomy and partial or total pancreatectomy must be considered. In cases with severe peritonitis, open abdominal drainage after celiotomy may be considered.

References

Jacobs RM, Murtaugh RJ, DeHoff WD. Review of the clinicopathological findings of acute pancreatitis in the dog: use of an experimental model. JAAHA 1985; 21:795.

Kleine LJ, Hornbuckle WE. Acute pancreatitis: the radiographic findings in 182 dogs. Vet Radiol 1978; 19(4):102.

Mulvany MH, Feinberg CK, Tilson DL. Clinical characterization of acute necrotizing pancreatitis. Comp Cont Ed 1982; 4(5):394.

Orsher RJ, Rosin E. Open peritoneal drainage in experimental peritonitis in dogs. Vet Surg 1984; 13(4):222.

Parks J, Greene RW. Peritoneal lavage for peritonitis and pancreatitis in 22 dogs. JAAHA 1973; 9:442.

Ranson JHC, Spencer FC. The role of peritoneal lavage in severe acute pancreatitis. Ann Surg 1978; 187(5):565.

Schaer M. A clinicopathologic survey of acute pancreatitis in 30 dogs and five cats. JAAHA 1979; 15:681.

Wolfson P. Surgical management of inflammatory disorders of the pancreas. Surg Gynecol Obstet 1980; 151:689.

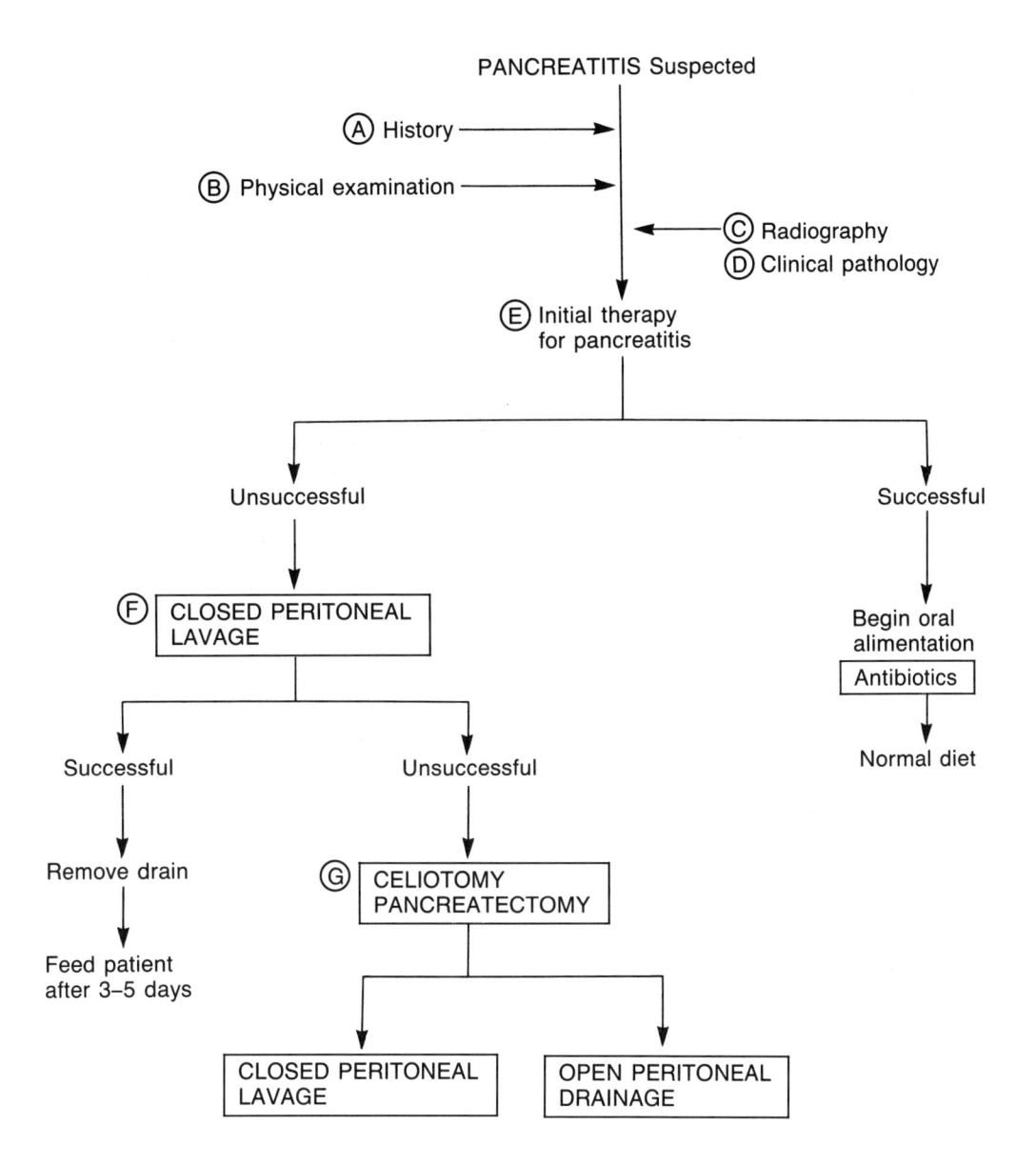

```
                    PANCREATITIS Suspected
                              │
            Ⓐ History ────────▶│
                              │
            Ⓑ Physical examination ──▶│
                              │◀──── Ⓒ Radiography
                              │      Ⓓ Clinical pathology
                              ▼
                        Ⓔ Initial therapy
                          for pancreatitis
                              │
              ┌───────────────┴───────────────┐
              ▼                               ▼
         Unsuccessful                     Successful
              │                               │
              ▼                               ▼
         ┌─────────────────┐             Begin oral
         │Ⓕ CLOSED PERITONEAL│            alimentation
         │   LAVAGE        │             ┌──────────┐
         └─────────────────┘             │Antibiotics│
              │                          └──────────┘
      ┌───────┴───────┐                       │
      ▼               ▼                       ▼
  Successful     Unsuccessful              Normal diet
      │               │
      ▼               ▼
  Remove drain   ┌─────────────────┐
      │          │Ⓖ CELIOTOMY      │
      ▼          │  PANCREATECTOMY │
  Feed patient   └─────────────────┘
  after 3–5 days         │
                 ┌───────┴────────┐
                 ▼                ▼
         ┌──────────────┐  ┌──────────────┐
         │CLOSED PERITONEAL│ │OPEN PERITONEAL│
         │   LAVAGE     │  │   DRAINAGE   │
         └──────────────┘  └──────────────┘
```

PANCREATIC NEOPLASIA

Elizabeth J. Laing

Pancreatic neoplasms are primarily of endocrine or exocrine epithelial origin. Islet cell carcinoma, or insulinoma, is the most common endocrine tumor. Pancreatic adenocarcinoma is the most common exocrine tumor. In both tumors, metastasis to mesenteric lymph nodes and liver is common; this results in clinical signs of liver disease or biliary stasis.

A. Pancreatic neoplasia should be considered in patients with a history of weight loss, anorexia, chronic vomiting, depression, or jaundice. Functional islet cell tumors may also cause polyuria-polydipsia, weakness, muscle tremors, disorientation, and seizures.

B. Examination may reveal tenderness in the cranial abdomen, but the tumor itself is rarely palpable. Jaundice may occur from bile duct obstruction.

C. Laboratory data base should include CBC, urinalysis, liver enzymes, bilirubin, amylase, and blood glucose. If the blood glucose is low (<60 mg per deciliter) or clinical signs suggest hypoglycemia, check fasting serum insulin levels and determine the insulin:glucose ratio. Hypoglycemia with concomitant hyperinsulinemia, in the absence of liver disease or sepsis, is suggestive of a functional islet cell carcinoma.

D. Other diseases with similar signs include chronic pancreatitis, pancreatitic hyperplasia, extrapancreatic abdominal tumors, and primary gastrointestinal or liver disease. Exploratory celiotomy and biopsy are usually needed for a definitive diagnosis. Regional lymph node and liver biopsies are used to determine the extent of disease.

E. The clinical signs of a functional islet cell carcinoma are usually caused by the associated paraneoplastic syndrome, rather than the tumor mass. Two functional pancreatic tumors occur in small animals, the most common is insulinoma or functional beta cell carcinoma, in which increased insulin secretion causes clinical signs of hypoglycemia. The less common gastrin-secreting tumors (gastrinomas) cause Zollinger-Ellison syndrome with diarrhea, weight loss, and gastric ulceration. In both cases, functional liver or lymph node metastases are present at diagnosis in 50 percent of cases.

F. Adenocarcinoma is the most common type of nonfunctional pancreatic tumor. Others include nonfunctional islet cell carcinomas or nonepithelial tumors. Liver or lymph node metastasis is often present at diagnosis. Metastasis may also occur to the lung, duodenum, kidney, adrenal gland, and retroperitoneum.

G. Partial pancreatectomy is recommended for solitary pancreatic lesions (Fig. 1). If the mass is causing bile duct obstruction, a cholecystojejunostomy is indicated. Occasionally, the primary tumor is not clinically detectable; in this case, medical treatment is indicated. Total pancreatectomy or pancreaticoduodenal resection is no longer recommended and may, in fact, significantly increase postoperative morbidity. Following surgery, approximately 25 percent of patients develop transient hyperglycemia. Although blood glucose levels usually stabilize over the next 2 to 4 weeks, insulin therapy may be needed. Persistent hypoglycemia suggests incomplete excision or metastatic disease.

H. For diffuse or metastatic lesions, surgery is usually limited to biopsy for diagnosis. Medical therapy is used to control the paraneoplastic signs. For insulinomas, frequent (four to six times per day) feedings of a high protein, low

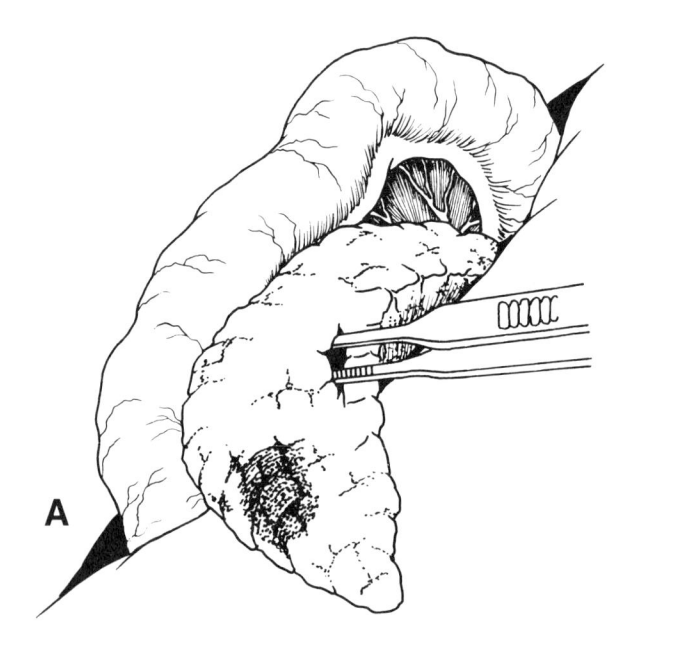

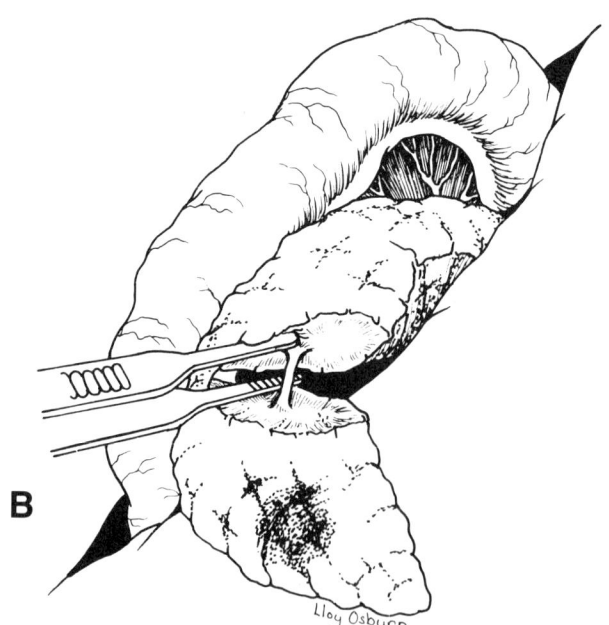

Figure 1 Partial pancreatectomy: *A*, separation of pancreatic lobules; and *B*, preparation of central duct for ligation.

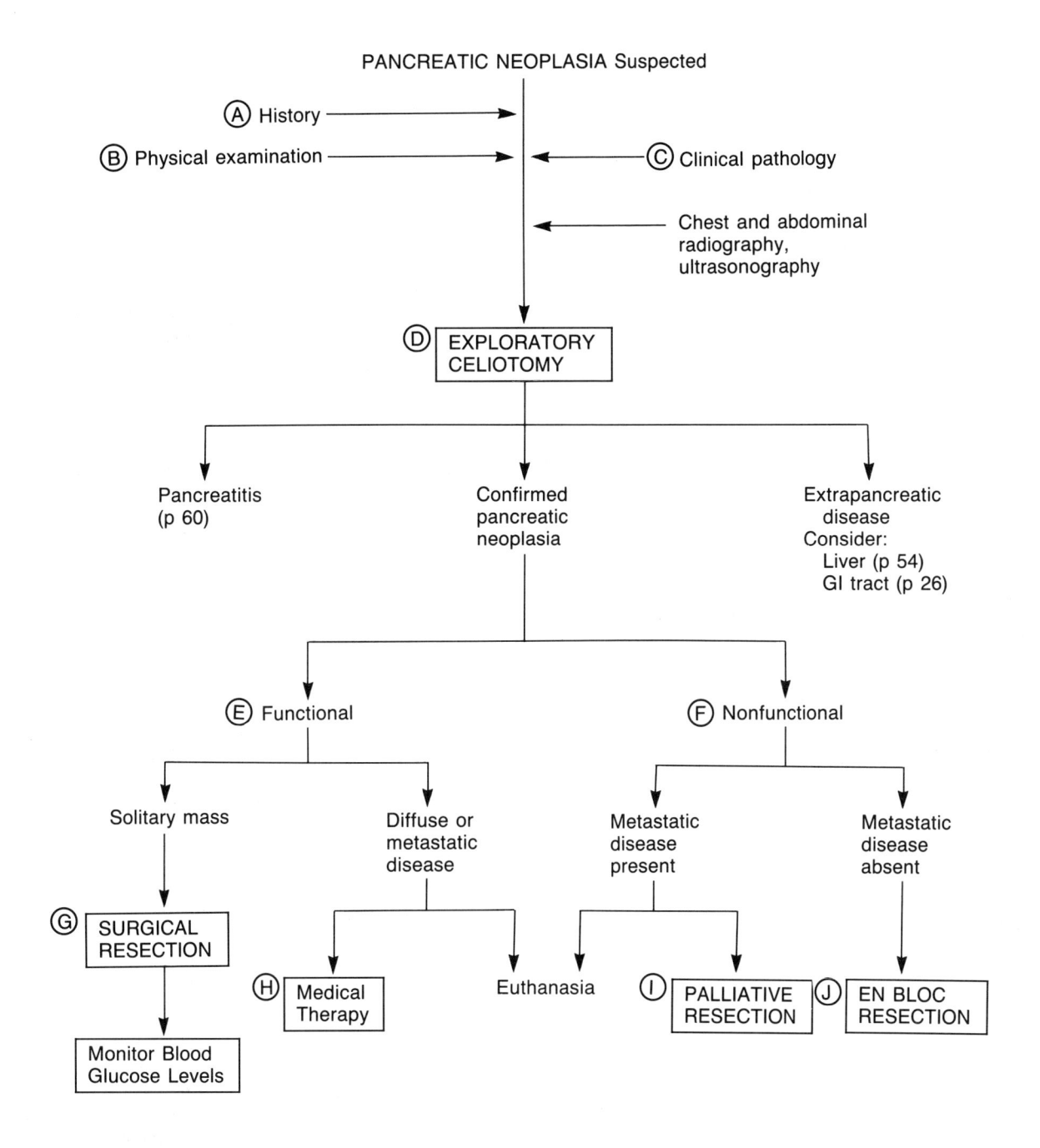

```
                    PANCREATIC NEOPLASIA Suspected
                                │
        Ⓐ History ──────────────→│
                                 │
        Ⓑ Physical examination ─→│←── Ⓒ Clinical pathology
                                 │
                                 │←── Chest and abdominal
                                 │    radiography,
                                 │    ultrasonography
                                 ↓
                        Ⓓ ┌─────────────┐
                          │ EXPLORATORY │
                          │  CELIOTOMY  │
                          └─────────────┘
                    ┌───────────┼───────────┐
                    ↓           ↓           ↓
              Pancreatitis  Confirmed   Extrapancreatic
                 (p 60)     pancreatic     disease
                            neoplasia    Consider:
                                         Liver (p 54)
                                         GI tract (p 26)
                            ┌──────┴──────┐
                            ↓             ↓
                        Ⓔ Functional   Ⓕ Nonfunctional
                         ┌───┴───┐      ┌────┴────┐
                         ↓       ↓      ↓         ↓
                    Solitary  Diffuse or  Metastatic  Metastatic
                     mass     metastatic   disease    disease
                              disease     present     absent
                       ↓       ┌─┴─┐         ↓         ↓
                    Ⓖ┌──────┐  ↓   ↓      Ⓘ┌─────────┐ Ⓙ┌──────────┐
                     │SURGICAL│ Ⓗ Medical   │PALLIATIVE│ │ EN BLOC  │
                     │RESECTION│  Therapy  │RESECTION │ │RESECTION │
                     └────────┘  Euthanasia└─────────┘ └──────────┘
                        ↓
                    Monitor Blood
                    Glucose Levels
```

carbohydrate diet is indicated. Blood glucose levels may also be maintained by the use of insulin antagonists such as diazoxide (3 to 12 mg per kilogram orally three times a day) and prednisolone (0.25 to 0.5 mg per kilogram daily by mouth). Various antineoplastic agents have been used in human medicine, including doxorubicin, cyclophosphamide, and 5-fluorouracil.

I. Palliative surgery may be used to temporarily alleviate clinical signs of biliary or gastrointestinal obstruction. More commonly, however, euthanasia is recommended because of the poor long-term prognosis.

J. If no gross evidence of metastatic disease is present, en bloc resection is used to remove both tumor and draining lymph nodes. This procedure frequently necessitates gastric outlet and biliary tract reconstruction. If possible, 10 percent of normal pancreas should be preserved in order to maintain endocrine function.

References

Caywood DD. Surgery of the pancreas. In: Bojrab MJ, ed. Current techniques in small animal surgery. 2nd ed. Philadelphia: Lea & Febiger, 1983:232.

Drazner FH. Canine gastrinoma: a condition analogous to the Zollinger-Ellison syndrome in man. Calif Vet 1981; 11:6.

Klausner JS, Hardy RM. Pancreatic neoplasia. In: Slatter DH, ed. Textbook of small animal surgery. Toronto: WB Saunders, 1985:2464.

Rogers KS, Luttgen PJ. Hyperinsulinism. Comp Cont Ed 1985; 7:829.

COUGHING

Dennis A. Jackson

A. The history should review past medical problems as well as the current problem and its response to treatment. Coughing is a term often misunderstood and confused by the owners with gagging, retching, vomiting, or reverse sneezing. Careful questioning should confirm a history of coughing and characterize the nature of the cough. Nocturnal coughing is usually associated with cardiac disease, but may also be seen with collapsing trachea or severe pneumonia. Most infectious, allergic, and neoplastic diseases, as well as parasitic infestations, present initially with daytime coughing. Paroxysmal coughing caused by tracheal irritation or trauma is often precipitated by excitement or pulling on a leash.

B. The nature of the cough can be valuable in determining etiology. Moist coughing suggests the presence of bronchiectasis, pneumonia, or pulmonary edema. Dry sounds suggest conditions such as bronchitis, tracheobronchitis, tonsillitis, most allergic coughs, early neoplasia, and nonfailure cardiac coughing. Dry, goose-honk coughs are typically associated with collapsing or hypoplastic trachea, collapsing mainstem bronchi, and segmental tracheal injuries. Conditions in which edema, mucus, mucopurulent material, and hemorrhage are present usually result in productive material being expectorated following a coughing bout. Expectorated material can be useful in indicating the nature of the underlying disease process, although the animal may swallow the expectorant before it can be gagged out of the mouth.

C. A complete blood count (CBC), blood chemistry, and urinalysis give an indication of any systemic reaction to the respiratory condition. Blood gas analysis may provide valuable information regarding hypoxia, hypercapnia, and acid-base imbalances. Radiographic evaluation is useful in assessing the extent and character of the disease process. Plain radiographs of the cervical and thoracic regions, with or without special positioning, and fluoroscopy and contrast studies such as bronchography and pleurography may be necessary to provide additional information. Diagnostic transtracheal wash and aspiration often provides material for cytology or culture (Fig. 1). Endoscopy may localize the inciting cause of unexplained coughing. It should be performed after transtracheal wash in order to prevent translocation of upper respiratory organisms to the tracheobronchial area. In cases with pleural effusion, thoracocentesis can be performed to obtain fluid for cytology and culture and to allow improved viscera visualization on thoracic radiographs.

D. Conduct fecal and heartworm examinations if parasitic disease is suspected. An electrocardiogram is indicated if underlying heart disease is suspected.

E. Inflammatory disease may be divided into medically and surgically treatable conditions. Medical diseases include pharyngitis, tonsillitis, tracheobronchitis, chronic bronchitis, bronchiectasis, viral, bacterial and mycotic pneumonias, and tracheal collapse. Medical conditions also include allergic diseases, such as bronchial asthma and eosinophilic pneumonia. Treatment is usually symptomatic, with specific drug therapy directed at the underlying etiology. Surgical diseases include pneumonia that has not responded to medical therapy, lung lobe granuloma or abscess, and tracheal collapse not controlled by conservative treatment. Treatment varies with the specific case, but can include exploratory thoracotomy, combined with lobectomy for pulmonary disease or implantation of tracheal ring prostheses combined with medical therapy for tracheal collapse.

F. Neoplasia involving the larynx, trachea, mediastinum, or thoracic wall may present with coughing. Diagnostic tests are used to localize the lesion and determine the extent of the process. Treatment is determined by the individual case, but may include surgical resection with combined immuno-, chemo-, or radiation therapy depending on the tumor type.

G. Mechanical causes of coughing include esophageal, tracheal, or bronchial foreign bodies; collapsed or hypoplastic trachea; and traumatic injury to the airway. Treatment can involve foreign body removal, surgical repair of traumatic injuries, tracheal ring prostheses for tracheal collapse, or tracheal resection with anastomosis for isolated tracheal hypoplasia or stricture (p 70).

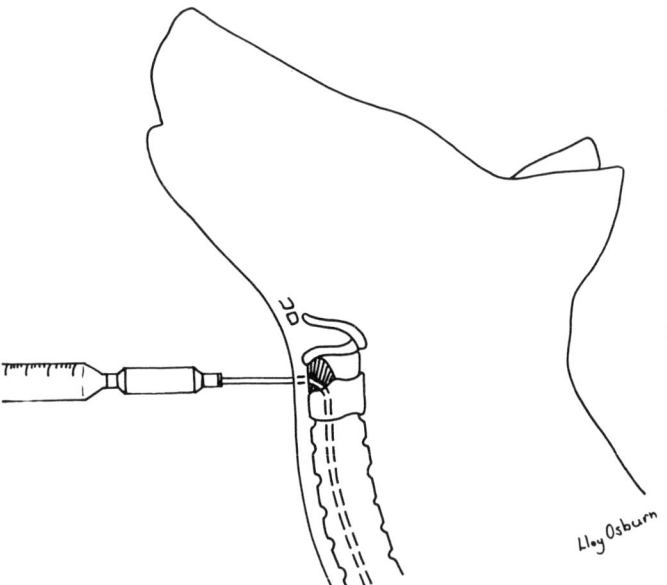

Figure 1 Position of animal for transtracheal aspiration. The catheter passes through a needle inserted in the cricothyroid membrane and down trachea.

References

Creighton SR, Wilkins RJ. Transtracheal aspiration biopsy: technique and cytologic evaluation. JAAHA 1974; 10:219.

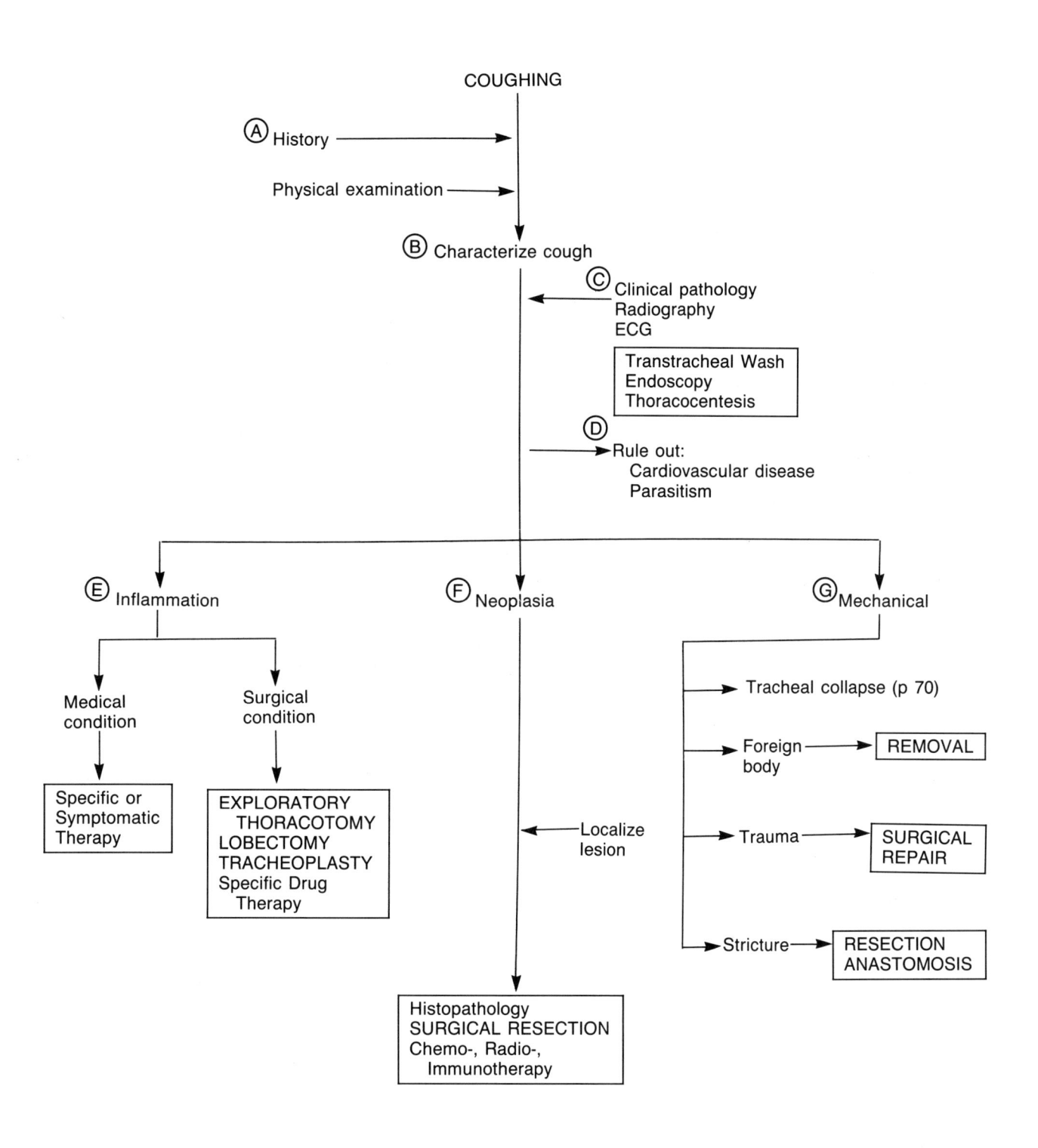

```
                          COUGHING
                              │
         Ⓐ History ──────────→│
                              │
            Physical examination ──→│
                              ↓
                    Ⓑ Characterize cough
                              │
              Ⓒ Clinical pathology
                 Radiography ────→│
                 ECG
                         ┌─────────────────────┐
                         │ Transtracheal Wash  │
                         │ Endoscopy           │
                         │ Thoracocentesis     │
                         └─────────────────────┘
                    Ⓓ
                     ──→ Rule out:
                         Cardiovascular disease
                         Parasitism
```

```
        ┌─────────────────────┼─────────────────────┐
        ↓                     ↓                     ↓
   Ⓔ Inflammation        Ⓕ Neoplasia           Ⓖ Mechanical
        │                                             │
   ┌────┴────┐                                        ├──→ Tracheal collapse (p 70)
   ↓         ↓                                        │
Medical   Surgical                                    ├──→ Foreign ──→ ┌─────────┐
condition condition                                   │    body        │ REMOVAL │
   │         │                                        │                └─────────┘
   ↓         ↓                         ←── Localize   │
┌────────┐ ┌──────────────┐                lesion     ├──→ Trauma ───→ ┌──────────┐
│Specific│ │ EXPLORATORY  │                           │                │ SURGICAL │
│   or   │ │ THORACOTOMY  │                           │                │  REPAIR  │
│Sympto- │ │ LOBECTOMY    │                           │                └──────────┘
│matic   │ │ TRACHEOPLASTY│                           │
│Therapy │ │ Specific Drug│                           └──→ Stricture ─→┌───────────┐
└────────┘ │  Therapy     │                                            │ RESECTION │
           └──────────────┘                                            │ANASTOMOSIS│
                                                                       └───────────┘
                                    ↓
                          ┌──────────────────────┐
                          │ Histopathology       │
                          │ SURGICAL RESECTION   │
                          │ Chemo-, Radio-,      │
                          │   Immunotherapy      │
                          └──────────────────────┘
```

Douglas SW. The interpretation of canine bronchograms. J Am Vet Rad Soc 1974; 15:18.

McKiernan BC. Lower respiratory tract disease. In: Ettinger SJ, ed. Veterinary internal medicine. Philadelphia: WB Saunders, 1983:760.

Venker-van Haagen AJ. Bronchoscopy of the normal and abnormal canine. JAAHA 1979; 15:397.

NASAL DISCHARGE

Dennis A. Jackson

A. The historical and physical findings may provide the most diagnostic information. The age of the patient, the chronicity of the disease, and the extent to which the clinical signs are intermittent, persistent, or progressive should be ascertained. The history should include general information on the patient's environment, vaccination status, and previous medical problems. The discharge may be unilateral or bilateral and may vary in character from serous to purulent or hemorrhagic. The presence of nasal or skull deformity, dental or oral involvement, and nasal obstruction should be noted.

B. With chronic nasal discharge, it is useful to classify the animal by age, type of discharge, and whether the process is unilateral or bilateral. Older animals, presented with a unilateral, bloody discharge, frequently have underlying nasal or paranasal sinus tumors. Animals of any age that are presented with bilateral, copious, tenacious nasal discharge should be suspected of having mycotic infection.

C. A complete radiographic study (lateral, dorsoventral, occlusal, and frontal sinus projections) is necessary in order to fully evaluate the nasal passages and frontal sinuses. General anesthesia is required to position the animal correctly, in order to obtain high quality diagnostic radiographs. Perform anterior and posterior rhinoscopy with the animal under general anesthesia. Radiographs should be obtained prior to the rhinoscopic study as scoping may cause intranasal hemorrhage, which may result in confusion when interpreting the radiographs. Without the use of fibre optics, rhinoscopic examination is restricted to, at most, the anterior and posterior thirds of the nasal cavity in most animals. Radiographs are necessary in order to fully evaluate the middle third of the nasal passages. Nasal biopsy is performed by means of a cutting plastic catheter or biopsy needle, combined with a nasal flushing technique (Fig. 1). Avoid penetration of the cribriform plate during biopsy.

D. Adenocarcinoma is the most common neoplasm of the nasal and paranasal sinus areas of the dog. Squamous cell carcinoma, fibrosarcoma, chondrosarcoma, and osteosarcoma may also occur. Malignant nasal neoplasia is seen occasionally in the cat. Malignant tumors have rapid local invasion; metastasis to local lymph nodes or the lungs is rare. Benign nasal polyps rarely occur in the dog; however, inflammatory nasopharyngeal polyps are occasionally seen in cats. With advanced malignancy, radiographic findings may include increased nasal or frontal sinus radiodensity, accompanied by turbinate lysis and vomer bone destruction or displacement. Nasal flushing and cytologic examination may provide a diagnosis; however, definitive diagnosis often requires biopsy at the time of surgical exploration. Surgery alone does not provide effective treatment and is usually considered a diagnostic procedure and a method of reducing the tumor mass. Combination therapy that consists of rhinotomy, surgical curettage, and radiation treatment provides the most effective way to manage malignant nasal tumors.

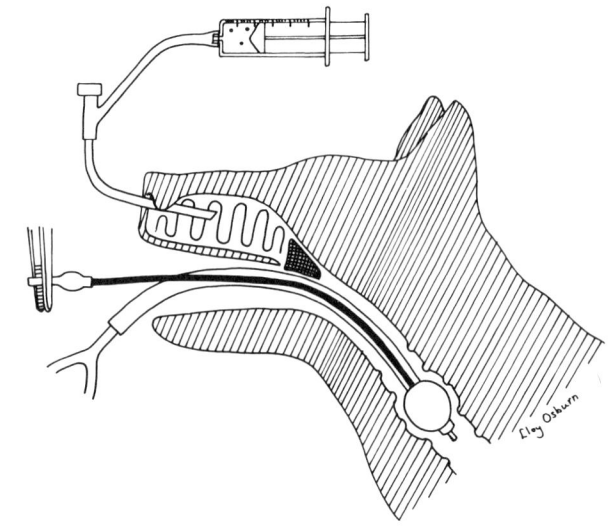

Figure 1 Obtaining cytologic material from the nasal cavity. Under general anesthesia, a cuffed endotracheal tube is inserted, and the nasopharynx is packed with gauze. A catheter or stiff IV tubing cut at a 45 degree angle is moved in and out rapidly in order to dislodge cytologic material. Saline flushes wash material from the external nares.

E. The most common mycotic organisms are *Aspergillus* and *Penicillium*. Rarely, saprophytic opportunistic fungi, such as *Rhizopus* and *Mucor*, or systemic mycoses may be causative. *Actinomycosis* and *Actinobacillosis* are seen very rarely and are usually subsequent to nasal or frontal sinus trauma. Diagnosis is based on radiographs, direct smears, fungal culture, immunodiffusion tests or complement fixation titers, and histology. Surgical exploration with partial or total turbinectomy and curettage of diseased tissue is required in all but very early cases (Fig. 1, p 68). A surgical drain should be placed to provide drainage and to allow local flushing of antimycotic drugs. Systemic antimycotic therapy is often necessary for several weeks. Tissue taken at surgery is submitted for histopathology and culture in order to confirm the disease. Prognosis in advanced cases is guarded.

F. Chronic bacterial or traumatic rhinitis often includes a history of hunting in long grass or in foxtail or pine needle country. Allergic rhinitis usually is seen in young animals and may have a seasonal occurrence. Recurrent rhinitis and sinusitis in the cat often follows feline viral rhinotracheitis or calicivirus infections.

G. Trauma may result in sequestrum formation or turbinate osteomyelitis. Unilateral chronic nasal discharge may occur secondary to an upper canine or carnassial tooth root abscess. Following tooth extractions, older dogs may present with nasal discharge secondary to an oronasal fistula. Specific surgical treatment depends on the underlying cause of the disease.

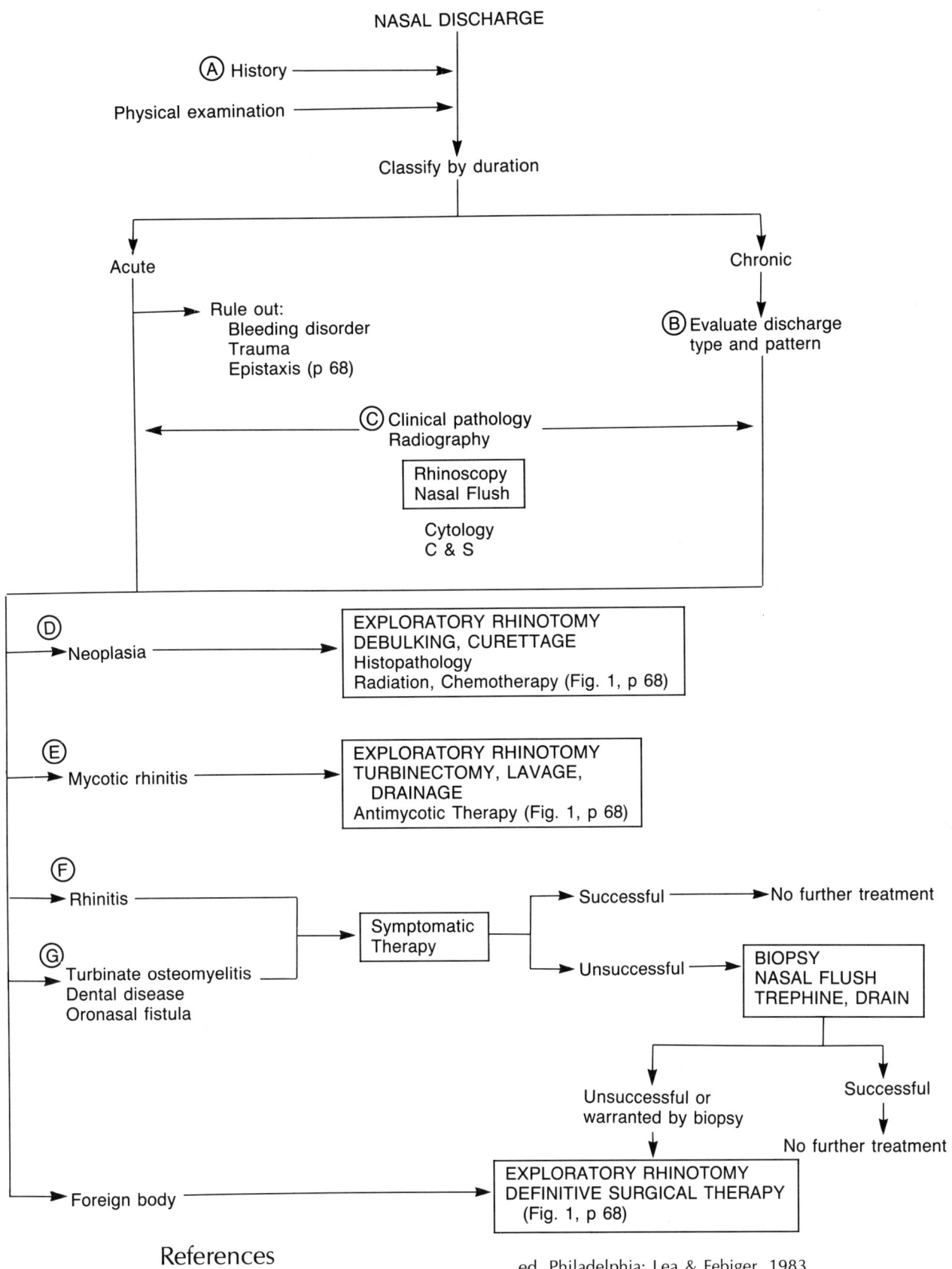

```
                            NASAL DISCHARGE
                       Ⓐ History ─────────►
                         Physical examination ─►
                                 │
                                 ▼
                          Classify by duration
                           ┌─────┴─────┐
                           ▼           ▼
                         Acute       Chronic
                           │           │
                           │           ▼
                           ├──► Rule out:    Ⓑ Evaluate discharge
                           │    Bleeding disorder   type and pattern
                           │    Trauma
                           │    Epistaxis (p 68)
                           │
                      ◄──────── Ⓒ Clinical pathology ────────►
                                  Radiography
                               ┌──────────────┐
                               │  Rhinoscopy  │
                               │  Nasal Flush │
                               └──────────────┘
                                   Cytology
                                   C & S
```

Ⓓ ► Neoplasia ─────────►	**EXPLORATORY RHINOTOMY** **DEBULKING, CURETTAGE** Histopathology Radiation, Chemotherapy (Fig. 1, p 68)
Ⓔ ► Mycotic rhinitis ──►	**EXPLORATORY RHINOTOMY** **TURBINECTOMY, LAVAGE, DRAINAGE** Antimycotic Therapy (Fig. 1, p 68)

```
  Ⓕ
  ► Rhinitis ──────────┐
                       │        ┌──────────┐  ──► Successful ──► No further treatment
  Ⓖ                    ├───────►│Symptomatic│
  ►Turbinate osteomyelitis      │ Therapy  │  ──► Unsuccessful ──► ┌─────────────┐
    Dental disease     │        └──────────┘                       │   BIOPSY    │
    Oronasal fistula   │                                           │ NASAL FLUSH │
                                                                   │TREPHINE,DRAIN│
                                                                   └──────┬──────┘
                                                              ┌───────────┴─────────┐
                                                              ▼                     ▼
                                                         Unsuccessful or        Successful
                                                         warranted by biopsy        │
                                                              │                     ▼
                                                              │              No further treatment
                                                              ▼
                                                     ┌─────────────────┐
  ► Foreign body ────────────────────────────────────►│ EXPLORATORY RHINOTOMY │
                                                     │ DEFINITIVE SURGICAL THERAPY │
                                                     │       (Fig. 1, p 68)  │
                                                     └─────────────────┘
```

References

Gibbs C, Lane JG, Denny HR. Radiological features of intranasal lesions in the dog. A review of 100 cases. J Small Anim Pract 1979; 20(9):515.

Harvey CE. Surgery of the nasal cavity and sinuses. In: Bojrab MJ, ed. Current techniques in small animal surgery. 2nd ed. Philadelphia: Lea & Febiger, 1983.

MacEwen EG, Withrow SJ, Patnaik AK. Nasal tumors in the dog. Retrospective evaluation of diagnosis, prognosis, and treatment. JAVMA 1977; 170(1):45.

Withrow SJ. Diagnostic and therapeutic nasal flush in small animals. JAAHA 1977; 13:704.

EPISTAXIS

Dennis A. Jackson

A. The history is very important in order to determine the etiology in patients with epistaxis. Unilateral epistaxis usually suggests an anatomic lesion, whereas bilateral epistaxis is more likely to occur with a systemic disorder. Failure to easily control the hemorrhage, accompanied by poor clotting and recurrent bleeding episodes, suggests a bleeding disorder. Certain medications such as anti-inflammatory agents, estrogens, and anticoagulants may predispose to bleeding.

B. There may be evidence of external trauma or recent surgery. A general physical examination may reveal an underlying cause. Perform complete examination of the head, oral cavity, and neck, and localize the site of hemorrhage, if possible. In cats with "High rise" syndrome, the hard palate and lower mandible should be examined for evidence of traumatic cleft palate or symphyseal separation caused by falling from an upper-story apartment.

C. Patients presented with signs of hypovolemic shock secondary to blood loss require intravenous fluids or blood. The hemorrhage can usually be controlled by icepacks, gentle tamponade, and cage rest.

D. A complete blood count (CBC) and clotting profile may be indicated and can reveal pertinent abnormalities. Nasal and frontal sinus radiographs can differentiate intranasal masses from destructive or traumatic bone lesions.

E. A detailed medical history and physical examination may suggest a bleeding disorder (e.g., spontaneous bleeding, prolonged bleeding, or bleeding from multiple sites). Difficulty in formation of the primary platelet plug (primary bleeding) often is evidenced by immediate-onset capillary bleeding, characterized by petechiation or ecchymosis of skin and mucous membranes. In contrast, problems forming a definitive hemostatic plug (secondary bleeding) often result in deep intramuscular or subcutaneous hematomas (delayed-onset bleeding). The history should be reviewed for evidence of a subclinical bleeding diathesis (periodic weakness, hematuria, lameness) or for a history of bleeding that occurred early in life or in related animals. Detailed physical and laboratory examination of the gastrointestinal, hepatic, renal, and cardiovascular systems is necessary. Assessment of the spleen and bone marrow may be indicated. Review all previously administered drugs for anticoagulant activity, and explore the possibility of exposure to rodenticides. Perform appropriate laboratory tests in order to confirm the presence of a specific bleeding disorder.

F. Malignant neoplasia and fungal infections may cause erosion into major vessels as well as turbinate destruction. Although the history is usually one of chronic nasal disease, acute episodes of epistaxis can occur with neoplasia (p 66).

G. Blunt trauma secondary to vehicular accident, falling, penetrating trauma (bullet wounds or animal fights), severe sneezing (allergic rhinitis), or nasal surgery can cause epistaxis. The bleeding is usually easily controlled, even though initially it may be severe. A detailed physical examination and radiographs of the skull often reveal fractures of the nasal cavity, skull, and mandible or a penetrating foreign body. Trauma to the nose and sinuses may result in chronic nasal disease (p 66). Osteomyelitis of the turbinates, bacterial or fungal infections, chronic osteomyelitis bone sequestrum, and blockage of the frontal sino-nasal opening, causing a frontal mucocele, can all occur as a result of nasal trauma.

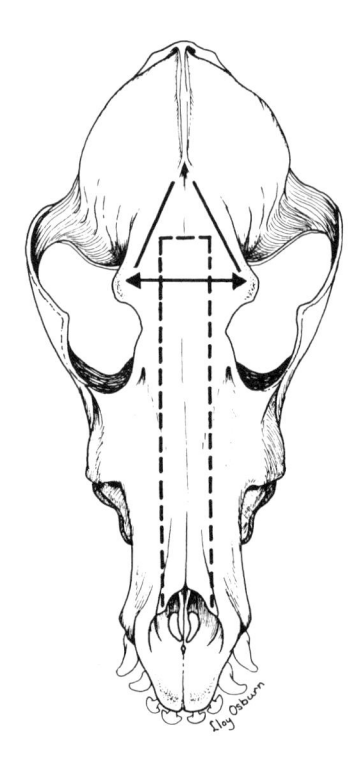

Figure 1 Exposure of frontal sinuses and nasal cavity: triangle - frontal sinuses; rectangle - nasal cavity.

References

Green RA. Bleeding disorders. In: Ettinger SJ, ed. Textbook of veterinary internal medicine. 2nd ed. Philadelphia: WB Saunders, 1983: 2076.

Harvey CE, O'Brien JA. Management of respiratory emergencies in small animals. Vet Clin North Am 1972; 2(2):243.

McDougal BJ. Allergic rhinitis—a cause of recurrent epistaxis. JAVMA 1977; 171(6):545.

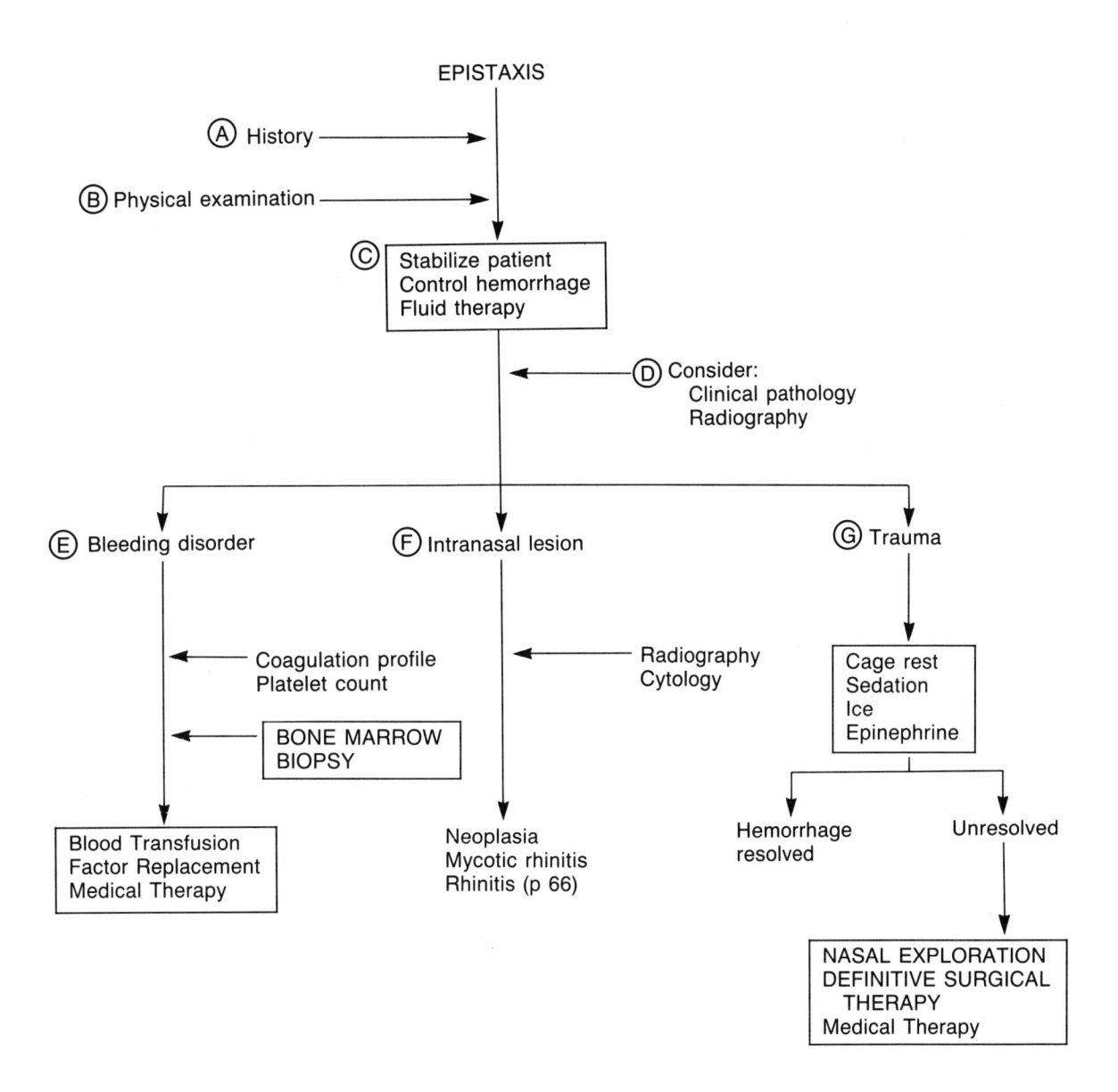

EPISTAXIS

- (A) History
- (B) Physical examination

(C) Stabilize patient
Control hemorrhage
Fluid therapy

(D) Consider:
Clinical pathology
Radiography

(E) Bleeding disorder
- Coagulation profile
- Platelet count
- BONE MARROW BIOPSY
- Blood Transfusion
  Factor Replacement
  Medical Therapy

(F) Intranasal lesion
- Radiography
- Cytology
- Neoplasia
  Mycotic rhinitis
  Rhinitis (p 66)

(G) Trauma
- Cage rest
  Sedation
  Ice
  Epinephrine
- Hemorrhage resolved
- Unresolved
  - NASAL EXPLORATION
    DEFINITIVE SURGICAL THERAPY
    Medical Therapy

AIRWAY OBSTRUCTION

Dennis A. Jackson

A. The history and clinical signs vary with the rate of onset and degree of obstruction. Upper airway auscultation usually localizes stridor to a specific anatomic site.

B. When emergency intubation is impossible, administer supplemental oxygen through a small-diameter catheter inserted through the rima glottidis or by direct tracheal needle puncture. Emergency intubation or tracheostomy can then be performed and corticosteroids administered. Correct any fluid and acid base imbalances (p 190).

C. Stabilize the animal and obtain plain thoracic and cervical radiographs. Radiographs are examined for stridor-producing intrathoracic or cervical airway lesions as well as any concurrent cardiopulmonary disease.

D. Definitive diagnosis of airway obstruction requires direct laryngoscopy and tracheoscopy under light anesthesia. Methodically examine the oropharynx, larynx, and trachea for redundant soft palate or pharyngeal mucosa, paralysis of the vocal cords, arytenoid cartilages, proliferative granulation tissue, or neoplasia. Evaluate the upper airway for evidence of previous trauma, everted laryngeal saccules, tracheal foreign bodies, or neoplasia.

E. Unilateral laryngeal paralysis is not usually associated with clinical signs. Acquired bilateral laryngeal paralysis most commonly affects old, giant or large breed dogs. Congenital unilateral or bilateral laryngeal paralysis is reported in Siberian Huskies, in racing sled dogs, and in Bouviers. A relationship may exist between hypothyroidism and laryngeal paralysis, and thyroid supplementation may be indicated. However, surgery provides the best method of management (Fig. 1).

F. Tumors of the larynx are uncommon. Endolaryngeal surgical excision may prove curative for benign lesions, but only palliative for malignant disease. Chemotherapy, radiation therapy, and total laryngectomy may be of value with malignant disease and can be considered in selected cases.

G. Most cases of acute laryngitis in dogs and cats are part of a general systemic disorder or widespread viral respiratory disease. Acute traumatic laryngitis may be caused by endotracheal intubation or laryngeal surgery and is best resolved with antibiotics, supplemental oxygen, and steroid therapy. Chronic proliferative laryngitis is serious, albeit rare, in the dog and cat. It is usually bilateral and involves the supraglottal and glottal surfaces of the arytenoid cartilages and aryepiglottic folds. Fungal smears and cultures of the lesion are usually negative. The etiology is unclear. The prognosis is generally guarded; treatment often requires staged surgical resection with combined local and systemic steroid therapy.

H. Obstructive laryngeal webbing secondary to laryngeal surgery may present as a focal or circumferential web.

I. The brachycephalic syndrome is seen most frequently in English and French Bulldogs, Boxers, Boston Terriers, Pugs, Pekinese, and the Shih Tzu. Obstruction results

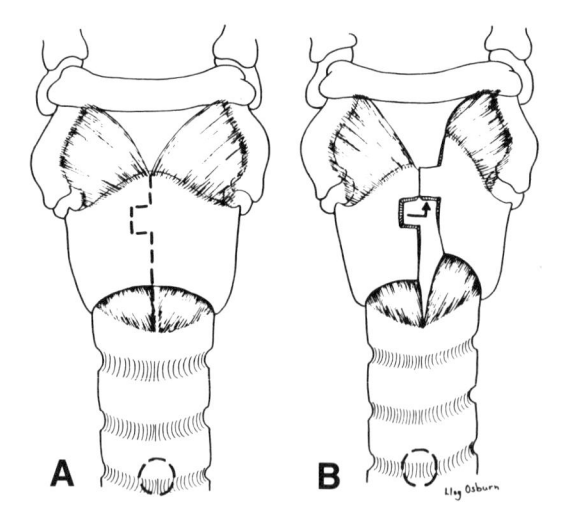

Figure 1 A castellated laryngofissure: *A*, dotted line indicates cut in ventral thyroid cartilage; *B*, arrow shows direction of cartilage advancement for widening laryngeal airway. Circle indicates site of tracheostomy tube placement, if it is necessary.

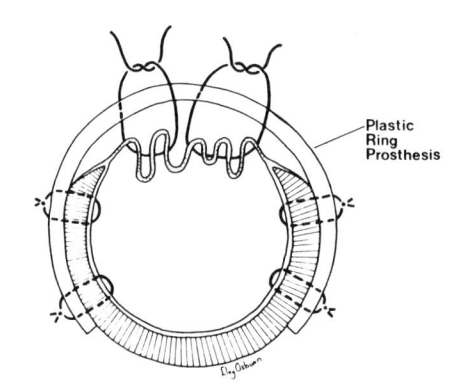

Figure 2 Attachment of plastic ring prosthesis with sutures to support collapsing trachea.

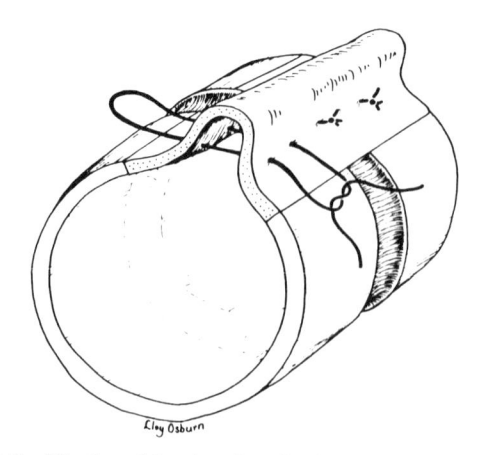

Figure 3 Plication of the dorsal trachealis muscle using a mattress suture in order to prevent tracheal collapse.

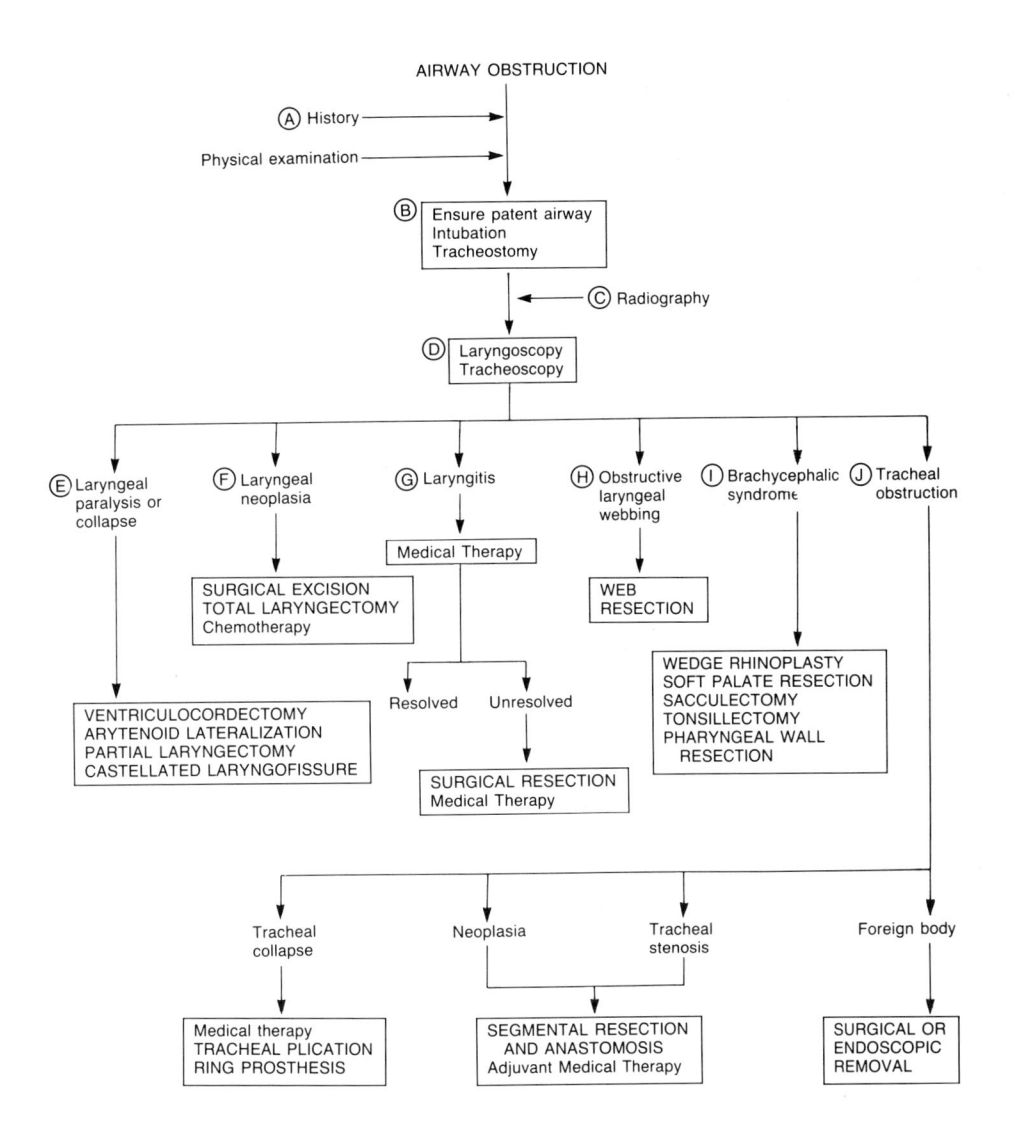

```
                        AIRWAY OBSTRUCTION
                                │
         (A) History ──────────►│
                                │
         Physical examination ─►│
                                ▼
                        (B) ┌─────────────────────┐
                            │ Ensure patent airway│
                            │ Intubation          │
                            │ Tracheostomy        │
                            └─────────────────────┘
                                │
                                ◄──── (C) Radiography
                                ▼
                        (D) ┌─────────────────┐
                            │ Laryngoscopy    │
                            │ Tracheoscopy    │
                            └─────────────────┘
                                │
   ┌──────────┬──────────┬──────┼──────────┬──────────┬──────────┐
   ▼          ▼          ▼                 ▼          ▼          ▼
 (E)        (F)        (G)               (H)        (I)        (J)
Laryngeal  Laryngeal  Laryngitis      Obstructive Brachycephalic Tracheal
paralysis  neoplasia                  laryngeal   syndrome     obstruction
or                                    webbing
collapse
                      Medical Therapy
           ┌──────────────┐     │      ┌──────────┐
           │SURGICAL      │     │      │  WEB     │
           │EXCISION      │     │      │RESECTION │
           │TOTAL         │     │      └──────────┘
           │LARYNGECTOMY  │     │                  ┌──────────────┐
           │Chemotherapy  │     │                  │WEDGE RHINOPLASTY│
           └──────────────┘     │                  │SOFT PALATE RESECTION│
                                │                  │SACCULECTOMY  │
┌──────────────────┐      Resolved  Unresolved     │TONSILLECTOMY │
│VENTRICULOCORDECTOMY│                              │PHARYNGEAL WALL│
│ARYTENOID LATERALIZATION│                          │RESECTION     │
│PARTIAL LARYNGECTOMY│         ┌──────────────┐    └──────────────┘
│CASTELLATED LARYNGOFISSURE│   │SURGICAL RESECTION│
└──────────────────┘           │Medical Therapy│
                               └──────────────┘

        ┌──────────┬──────────┬──────────┬──────────┐
        ▼          ▼          ▼                     ▼
    Tracheal   Neoplasia   Tracheal            Foreign body
    collapse               stenosis
   ┌──────────┐  ┌──────────────────┐         ┌──────────┐
   │Medical   │  │SEGMENTAL RESECTION│         │SURGICAL OR│
   │therapy   │  │AND ANASTOMOSIS   │         │ENDOSCOPIC│
   │TRACHEAL  │  │Adjuvant Medical  │         │REMOVAL   │
   │PLICATION │  │Therapy           │         └──────────┘
   │RING      │  └──────────────────┘
   │PROSTHESIS│
   └──────────┘
```

from a combination of stenotic external nares, infolding of the pharyngeal wall, elongation and thickening of the soft palate, and everted laryngeal saccules. Tonsillar hyperplasia and laryngeal collapse may further complicate the condition. In English Bulldogs, respiratory difficulty may be further aggravated by the presence of a hypoplastic trachea. Increasing severity of obstructive signs, especially at an early age, is a clear indication for surgical intervention. Surgical treatment involves soft palate resection in order to achieve a normal anatomic relationship between the soft palate and the epiglottis. The tonsils and lateral pharyngeal wall are resected if redundant. Everted laryngeal saccules are removed by endolaryngeal resection. Stenotic external nares are treated by means of a wedge resection technique in order to enlarge the external openings.

J. Tracheal obstruction may be caused by foreign bodies, traumatic injuries that lead to stenosis, congenital stenosis, neoplasia, or tracheal collapse. In certain instances, foreign bodies may be retrieved by tracheoscopy. If this fails, surgical removal through thoracotomy, open tracheotomy, or lobar excision is required. Traumatic injury to the trachea with secondary or congenital stenosis requires segmental tracheal resection and anastomosis. Tracheal neoplasia is uncommon, and tumor resection and tracheal anastomosis provide the best treatment. Tracheal collapse is a common cause of incomplete airway obstruction, especially in toy and miniature breed dogs. Tracheoscopy, inspiratory and expiratory cervical and thoracic radiographs, or fluoroscopy are necessary in order to fully evaluate these cases. Most can be successfully treated symptomatically with bronchodilators, expectorants, sedatives, corticosteroids, antibiotics, nebulization, and weight reduction. Surgery is indicated for unresponsive cases. Tracheal ring prostheses (Fig. 2) or tracheal plication (Fig. 3), combined with medical therapy, usually provide good results in selected cases.

References

Harvey HJ, Irby NL, Watrous BJ. Laryngeal paralysis in hypothyroid dogs. In: Kirk RW, ed. Current veterinary therapy VIII. Philadelphia: WB Saunders, 1983:694.

O'Brien JA, Harvey CE. Disease of the upper airway. In: Ettinger SJ, ed. Textbook of veterinary internal medicine. 2nd ed. Philadelphia: WB Saunders, 1983:692.

Walshaw R, Ford RB. Upper respiratory disease in brachycephalic dogs. In: Kirk RW, ed. Current veterinary therapy VII. Philadelphia: WB Saunders, 1980:221.

PLEURAL FILLING DEFECTS

Dennis A. Jackson

A. History and clinical signs vary with the severity of the filling defect and the degree of subsequent lung collapse. The most consistent sign is dyspnea. With severe disease, abdominal breathing, and mouth breathing accompanied by extension of the head and neck, may become evident. Some animals stand with their elbows abducted and are reluctant to lie down. In these animals, even the slightest stress may result in respiratory arrest. Coughing may occasionally be seen and is usually nonproductive. Auscultation often reveals muffled heart and lung sounds.

B. Use careful restraint in order to avoid any undue stress in animals with severe signs. Emergency thoracocentesis, supplemental oxygen, cardiac antiarrhythmics, and intravenous fluids are often necessary.

C. A routine hemogram, urinalysis, and biochemical screen are indicated in animals presented with pleural filling defects. A clotting profile is indicated if a bleeding disorder is considered to be the underlying cause of the pleural effusion. Obtain an ECG if concurrent or primary heart disease is suspected.

D. Examination of the thorax should include dorsoventral and lateral projections. Special radiographic studies such as standing lateral or lateral decubitus projections can differentiate freely moveable, trapped, or encapsulated fluid. With severe pleural effusions, thoracocentesis should be performed and the radiographs repeated in order to provide better visualization of the thoracic viscera.

E. Thoracocentesis can be used to differentiate air or fluid pleural filling defects. Aseptically collected fluid should be submitted for laboratory evaluation as soon as possible. Determination of the specific gravity and total protein content can classify the fluid as a transudate or exudate, and the pleural effusion can be further classified by its cytologic characteristics.

F. Pleural filling defects can also result from trauma and may present as pneumothorax, hemothorax, or diaphragmatic hernia (p 76).

G. Infectious inflammatory disease may gain access to the pleural space by several routes. Infections may extend from the lung, mediastinum, or diaphragm; from thoracic, esophageal, or neck wounds; or may result from secondary infection of an existing pleural effusion.

H. Chylous and pseudochylous effusions are differentiated on the basis of cytologic features and the presence or absence of chylomicrons. True chylous effusion may be (1) caused by thoracic trauma or tumors that invade or obstruct lymphatics; (2) a complication of thoracic surgery; (3) from thrombosis of the anterior vena cava; or (4) secondary to a congenital defect of the thoracic duct. In cats, pseudochylous effusions may be caused by acquired cardiomyopathy and lymphosarcoma. In most cases of pseudochylous effusion are either idiopathic or occur following surgery for chylothorax.

I. Neoplastic effusion may be produced by a primary or metastatic tumor in the thoracic cavity. Exfoliated mesothelial cells may become reactive and undergo morphologic changes that suggest neoplasia. As a result, diagnosis of neoplastic disease based on cytology can be difficult.

J. Most hemorrhagic effusions are seen following thoracic surgery or trauma. Other causes include bleeding disorders, intrathoracic tumors, or lung lobe torsion.

K. Obstructive effusions occur as a result of obstruction, constriction, or congestion of lymph or blood vessels. The most common cause of obstructive effusion is heart failure. Other causes include lung collapse, diaphragmatic hernia with liver herniation, or tumors that compress vessels and lymphatics.

References

Cantwell HD, Rebar AH, Allen AR. Pleural effusion in the dog: principles for diagnosis. JAAHA 1983; 19:227.

Creighton SR, Wilkins RJ. Thoracic effusions in the cat. Etiology and diagnostic features. JAAHA 1975; 11:66.

Holmberg DL. Management of pyothorax. Vet Clin North Am 1979; 9:357.

Kagan KG, Breznock EM. Variations in the canine thoracic duct system and the effects of surgical occlusion demonstrated by rapid aqueous lymphography, using an intestinal lymphatic trunk. Am J Vet Res 1979; 40:948.

Lindsay FEF. Chylothorax in the domestic cat — a review. J Small Anim Pract 1974; 15:241.

PLEURAL FILLING DEFECT Suspected

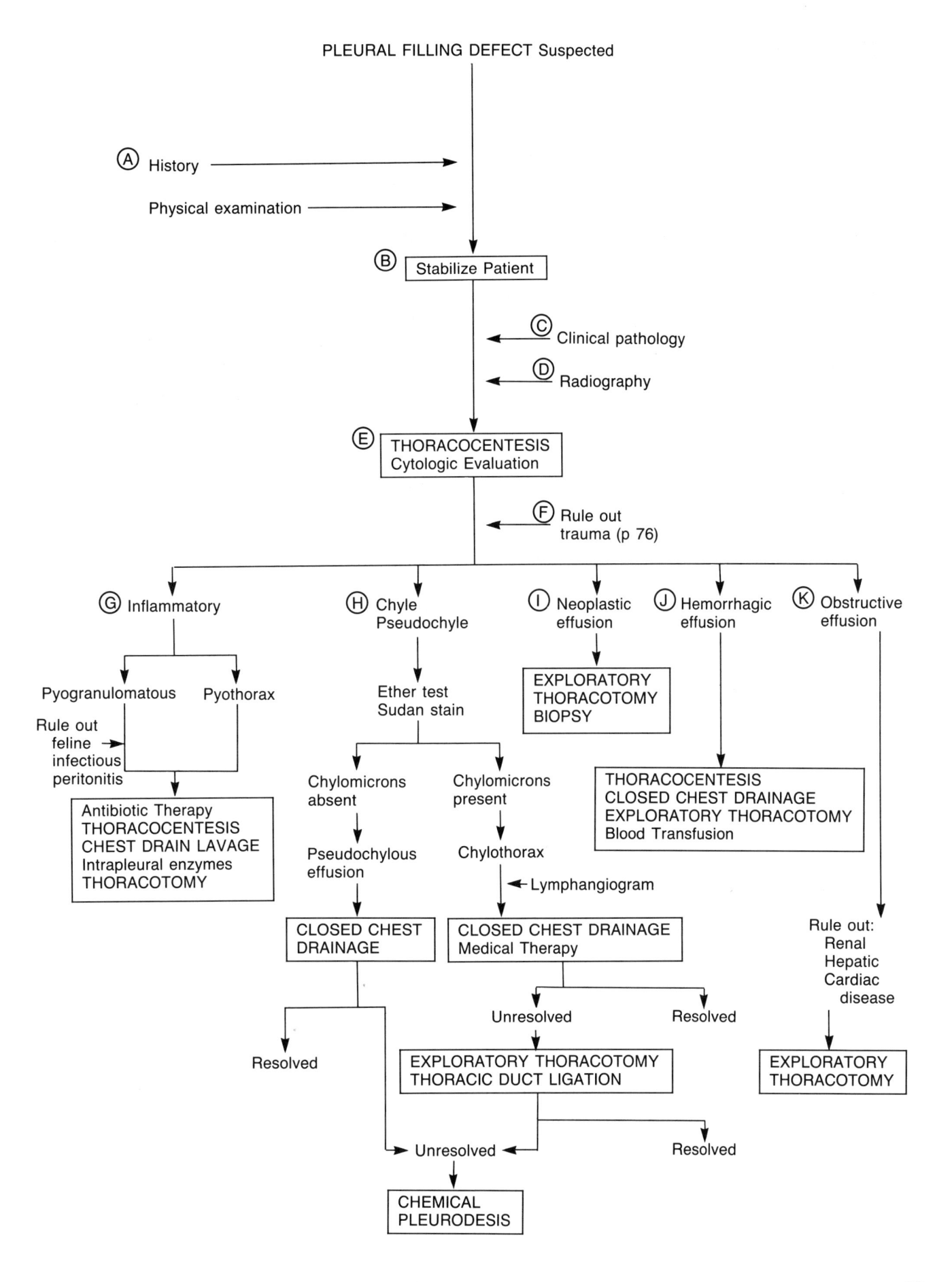

- Ⓐ History
- Physical examination
- Ⓑ Stabilize Patient
- Ⓒ Clinical pathology
- Ⓓ Radiography
- Ⓔ THORACOCENTESIS Cytologic Evaluation
- Ⓕ Rule out trauma (p 76)

Ⓖ Inflammatory
- Pyogranulomatous
- Pyothorax
- Rule out feline infectious peritonitis

Antibiotic Therapy
THORACOCENTESIS
CHEST DRAIN LAVAGE
Intrapleural enzymes
THORACOTOMY

Ⓗ Chyle Pseudochyle
- Ether test Sudan stain
  - Chylomicrons absent → Pseudochylous effusion → CLOSED CHEST DRAINAGE
  - Chylomicrons present → Chylothorax ← Lymphangiogram → CLOSED CHEST DRAINAGE Medical Therapy
    - Resolved
    - Unresolved → EXPLORATORY THORACOTOMY THORACIC DUCT LIGATION
      - Resolved
      - Unresolved → CHEMICAL PLEURODESIS

Ⓘ Neoplastic effusion → EXPLORATORY THORACOTOMY BIOPSY

Ⓙ Hemorrhagic effusion → THORACOCENTESIS CLOSED CHEST DRAINAGE EXPLORATORY THORACOTOMY Blood Transfusion

Ⓚ Obstructive effusion → Rule out: Renal Hepatic Cardiac disease → EXPLORATORY THORACOTOMY

PULMONARY MASS

Dennis A. Jackson

A. Valuable diagnostic information can be gained by obtaining a full history, including the use of the animal (e.g., showdog, field-trial or hunting dog), exposure to regional disease (secondary to travel), and response to previous therapy. Specific characteristics of a cough, if present, should be noted as certain diseases have typical sounds and patterns of occurrence. Exercise intolerance may relate to many organ systems other than the respiratory tract. Rule out cardiovascular and neuromuscular diseases and metabolic and endocrine disorders as possible underlying causes.

B. A general physical examination of all systems should precede specific examination of the respiratory tract. Note the animal's breathing pattern. Careful auscultation of the respiratory tract can provide the clinician with significant information concerning underlying lung disease. Percussion may detect alterations in the density of the underlying lung tissue and pleural space.

C. An extensive diagnostic work-up may be required; the choice and combination of diagnostic tests depends on the specific case and disease entity. An electrocardiogram may be indicated to exclude the heart as a contributing factor. Perform fecal examination for parasites as well as heartworm testing in endemic geographic areas.

D. Obtain peak-inspiration exposures with right and left lateral, ventrodorsal, and dorsoventral projections for optimal visualization and interpretation. Bronchography and fluoroscopy can be used to supplement plain thoracic radiographs.

E. A fine-needle aspirate of a lung mass may yield material for cytology and culture; however, the risk of pneumothorax precludes this procedure in animals with cystic or bullous lung disease. Significant diagnostic information may be gained by direct endoscopic visualization of the bronchial tree, combined with bronchial brushing, washing, or biopsy.

F. Mycotic pulmonary infections can be in the form of deep mycoses or caused by opportunistic fungi such as *Aspergillus*. Surgery plays only a diagnostic role as treatment requires antifungal therapy. Failure of bacterial lobar pneumonia or aspiration pneumonia to respond to appropriate medical therapy usually indicates lung abscess or granuloma formation and requires thoracotomy and lung lobectomy.

G. Hunting and field-trial dogs are at higher risk for aspiration of foreign bodies such as small sticks and plant awns. Temporary response to previous antibiotic and symptomatic treatment is common. Bronchoscopy is useful in identifying the bronchus involved and can be therapeutic if the foreign body is retrieved. However, most cases of bronchial foreign body require thoracotomy with partial or complete lobectomy for resolution of the problem.

H. Solitary lung lesions are a relatively common finding with primary lung tumors. Up to one third of cases of pulmonary neoplasia have no clinical signs and are found incidentally on thoracic radiographs. The prognosis is generally unfavorable. Surgical lobectomy of the involved lobe, with combined immuno- and chemotherapy in selected cases, provides the best treatment.

I. Congenital pulmonary cysts, as well as acquired cysts and congenital and acquired bullae or blebs, occur in dogs and cats. Most cysts or blebs cause no overt clinical signs. However, complications can occur and present as repeated infection or sudden rupture, which causes spontaneous pneumothorax. Pulmonary cysts that cause clinical signs are best treated by surgical removal of the involved lobe.

J. Lung lobe torsion is an uncommon finding in the dog and cat. It usually occurs after trauma, or spontaneously in large-breed dogs, and usually involves the right middle lobe. Diagnosis is best confirmed with plain radiographs and contrast bronchography. Hydrothorax may be present. Once the animal's condition has been stabilized, removal of the affected lobe usually resolves the problem.

K. Pulmonary thrombosis may occur secondary to primary thrombosis or pulmonary thromboembolism. Most cases of pulmonary thrombosis cause no outward clinical signs. However, extensive thrombosis or secondary complications such as infarction, infection, or secondary or recurrent thrombosis can cause clinical signs. Therapy for pulmonary thrombosis is supportive, symptomatic, and usually nonsurgical.

References

Burns MG, Kelly AB, Hornof W, Howerth EW. Pulmonary artery thrombosis in three dogs with hyperadrenocorticism. JAVMA 1981; 178:388.

Lewis RE, Kleine LJ. Radiographic diagnosis of solitary densities of the canine and feline thorax. JAAHA 1969; 5:195.

Lord PF, Greiner TP, Greene RW, DeHoff WD. Lung lobe torsion in the dog. JAAHA 1973; 9:473.

Silverman S, Poulus PW, Suter PF. Cavitary pulmonary lesions in animals. J Am Vet Radiol Soc 1976; 17:134.

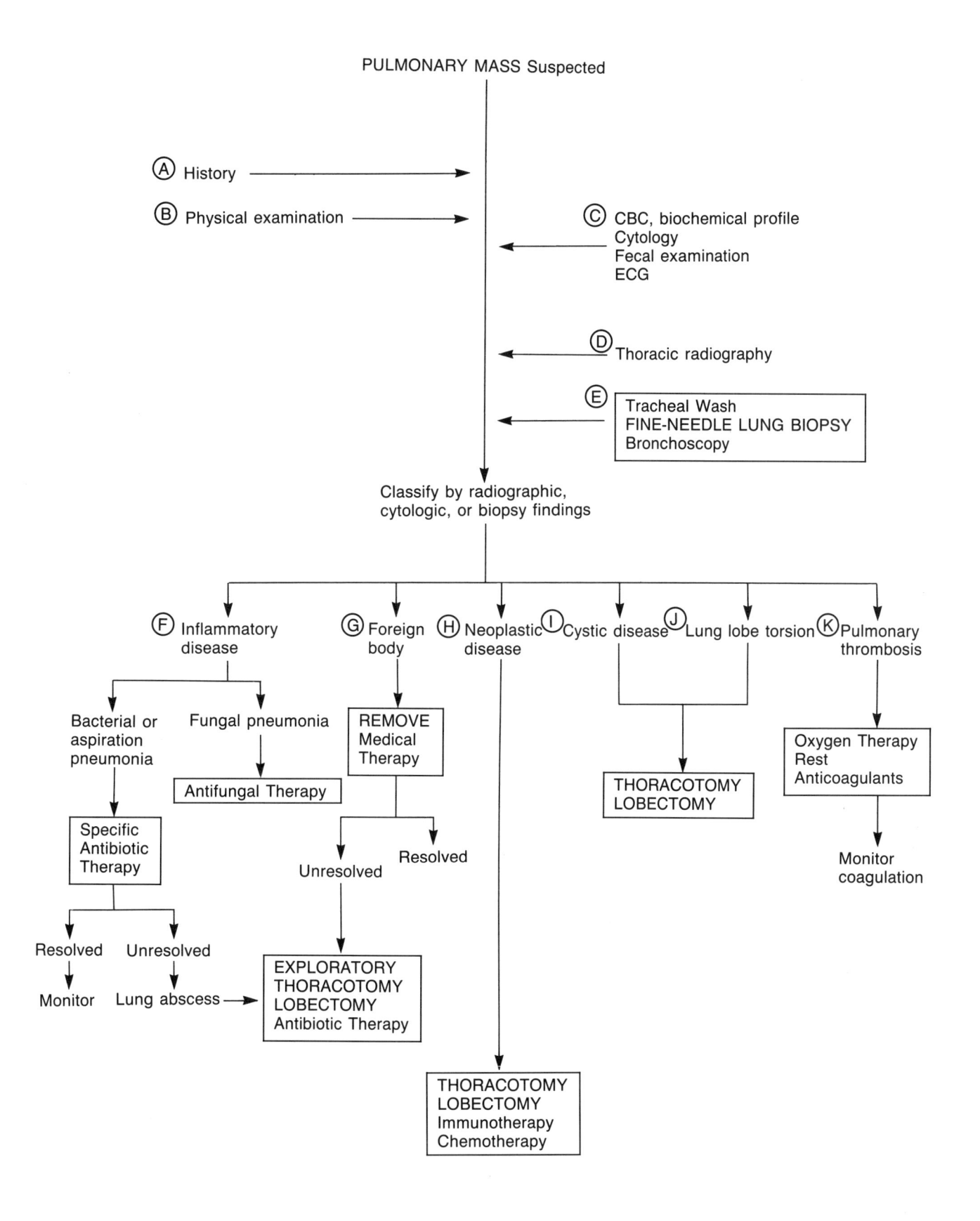

PULMONARY MASS Suspected

- **A** History
- **B** Physical examination
- **C** CBC, biochemical profile / Cytology / Fecal examination / ECG
- **D** Thoracic radiography
- **E** Tracheal Wash / FINE-NEEDLE LUNG BIOPSY / Bronchoscopy

Classify by radiographic, cytologic, or biopsy findings

- **F** Inflammatory disease
  - Bacterial or aspiration pneumonia → Specific Antibiotic Therapy
    - Resolved → Monitor
    - Unresolved → Lung abscess → EXPLORATORY THORACOTOMY LOBECTOMY / Antibiotic Therapy
  - Fungal pneumonia → Antifungal Therapy
- **G** Foreign body → REMOVE / Medical Therapy
  - Resolved
  - Unresolved → EXPLORATORY THORACOTOMY LOBECTOMY / Antibiotic Therapy
- **H** Neoplastic disease → THORACOTOMY LOBECTOMY / Immunotherapy / Chemotherapy
- **I** Cystic disease → THORACOTOMY LOBECTOMY
- **J** Lung lobe torsion → THORACOTOMY LOBECTOMY
- **K** Pulmonary thrombosis → Oxygen Therapy / Rest / Anticoagulants → Monitor coagulation

THORACIC TRAUMA

Dennis A. Jackson

A. A description of the traumatic event may assist in predicting the sites and degree of injury sustained and may guide the clinician's initial emergency therapy and workup. Diaphragmatic hernia or chylothorax may cause acute onset of clinical signs some time after the traumatic incident.

B. Although immediate attention should be given to assessment of vital signs and cardiopulmonary function, a detailed physical examination is mandatory in order to detect concurrent injuries.

C. The immediate objective is to restore and maintain cardiopulmonary function until the condition can be diagnosed and properly treated. This may include establishing and maintaining a patent airway, administering intravenous fluids or blood, controlling hemorrhage, and administering supplemental oxygen. Thoracocentesis to remove fluid or air is often required (Fig. 1). The thoracic wall may need stabilization or sealing in order to allow effective lung expansion. Positive-pressure ventilation and general anesthesia may be necessary in some animals. Closely monitor the vital signs of patients with thoracic trauma as these patients may deteriorate rapidly.

D. Thoracic radiographs are useful provided that they can be obtained without further stress on the animal. If standard lateral and dorsoventral views are not possible, other radiographic views, such as standing laterals, should be substituted. If fluid or air is present within the pleural space, repeat the radiographs following thoracocentesis. Serial hematocrits are valuable in assessing blood loss, as is blood chemistry in evaluating concurrent internal organ injury. If available, determinations of arterial Po_2, Pco_2, and pH can aid in assessing ventilatory and circulatory function. Obtain an electrocardiogram (ECG) in order to detect traumatic cardiomyopathy.

E. Airway obstruction may arise from trauma to the larynx or trachea. Tracheal laceration or rupture may occur following fight injuries, penetration by foreign bodies, or overinflation of endotracheal tube cuffs. These animals may present with progressive dyspnea, subcutaneous emphysema, soft tissue swelling, or external neck wounds. Utilize endoscopy and plain cervical and thoracic radiography, as well as contrast tracheography, to localize the site and determine the extent of the injury.

F. Pneumothorax may arise from penetrating thoracic wall injury, thoracic surgery, tears of the lung or tracheobronchial tree, and alveolar rupture from blunt trauma. Pneumothorax may also arise iatrogenically, following thoracocentesis or overzealous lung inflation. Confirm the diagnosis by radiography and thoracocentesis. Serial radiographs are useful for evaluating the progression of the pneumothorax. Most cases of pneumothorax can be managed by nonsurgical methods. Persistent pneumothorax or rapidly progressive tension pneumothorax requires surgical exploration and repair of the damaged tissue.

G. Traumatic hemothorax may occur with penetrating chest injuries, with fractured ribs causing lung laceration or intercostal vessel tears, with hepatic and diaphragmatic hemorrhage associated with diaphragmatic hernia, or following thoracic surgery. Confirm the diagnosis by thoracocentesis and radiography. Serial radiographs and packed cell volumes are useful in ascertaining whether the hemothorax is progressive. Fluid cytology is useful in determining if other disease processes are involved.

Figure 1 Thoracentesis sites.

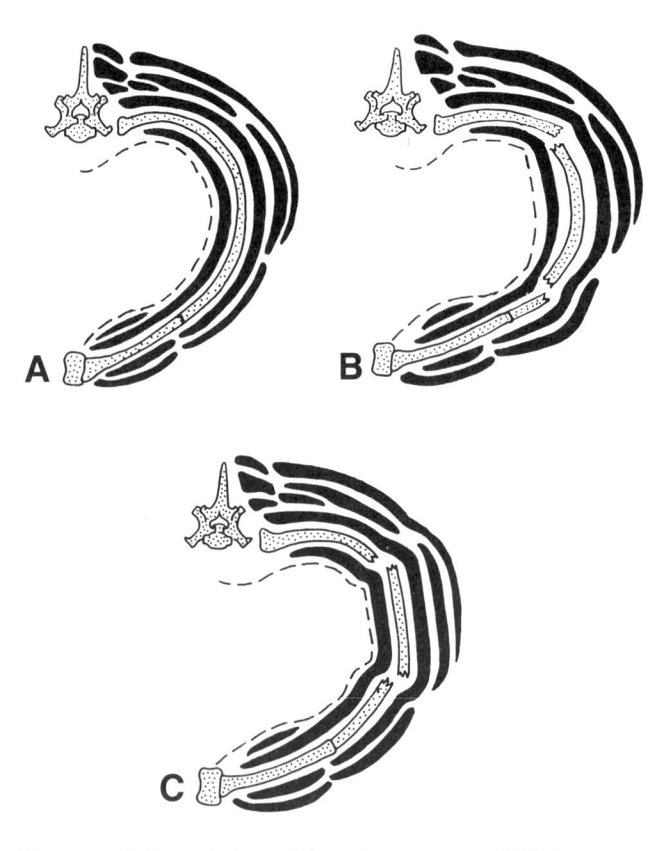

Figure 2 *A*, Normal chest; *B*, Inward movement of flail chest segment on inspiration; *C*, Outward movement of flail chest segment on expiration.

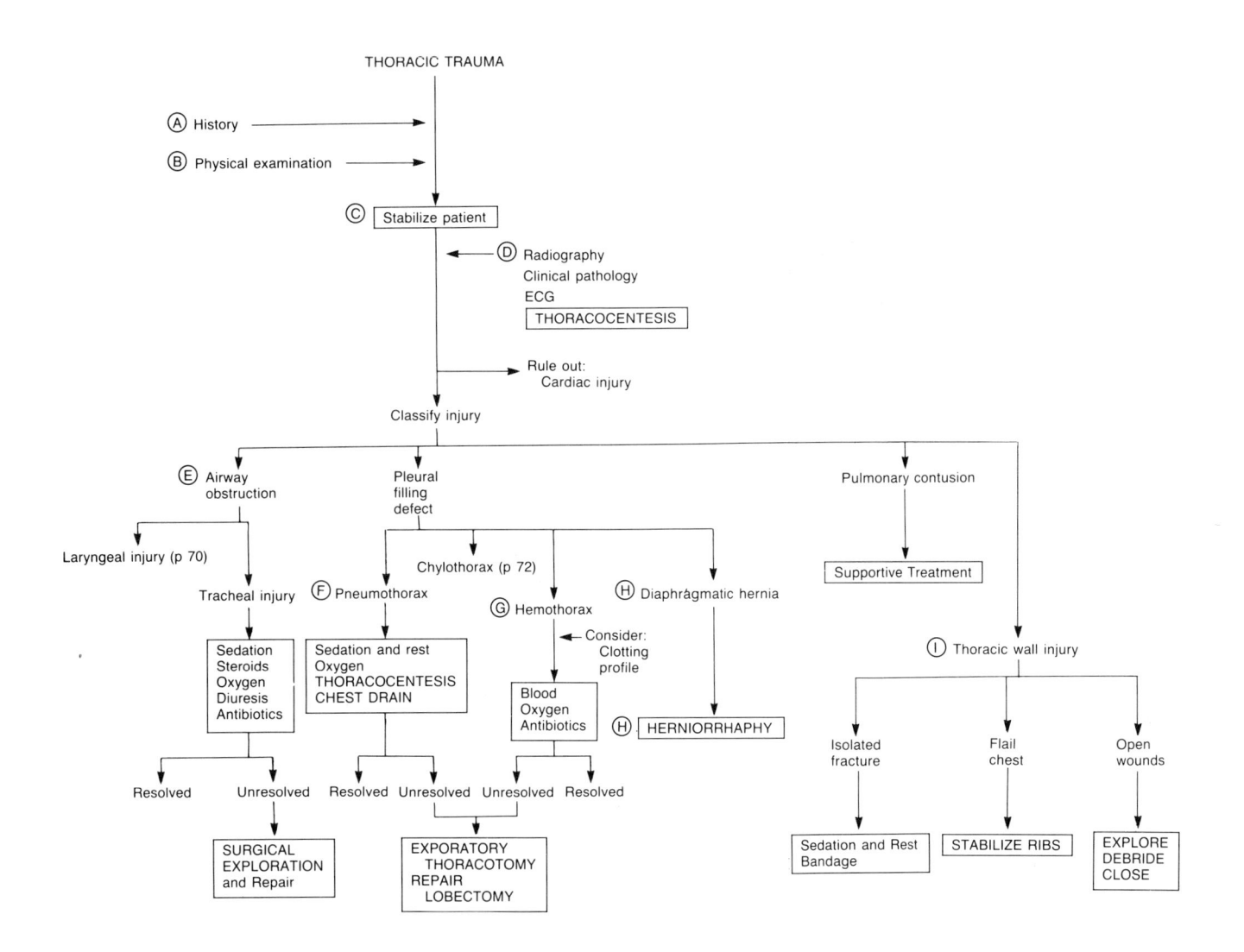

```
                                    THORACIC TRAUMA
                                          │
                    Ⓐ History ────────────→│
                    Ⓑ Physical examination →│
                                          ▼
                                    Ⓒ ┌──────────────┐
                                      │Stabilize patient│
                                      └──────────────┘
                                          │
                                          │←── Ⓓ Radiography
                                          │      Clinical pathology
                                          │      ECG
                                          │      ┌──────────────┐
                                          │      │THORACOCENTESIS│
                                          │      └──────────────┘
                                          │──→ Rule out:
                                          │      Cardiac injury
                                          ▼
                                    Classify injury
```

┌────────────┬────────────────────┬──────────────────┐
Ⓔ Airway   Pleural   Pulmonary
  obstruction filling   contusion
              defect

Laryngeal injury (p 70)   Supportive Treatment

Tracheal injury Chylothorax (p 72)   Ⓘ Thoracic wall injury
  Ⓕ Pneumothorax Ⓖ Hemothorax Ⓗ Diaphragmatic hernia
                                ← Consider:
                                   Clotting
                                   profile
  Sedation   Sedation and rest   Blood
  Steroids   Oxygen   Oxygen
  Oxygen   THORACOCENTESIS   Antibiotics
  Diuresis   CHEST DRAIN   Ⓗ HERNIORRHAPHY
  Antibiotics

Resolved Unresolved Resolved Unresolved Unresolved Resolved

  SURGICAL   EXPORATORY   Isolated   Flail   Open
  EXPLORATION   THORACOTOMY   fracture   chest   wounds
  and Repair   REPAIR
                   LOBECTOMY   Sedation   STABILIZE EXPLORE
                                                   and Rest   RIBS   DEBRIDE
                                                   Bandage   CLOSE

Persistent hemorrhage that follows conservative medical management is a clear indication for exploratory thoracotomy in order to isolate and correct the hemorrhage.

H. The severity of clinical signs with diaphragmatic hernia varies with the viscera herniated. Diaphragmatic hernias of long duration are not uncommon and may cause intermittent symptoms as abdominal organs move in and out of the thorax. Diagnosis is confirmed by plain radiography or barium swallow. Treatment involves diaphragmatic herniorrhaphy, which is usually performed through a ventral abdominal or combined sternoabdominal approach.

I. Rib fractures and open wounds of the thorax are common injuries. Multiple and segmental rib fractures can cause instability of the chest wall and a resultant flail chest with paradoxic respiratory motion (Fig. 2). Diagnosis is based on palpation and radiography. Minor injuries may be managed conservatively, whereas flail chest or open thoracic wounds require surgical intervention (p 78).

References

Alexander JW, Bolton GR, Koslow GL. Electrocardiographic changes in nonpenetrating trauma to the chest. JAAHA 1975; 11:160.

Crane SW. Evaluation and management of abdominal trauma in the dog and cat. Vet Clin North Am 1980; 10:655.

Kagan KG. Thoracic trauma. Vet Clin North Am 1980; 10:641.

Wilson GP, Newton CD, Burt JK. A review of 116 diaphragmatic hernias in dogs and cats. JAVMA 1971; 159:1142.

THORACIC WALL DISEASE

Dennis A. Jackson

A. Obtain a full history, including information on the duration and progression (if any) of clinical signs, details of any previous or recent thoracic trauma, and response to treatment.

B. Note the animal's breathing pattern, make a close visual examination, and palpate and auscultate the thorax. The presence of other abnormalities, such as fever or subcutaneous emphysema, may aid in categorizing the underlying disease process.

C. Carefully evaluate viscera within the thorax and abdomen for concurrent involvement. The ribs, vertebrae, and sternum are assessed for evidence of trauma or destructive or proliferative disease. External thoracic masses are examined for rib involvement or extension into the thoracic cavity. Fine-needle aspiration for cytology or culture can provide useful information.

D. Penetrating foreign bodies, bite wounds, surgical wounds, and traumatic lacerations can lead to infection of the thoracic wall. Careful evaluation is important in order to ascertain whether there is osteomyelitis of the ribs. Multiple fistulous tracts induced by foreign bodies or fungal infections may require contrast fistulography in order to determine their extent and location and to aid in their surgical treatment. This may include debridement, foreign body removal, drainage, and specific antibiotic or antifungal therapy.

E. Lipomas or benign cutaneous neoplasms may involve the thoracic wall. Most can be managed by local excision. Malignant neoplasms, including fibrosarcoma, osterosarcoma, chondrosarcoma, hemangiosarcoma, and mast cell tumor, can occur. Thoracic radiography usually determines whether rib involvement is present. Treatment involves en bloc resection followed by thoracic wall reconstruction. Depending on the tumor type, adjuvant chemotherapy or radiation therapy should be considered.

F. Thoracic wall injury may vary from blunt trauma with minimal injury to penetrating or crush injuries that are life threatening. Bite wounds of the thoracic wall are commonly seen with "big dog-little dog" encounters. Open thoracic wounds are serious injuries and require immediate sealing of the thorax, pleural evacuation, and patient stabilization. Flail chest can be stabilized initially with external splinting. Bite wounds or blunt trauma may cause intercostal muscle rupture, with subsequent thoracic viscera herniation. Repair involves direct surgical closure of the defects. Close large defects by utilizing latissimus dorsi and external abdominal oblique muscle flaps or synthetic mesh thoracoplasty techniques. Simple nondisplaced rib fractures are usually managed with cage rest only. Internal fixation is often required for multiple fractures of an unstable nature or for flail chest lesions. Once the patient is stabilized, the unstable segments are secured with orthopaedic wires or intramedullary pins and through soft tissue reconstruction. Sternebral luxations are occasionally seen with thoracic trauma; internal repair can usually be accomplished using orthopaedic wire.

G. Pectus excavatum is a rare congenital lesion. Surgical repair is indicated if cardiopulmonary impairment is significant or for esthetic reasons. Correction may involve multiple chondrotomies, cartilage resection, and internal reconstruction using internal synthetic supports.

References

Bjorling DE, Kolata RJ, DeNoro RC. Flail chest: review, clinical experience and new method of stabilization. JAAHA 1982; 18:269.

Brasmer TH. Thoracic wall reconstruction in dogs. JAVMA 1971; 159:1758.

Bright RM. Reconstruction of thoracic wall defects using Marlex Mesh. JAAHA 1981; 17:415.

Ellison GW, Trotter GW, Lumb WV. Reconstructive thoracoplasty using spinal fixation plates and polypropylene mesh. JAAHA 1981; 17:613.

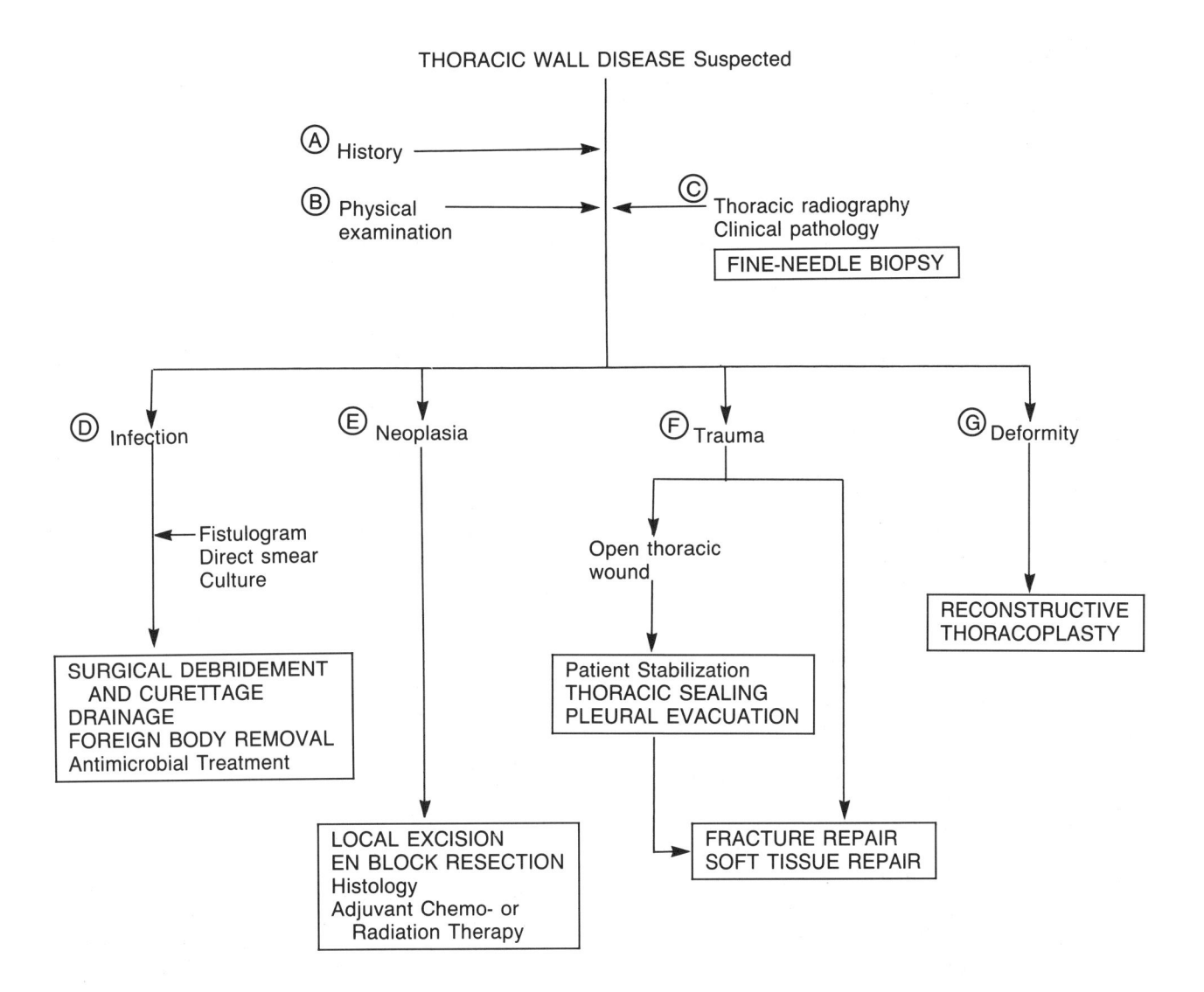

THORACIC WALL DISEASE Suspected

- Ⓐ History
- Ⓑ Physical examination
- Ⓒ Thoracic radiography
  Clinical pathology

  FINE-NEEDLE BIOPSY

- Ⓓ Infection
  - Fistulogram
  - Direct smear
  - Culture

  SURGICAL DEBRIDEMENT AND CURETTAGE
  DRAINAGE
  FOREIGN BODY REMOVAL
  Antimicrobial Treatment

- Ⓔ Neoplasia

  LOCAL EXCISION
  EN BLOCK RESECTION
  Histology
  Adjuvant Chemo- or Radiation Therapy

- Ⓕ Trauma
  - Open thoracic wound

  Patient Stabilization
  THORACIC SEALING
  PLEURAL EVACUATION

  FRACTURE REPAIR
  SOFT TISSUE REPAIR

- Ⓖ Deformity

  RECONSTRUCTIVE THORACOPLASTY

COMMON DIFFERENTIALS FOR CONGENITAL CARDIAC DEFECTS

David L. Holmberg

A. When a veterinarian auscultates a cardiac murmur in a young animal, a tentative diagnosis of congenital cardiac defect should be made. Acquired conditions such as cardiomyopathy or endocarditis/myocarditis do occur but are more often associated with arrhythmias. Clinical signs such as exercise intolerance, poor growth, syncope, or cyanosis are often mentioned in discussions of cardiopulmonary disease. Many animals with congenital heart defects present without evidence of disease, and the murmur is found during routine prevaccination examination. When dealing with the young animal it is often best to inform the owner of the physical findings and advise them of the prognosis, costs, and breeding considerations. Return of the animal to the place of purchase or partial refund of sale price because of "nonbreeder" status are options the owner may wish to pursue. Monthly reevaluation of the young asymtomatic patient should be advised until its future is decided. Occasionally, "innocent" murmurs change and/or disappear as the animal grows. If signs develop or if the murmur is still present as the animal approaches maturity, a cardiac work-up should be performed. Determination of whether correction is needed should be made prior to the development of permanent damage to the myocardium and vasculature. If the owner is not willing to consider surgical correction, advanced diagnostic tests are not indicated in the asymptomatic patient.

B. All of the common congenital defects have the potential for causing uncharacteristic murmurs. Figure 1 demonstrates phonocardiograms obtained from normal and abnormal hearts. Auscultation must include the entire cardiac area on both sides of the thorax, the thoracic inlet, midcervical area of the jugular furrow, and in some cases the occipital protuberance of the skull. The point of maximal intensity (PMI) of a murmur is the most reliable place to determine its characteristics. Secondary murmurs may also create confusion in the diagnosis of cardiac anomalies. Ventricular septal defects, which generally have a PMI on the right side of the chest, may cause a murmur in the pulmonic valve area due to the abnormally large amount of blood being ejected from the right ventricle. Similarly, a patent ductus arteriosus results in an increased volume of blood being returned to the left atrium and may cause a murmur of mitral insufficiency.

C. Palpation of the femoral arterial pulse during auscultation assists in determining the portion of the cardiac cycle in which the murmur occurs. Isolated diastolic murmurs are very uncommon in small animal practice and are not considered in this discussion. Systolic murmurs are the most common type and are usually associated with stenotic lesions of the pulmonary artery or aorta. Continuous murmurs are pathognomonic for arteriovenous fistulas, such as a patent ductus arteriosus. Arterial palpation often helps differentiate a systolic murmur from a continuous murmur in a patient with excitement tachycardia.

D. Although murmur location may help to decide whether a patient has a stenotic lesion of the pulmonic valve or aortic valve or a ventricular septal defect, thoracic radiography and/or electrocardiography help to determine which side of the heart is most affected. The combination of auscultation, radiography, and electrocardiography should be adequate in most cases to diagnose the type of cardiac defect. Confirmation of this diagnosis and determination of its clinical significance in an asymptomatic patient often require cardiac catheterization, pressure monitoring, and oxymetry.

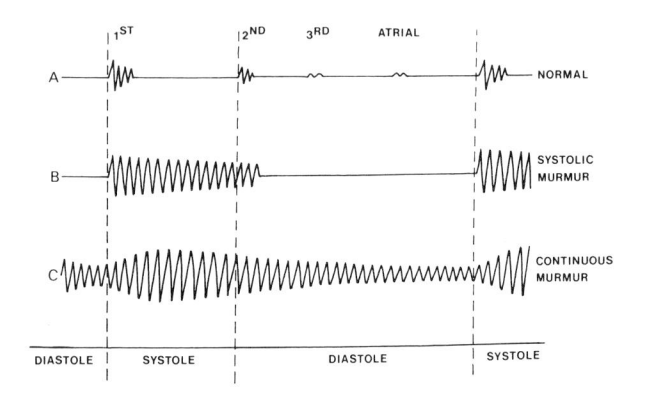

Figure 1 Phonocardiograms from normal and abnormal hearts.

References

Calvert CA, Greene CE. Cardiovascular infections in dogs: epizootiology, clinical manifestations, and prognosis. JAVMA 1985; 187:612.

Tilley LP, Si-Kwang L, Fox PP. Myocardial disease. In: Ettinger, S. Textbook of veterinary internal medicine. 2nd ed. Toronto: WB Saunders, 1983:1029.

CARDIAC MURMUR
↓
Ⓐ Auscultation

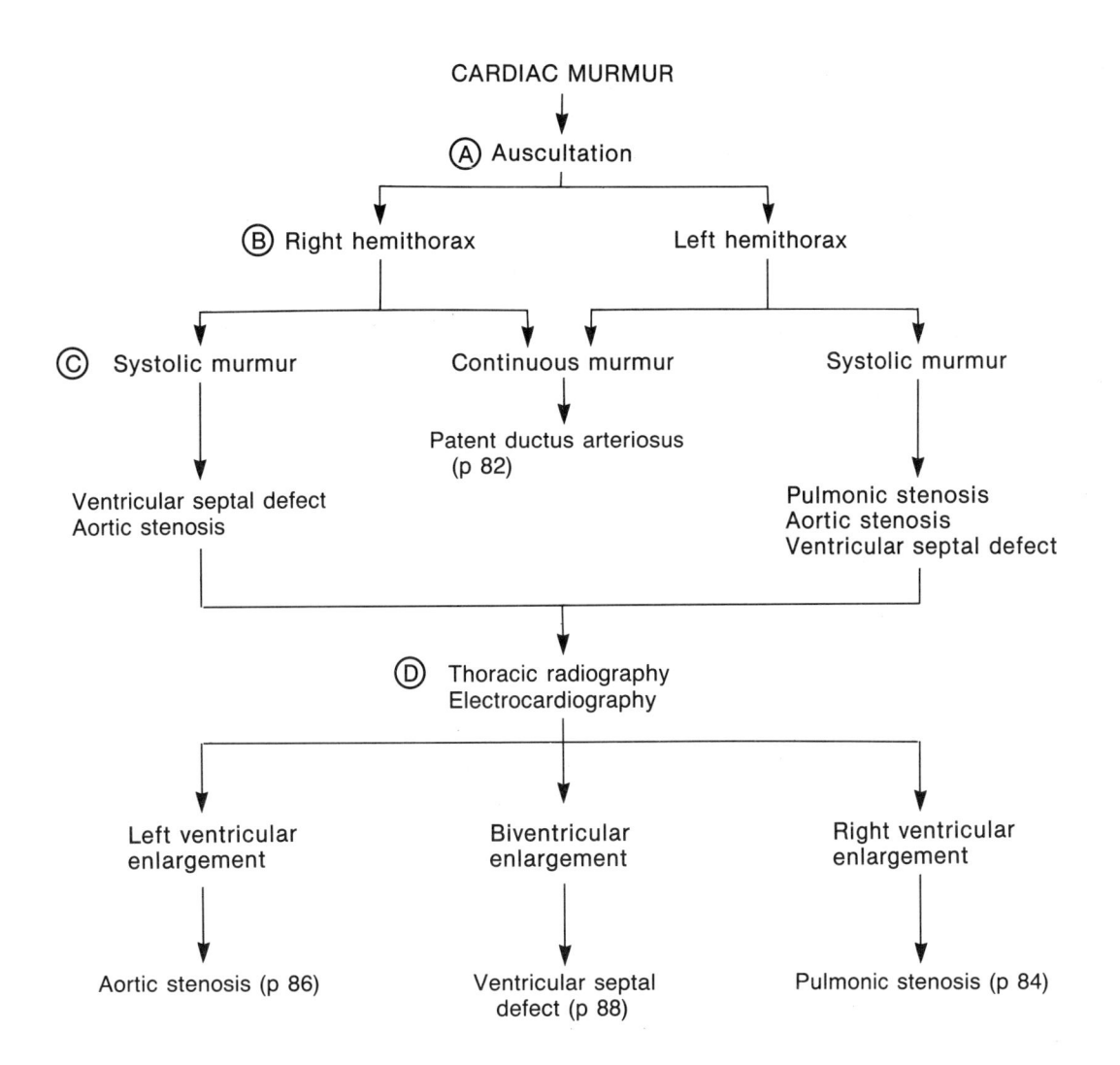

Ⓑ Right hemithorax → Left hemithorax

Ⓒ Systolic murmur | Continuous murmur | Systolic murmur

Continuous murmur → Patent ductus arteriosus (p 82)

Systolic murmur (Right) → Ventricular septal defect / Aortic stenosis

Systolic murmur (Left) → Pulmonic stenosis / Aortic stenosis / Ventricular septal defect

Ⓓ Thoracic radiography / Electrocardiography

- Left ventricular enlargement → Aortic stenosis (p 86)
- Biventricular enlargement → Ventricular septal defect (p 88)
- Right ventricular enlargement → Pulmonic stenosis (p 84)

81

PATENT DUCTUS ARTERIOSUS

David L. Holmberg

A. The most common congenital heart defect in dogs is patent ductus arteriosus (PDA). It is generally seen in very young female Poodles, Collies, and German Shepherds but may be encountered in any breed and either sex. Patients may present with histories of lethargy, exercise intolerance, and poor growth, but most cases are found during routine physical examination prior to vaccination. Auscultation of a continuous, systolic-diastolic murmur heard over the third, left intercostal space is diagnostic for PDA. Because the point of maximal intensity is usually located high under the foreleg and may not radiate widely, many murmurs are missed until the animal reaches several months of age. Older dogs with chronic PDAs are often of the larger breeds and may present with generalized emaciation or acute collapse.

B. The right ventricle hypertrophies to eject its normal stroke volume against an increased pulmonary artery pressure. The left ventricle dilates to accommodate the normal stroke volume from the right ventricle as well as the aliquot of blood "recycled" through the lungs via the PDA. The result of this biventricular enlargement is a normal mean electrical axis with tall R-waves. Atrial fibrillation may occur in dogs with chronic PDAs.

C. Thoracic radiography usually demonstrates biventricular enlargment of the heart. Dilatation of the aortic root, pulmonary artery, and left auricular appendage results in the appearance of bulges on the cardiac shadow at the 1, 2, and 3 o'clock positions in the dorsoventral projection. Overcirculation of the pulmonary vasculature is commonly seen and may lead to pulmonary edema or hypertension.

D. Cardiac catheterization is not needed to diagnose PDA if the characteristic murmur and radiographic findings are present. Catheterization may be of use in questionable cases and for ruling out other concomitant congenital defects. Injection of an iodinated contrast media into the aortic root gives the best visualization of an uncomplicated PDA and should show direct shunting of blood from the aorta into the pulmonary artery (Fig. 1). Blood gas analysis shows increasing amounts of dissolved oxygen in the right ventricular outflow tract, the pulmonary sinus of Valsalva, and the main pulmonary artery. Shunting of contrast from the pulmonary artery into the aorta indicates pulmonary hypertension and is associated with right ventricular hypertrophy, hind limb weakness, cyanosis of the caudal mucous membranes, and an elevated hematocrit. There is no characteristic murmur for these lesions.

E. Although patient size and vaccination status may delay the procedure, surgical correction of an uncomplicated PDA should be done as soon as possible after diagnosis to minimize secondary damage to the myocardium and vasculature. Closure of the shunt is performed through a left fourth intercostal incision and involves simple ligation in most cases. Partial occlusion, transection and oversewing of the great vessels may be needed if the defect is very short and wide. Right-to-left shunting PDAs should not be surgically closed as the ductus is acting as a safety valve for the right ventricle in these cases. Ligation of a reversed PDA results in acute right heart failure and death of the patient. Medical management is usually of no benefit in these cases, and euthanasia is generally recommended for animals showing significant clinical signs.

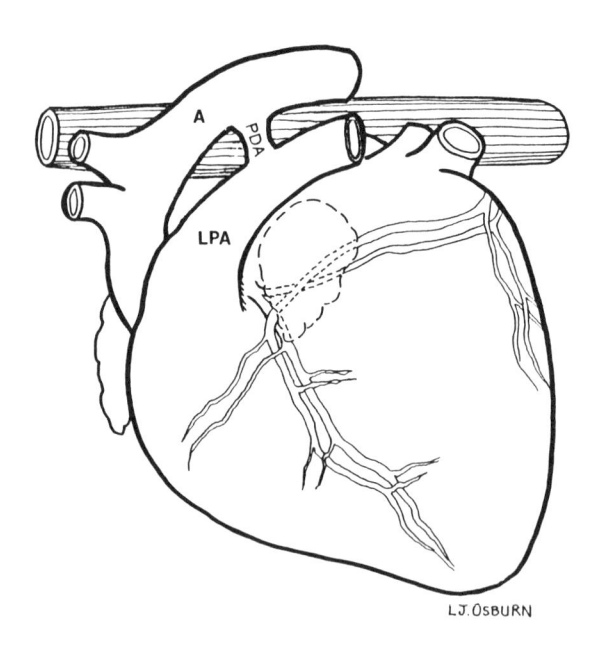

Figure 1 View of the heart from the left side showing left pulmonary artery *LPA*; patent ductus arteriosus *PDA*; and aorta *A*.

References

Buchanan JW. Radiographic aspects of patent ductus arteriosus in dogs before and after surgery. Br J Small Anim Pract 1968; 19: 271.

Eyster GE. Patent ductus arteriosus in the dog: characteristics of occurrence and results of surgery in one hundred consecutive cases. JAVMA 1976; 168:435.

Jackson WF, Henderson RA. Ligature placement in closure of patent ductus arteriosus JAAHA 1979; 15: 55.

INCIDENTAL FINDING
OF MURMUR

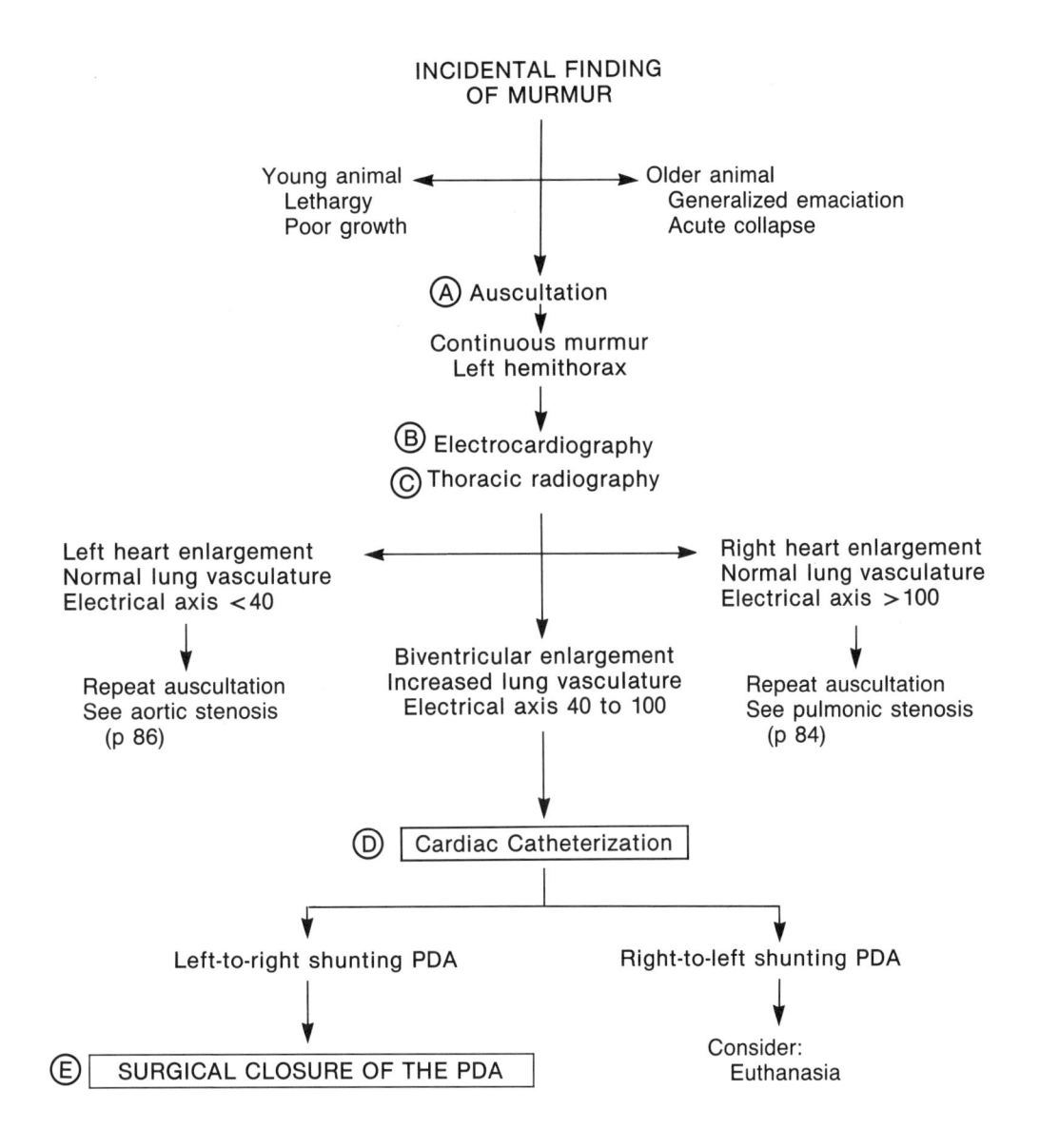

Young animal ← → Older animal
Lethargy   Generalized emaciation
Poor growth   Acute collapse

Ⓐ Auscultation

Continuous murmur
Left hemithorax

Ⓑ Electrocardiography
Ⓒ Thoracic radiography

Left heart enlargement ← → Right heart enlargement
Normal lung vasculature   Normal lung vasculature
Electrical axis <40   Electrical axis >100

Repeat auscultation   Repeat auscultation
See aortic stenosis   See pulmonic stenosis
(p 86)   (p 84)

Biventricular enlargement
Increased lung vasculature
Electrical axis 40 to 100

Ⓓ Cardiac Catheterization

Left-to-right shunting PDA   Right-to-left shunting PDA

Ⓔ SURGICAL CLOSURE OF THE PDA   Consider:
                                  Euthanasia

PULMONIC STENOSIS

David L. Holmberg

A. The second most common congenital heart defect in dogs is pulmonic stenosis (PS). Seen in many breeds, PS is most frequent in Collies, German Shepherds, and English Bulldogs. Some affected animals present with exercise intolerance, but the majority are asymptomatic, and the murmur is detected during routine physical examination. A systolic murmur is heard low on the chest wall over the pulmonic region (usually the third left intercostal space). Splitting of the second heart sound is occasionally present because of slowed emptying of the right ventricle and delayed closure of the pulmonic valve.

B. Right deviation of the mean electrical axis (>100 degrees) results from the increased work load and hypertrophy of the right ventricle. Thickening of the crista supraventricularis musculature in the pulmonary artery outflow tract produces S-waves in electrocardiogram leads I, II, and III. Severe cases may have P-pulmonale (P-wave amplitude >0.4 mv) and/or right bundle branch block (QRS complex negative in leads I, II, and III, and aVF with a duration >0.06 sec).

C. Radiographically, right ventricular enlargement is the most consistent finding with PS. The cardiac shadow takes the form of a reversed "D" in the dorsoventral view. There is an increased amount of contact between the heart and sternum in the lateral projection, and the main pulmonary artery is enlarged causing a loss of cranial waist. The peripheral pulmonary vasculature is normal.

D. Cardiac catheterization is helpful in determining an accurate diagnosis, prognosis, and treatment regimen for patients with PS. Recording of pressures within the heart and pulmonary artery permits localization and quantitation of the lesion. Injection of dye may also help determine the presence of secondary changes in the pulmonary artery and rule out the existence of additional cardiac defects, which are frequently associated with PS. Generally, the heart can tolerate stenotic lesions that create pressure gradients (pre- and poststenosis) of <50 mm Hg. Gradients >70 mm Hg, if untreated, result in unacceptable stress on the myocardium and cause heart failure. Immature patients with low gradients who have significant secondary vascular and electrocardiographic changes should be reevaluated at monthly intervals. Surgery should be considered if the changes appear to be progressive or if clinical signs develop.

E. The surgical technique used to correct PS depends on the location of the lesion and the size of the patient. Pulmonic stenosis may take four forms: valvular, subvalvular, supravalvular, and infundibular. Valvular stenosis, which is the most common form of the disease, is best treated by temporary venous occlusion, pulmonary arterotomy, and open valvulotomy (Fig. 1). This permits direct observation of the correction and minimizes postoperative valvular insufficiency. The small size of the pulmonary artery in patients <10 kg body weight makes the use of open valvulotomy technically very difficult. For very small patients, the use of a patch graft to increase the diameter of the vessel and outflow tract is preferable. Obstruction to outflow from the right ventricle commonly causes secondary hypertrophy of the myocardium in the infundibular area. This usually decreases spontaneously following removal of the obstruction. If, however, the primary lesion is in the subvalvular or infundibular areas, patch grafting this area can be done and is preferable to the more complicated myectomy procedures.

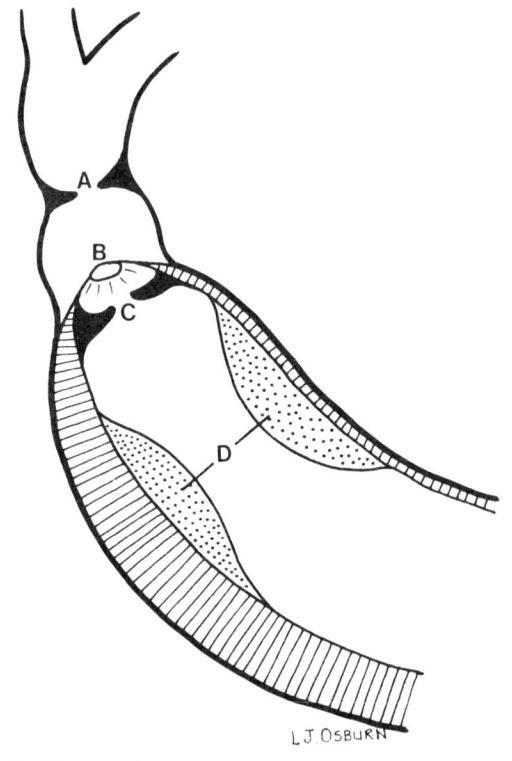

Figure 1 Diagram of pulmonary outflow tract showing *A*, supravalvular pulmonic stenosis, *B*, valvular pulmonic stenosis, *C*, subvalvular pulmonic stenosis and *D*, muscular infundibular pulmonic stenosis.

References

Breznock EM, Wood GL. A patch-graft technique for correction of pulmonic stenosis in dogs. JAVMA 1976; 169: 1090.

Eyster GE. Pulmonic stenosis. In: Bojrab, J. Current techniques in small animal surgery, 2nd ed. Philadelphia: Lea & Febiger, 1983: 462.

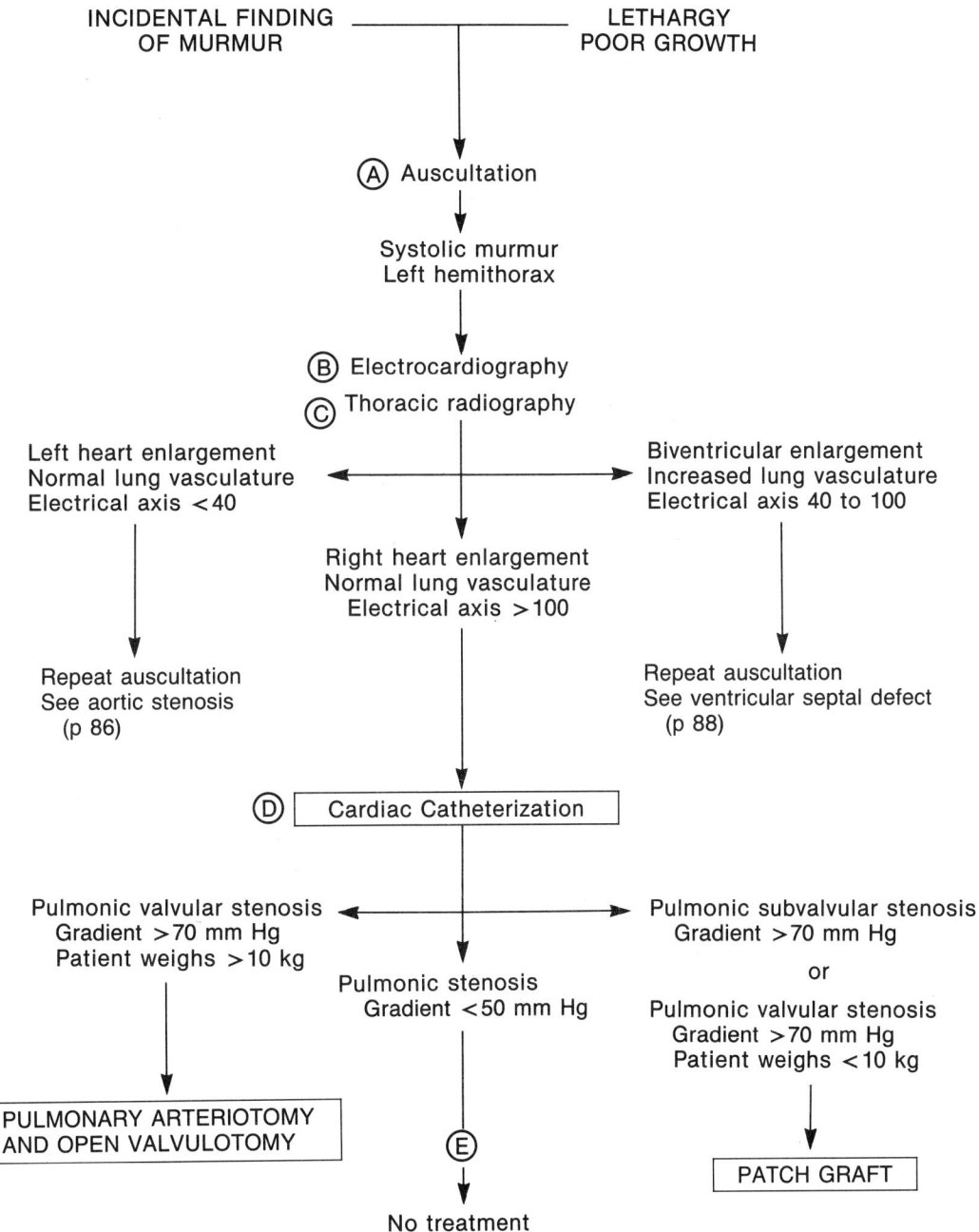

```
INCIDENTAL FINDING ─────────── LETHARGY
   OF MURMUR                    POOR GROWTH
                │
                ▼
           Ⓐ Auscultation
                │
                ▼
           Systolic murmur
           Left hemithorax
                │
                ▼
          Ⓑ Electrocardiography
          Ⓒ Thoracic radiography
```

Left heart enlargement	Right heart enlargement	Biventricular enlargement
Normal lung vasculature	Normal lung vasculature	Increased lung vasculature
Electrical axis <40	Electrical axis >100	Electrical axis 40 to 100

Repeat auscultation
See aortic stenosis
(p 86)

Repeat auscultation
See ventricular septal defect
(p 88)

Ⓓ Cardiac Catheterization

Pulmonic valvular stenosis
Gradient >70 mm Hg
Patient weighs >10 kg

Pulmonic stenosis
Gradient <50 mm Hg

Pulmonic subvalvular stenosis
Gradient >70 mm Hg
or
Pulmonic valvular stenosis
Gradient >70 mm Hg
Patient weighs <10 kg

PULMONARY ARTERIOTOMY AND OPEN VALVULOTOMY

Ⓔ

PATCH GRAFT

No treatment
Reevaluate monthly until the patient is mature

AORTIC STENOSIS

David L. Holmberg

A. The third most common congenital heart defect in dogs is aortic stenosis (AS). This defect is most frequently diagnosed in Boxers, Newfoundlands, and German Shepherds. Syncope and exercise intolerance can be seen in severe cases, but usually the systolic murmur is an incidental finding on physical examination. The murmur's point of maximal intensity is heard midthorax over the fourth left intercostal space. Often the murmur can be heard at the thoracic inlet and may be auscultated in the carotid arteries. Harsh turbulence may radiate up the vertebral arteries and produce an auscultatable murmur at the occiput of the head.

B. Left deviation of the mean electrical axis (<40 degrees) and an R-wave larger than 3.0 mv are indications of the left ventricular hypertrophy seen with this defect. Coving of the S-T segment suggests myocardial strain and ischemia, which occurs when the heart is forced to use increased ejection pressures.

C. Left heart enlargement is the major finding on thoracic radiographs. Increased contact between the heart and the diaphragm occurs as the overall cardiac shadow elongates. Dilatation of the ascending aortic arch is common, but the rest of the vasculature is usually normal.

D. Like stenosis of the pulmonary artery, AS may be valvular, supravalvular, subvalvular, or infundibular, with the subvalvular form being the most common type. Cardiac catheterization is required for accurate diagnosis, prognosis, and treatment of AS and should include measurement of the pressure gradient across the stenosis. Angiography should also be performed to demonstrate secondary vascular changes and to rule out additional cardiac defects. Gradients of less than 50 mm Hg are not considered significant, whereas those greater than 100 mm Hg require surgical correction. Immature patients with low gradients but having significant vascular and electrocardiographic changes should be reevaluated at monthly intervals. Surgical correction should be considered if the changes appear to be progressive or if clinical signs develop.

E. Surgical correction of three of the four forms of AS require full cardiopulmonary bypass and hypothermic cardioplegia. The stenotic lesion is resected under direct inspection through an aortic incision. A decrease of left ventricular pressure has also been achieved using valved conduits and may hold future promise. Correction of a significant AS must be done prior to 1 year of age to prevent irreversible myocardial damage. Ischemic myocardial contracture is not uncommon following cardioplegia or electric defibrillation of these patients and is a leading cause of intraoperative patient death. Supravalvular stenotic lesions may be corrected without cardiopulmonary bypass using vascular grafts; however, these cases are extremely rare.

References

Breznock EM, Whitting P, Pendray D, et al. Valved apico-aortic conduit of left ventricular hypertension caused by discrete subaortic stenosis in dogs. JAVMA 1983; 182:51.

Eyster GE, Hough JD, Evans AT, et al. Surgical repair of patent ductus arteriosus, aortic stenosis, and aortic regurgitation in a dog. JAVMA 1975; 167:942.

Pyle RL, Patterson DF, Chacko S. The genetics and pathology of discrete subaortic stenosis in the Newfoundland dog. Am Heart J 1976; 92:324.

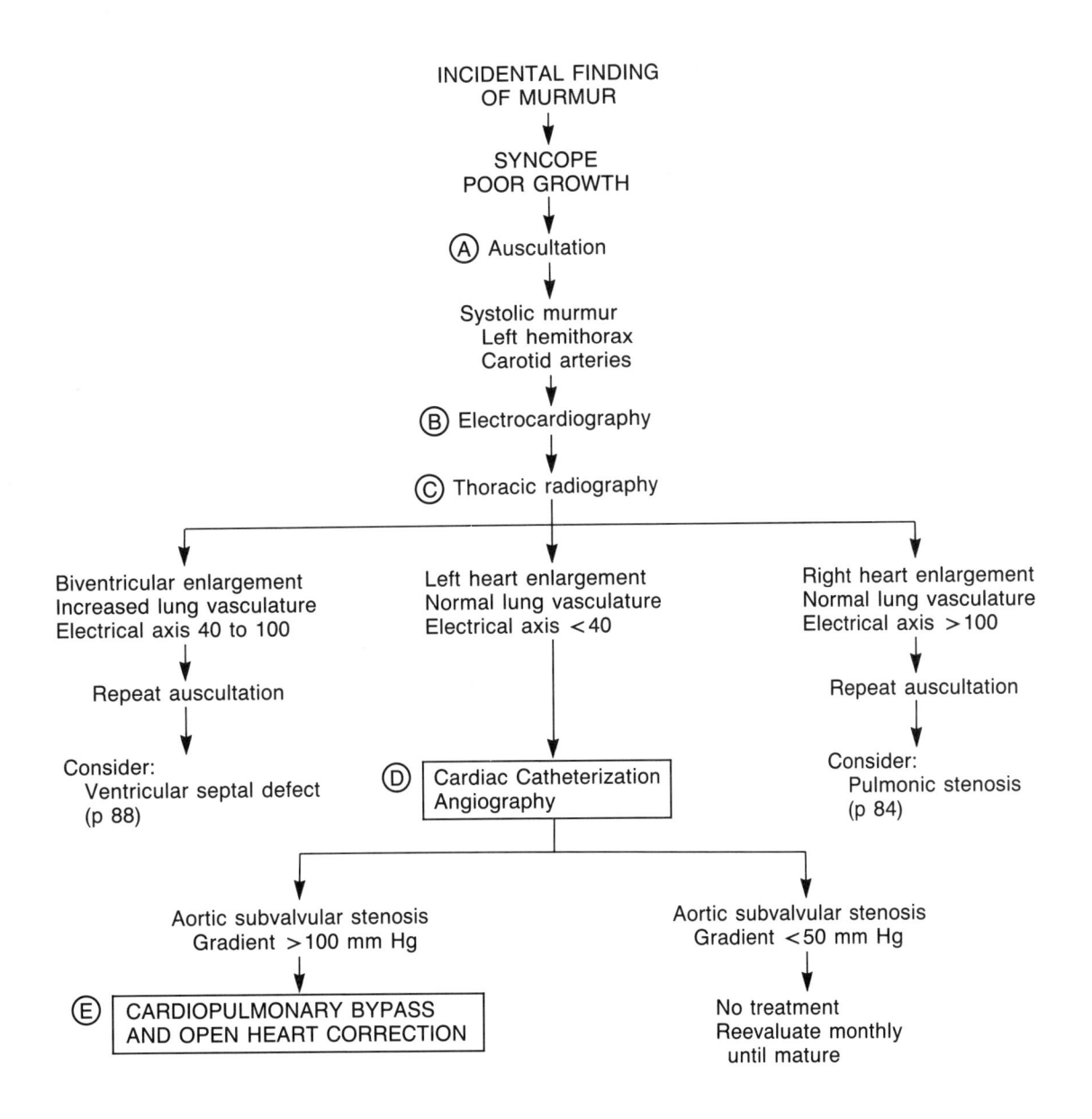

INCIDENTAL FINDING
OF MURMUR
↓
SYNCOPE
POOR GROWTH
↓
Ⓐ Auscultation
↓
Systolic murmur
Left hemithorax
Carotid arteries
↓
Ⓑ Electrocardiography
↓
Ⓒ Thoracic radiography
↓

- Biventricular enlargement
  Increased lung vasculature
  Electrical axis 40 to 100
  ↓
  Repeat auscultation
  ↓
  Consider:
  Ventricular septal defect
  (p 88)

- Left heart enlargement
  Normal lung vasculature
  Electrical axis <40
  ↓
  Ⓓ Cardiac Catheterization
  Angiography
  ↓
  - Aortic subvalvular stenosis
    Gradient >100 mm Hg
    ↓
    Ⓔ CARDIOPULMONARY BYPASS
    AND OPEN HEART CORRECTION
  - Aortic subvalvular stenosis
    Gradient <50 mm Hg
    ↓
    No treatment
    Reevaluate monthly
    until mature

- Right heart enlargement
  Normal lung vasculature
  Electrical axis >100
  ↓
  Repeat auscultation
  ↓
  Consider:
  Pulmonic stenosis
  (p 84)

VENTRICULAR SEPTAL DEFECT

David L. Holmberg

A. There is no breed predisposition for ventricular septal defect (VSD), but it is the most common congenital heart defect in cats. Auscultation usually reveals a systolic murmur, heard on both sides of the chest, which is loudest over the fourth right intercostal space. Occasionally large shunts result in a murmur over the pulmonic valve because of the increased blood flow across the valve.

B. Because of the difference in ventricular pressures, blood is ejected from the left to the right side of the heart during systole (Fig. 1). Hypertrophy of the right ventricle occurs to accommodate the increased pressure, and the left ventricle dilatates to accept the normal stroke volume from the right side as well as the aliquot of blood "recycled" through the right ventricle via the septal defect. The result is biventricular enlargement and a normal mean electrical axis. In cases with heart failure or pulmonary hypertension, the right ventricular changes are dominant and cause a right axis shift (>100 degrees).

C. Biventricular enlargement and overcirculation of the lungs are the usual radiographic findings with this condition. Dilatation of the main pulmonary artery is also common, and pulmonary edema can occur with large defects.

D. Although they create loud murmurs, most VSDs are small, do not require treatment, and may close spontaneously. Patients needing surgical correction usually present prior to 1 year of age with clinical signs of right heart failure. Although most defects occur in the upper membranous portion of the septum, ultrasonography and/or cardiac catheterization are required to confirm the position and size of the lesion. Injection of iodinated contrast media, blood gas analysis, and pressure monitoring are helpful in determining which surgical procedure, if any, is required. Relative pulmonary to systemic blood flow is calculated using the oxygen saturation level measured at various locations and equals:

$$\frac{\text{Aortic } O_2 - \text{Vena cava } O_2}{\text{Aortic } O_2 - \text{Pulmonary } O_2}$$

Usually pulmonary to systemic flows of 2 to 1 are required to cause clinical signs. If the flows are less than 2 to 1, the risks of surgical correction are generally greater than the risks of living with an untreated lesion. Some animals with pulmonary hypertension secondary to the increased flow shunt blood from the right into the left ventricle (Eisenmenger's syndrome). Surgical intervention is not indicated in these cases, since closure of the shunt leads to acute right heart failure, pulmonary edema, and death. Human patients with left-to-right shunting lesions and pulmonary vascular resistance greater than 60 percent of the systemic resistance die whether or not surgical correction is performed. This situation has not been well documented in veterinary medicine, but should be ruled out preoperatively when possible.

E. The surgical correction of VSDs can take two main forms: (1) Total correction requires full cardiopulmonary bypass and either direct suturing of the septum or placement of a patch graft across the defect; and (2) A more cost effective procedure for veterinary practice is pulmonary artery banding. This technique utilizes constriction of the pulmonary artery sufficient to decrease pulmonary arterial pressure by 50 percent, increase the right ventricular pressure, decrease the volume of shunted blood, and protect the lungs from high ejection pressures. Caution must be used so that a right-to-left shunt is not created.

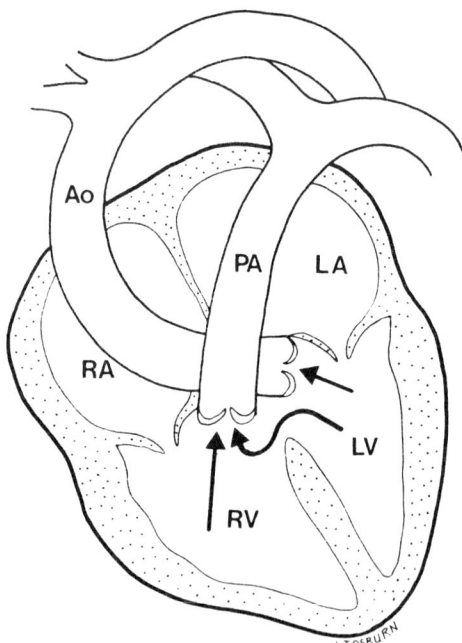

Figure 1 High-pressure blood from the left ventricle (LV) ejected into the aorta (Ao) and into the pulmonary artery (PA) through the ventricular septal defect.

References

Breznock EM. Spontaneous closure of ventricular septal defects in the dog. JAVMA 1973; 162:399.

Eyster GE, DeYoung B. Cardiac disorders. In: Slatter, DH. Textbook of small animal surgery. Toronto: WB Saunders, 1985:1076.

Eyster GE, Whipple RD, Anderson LK, et al. Pulmonary artery banding for ventricular septal defect in dogs and cats. JAVMA 1977; 170:434.

Feldman EC, Nimmo-Wilkie JS, Pharr JW. Eisenmenger's syndrome in the dog: case reports. JAAHA 1981; 17:477.

Plauth WH. Selection of the pediatric patient for heart surgery. In: Norman, JC. Cardiac surgery. New York: Appleton-Century-Crofts, 1972:245.

Weirich WE, Blevins WE. Ventricular septal defect repair. J Vet Surg 1978; 7:2.

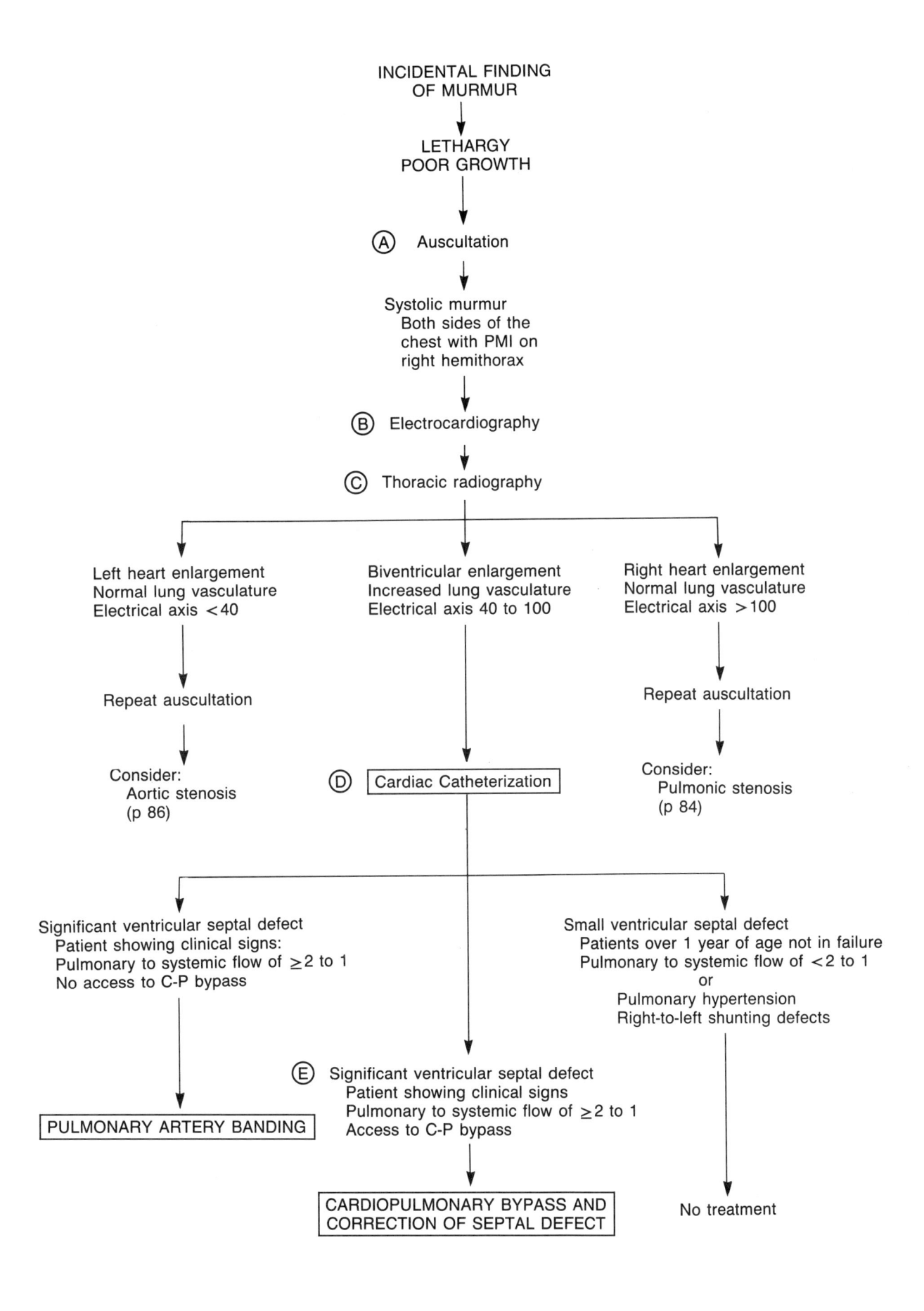

INCIDENTAL FINDING
OF MURMUR
↓
LETHARGY
POOR GROWTH
↓
Ⓐ Auscultation
↓
Systolic murmur
Both sides of the
chest with PMI on
right hemithorax
↓
Ⓑ Electrocardiography
↓
Ⓒ Thoracic radiography

- Left heart enlargement / Normal lung vasculature / Electrical axis <40
- Biventricular enlargement / Increased lung vasculature / Electrical axis 40 to 100
- Right heart enlargement / Normal lung vasculature / Electrical axis >100

Left branch:
Repeat auscultation
↓
Consider:
Aortic stenosis
(p 86)

Middle branch:
Ⓓ Cardiac Catheterization

Right branch:
Repeat auscultation
↓
Consider:
Pulmonic stenosis
(p 84)

Significant ventricular septal defect
Patient showing clinical signs:
Pulmonary to systemic flow of ≥2 to 1
No access to C-P bypass
↓
PULMONARY ARTERY BANDING

Ⓔ Significant ventricular septal defect
Patient showing clinical signs
Pulmonary to systemic flow of ≥2 to 1
Access to C-P bypass
↓
CARDIOPULMONARY BYPASS AND CORRECTION OF SEPTAL DEFECT

Small ventricular septal defect
Patients over 1 year of age not in failure
Pulmonary to systemic flow of <2 to 1
or
Pulmonary hypertension
Right-to-left shunting defects
↓
No treatment

TETRALOGY OF FALLOT

David L. Holmberg

Tetralogy of Fallot (TF) is formed by ventricular septal defect, stenosis of the pulmonary artery, overriding aorta, and hypertrophy of the right ventricle. Pulmonic stenosis prevents the blood of the right ventricle from exiting normally to the lungs. To successfully eject the blood through the septal defect against the high pressure generated in the left side of the heart, the right ventricle hypertrophies. The severity of the clinical signs is dependent on the relative amount of venous blood being passed through the lungs compared to the amount being shunted to the systemic circulation.

A. Patients with TF usually present before maturity with a history of exercise intolerance, depression, or syncope. The animal resists physical activity, and its mucous membranes are congested and can quickly become cyanotic if the examination is stressful. Little or no auscultatable murmur is present in these patients if blood flow is not turbulent. Occasionally a soft murmur of pulmonic stenosis is heard over the third left intercostal space.

B. Right ventricular hypertrophy is the major electrocardiographic finding in TF. Right deviation of the mean electrical axis (>100 degrees) and S-waves in leads I, II, and III are consistently present.

C. Stenosis of the pulmonary artery prevents the full ejection volume of the right ventricle from reaching the lungs. The pulmonary vasculature therefore appears decreased on thoracic radiographs, and the right ventricle and aortic shadow are prominent.

D. Cardiac catheterization is necessary to differentiate between TF and a ventricular septal defect with secondary pulmonary hypertension (Eisenmenger's syndrome). Both present with similar signs and have elevated hematocrits in response to the systemic circulation of venous blood. Injection of iodinated contrast media into the right ventricle demonstrates the shunt. The pulmonary artery and vasculature appear decreased with TF, but look normal or slightly increased with Eisenmenger's syndrome. Recording decreased pulmonary arterial pressures and right ventricular pressures in excess of those in the left ventricle confirms the diagnosis of TF.

E. The treatment of TF is aimed at increasing the amount of blood flowing through the patient's lungs. Although complete surgical correction of this defect is possible, adequate palliation of signs can be accomplished by anastomosing a systemic artery to the pulmonary artery. The left subclavian artery and the left internal thoracic artery have both been used in veterinary surgery.

F. Beta-adrenergic blocking agents are effective in improving pulmonary blood flow in 50 percent of cases because they cause dilation of the infundibular component of the stenosis. These agents can either be used as the final treatment or as a means to improve the patient's condition, thereby making the animal a better candidate for anesthesia and surgery. Generally, medical or surgical treatment does not "cure" TF, but can result in an acceptable house pet.

References

Eyster GE, Anderson LK, Sawyer DC, et al. Beta-adrenergic blockade for management of tetralogy of Fallot in a dog. JAVMA 1976; 169:637.

Eyster GE, Braden TD, Appleford M, et al. Surgical management of tetralogy of Fallot. J Small Anim Pract 1977; 18:387.

Feldman EC, Nimmo-Wilkie JS, Pharr JW. Eisenmenger's syndrome in the dog: case reports. JAAHA 1981; 17:477.

Miller CW, Holmberg DL, Bowen V, et al. Microsurgical management of tetralogy of Fallot in a cat. JAVMA 1985; 186:708.

Nimmo-Wilkie JS, Feldman EC. Pulmonary vascular lesions associated with congenital heart defects in three dogs. JAAHA 1981; 17:485.

GENERALIZED CYANOSIS
LETHARGY
POOR GROWTH

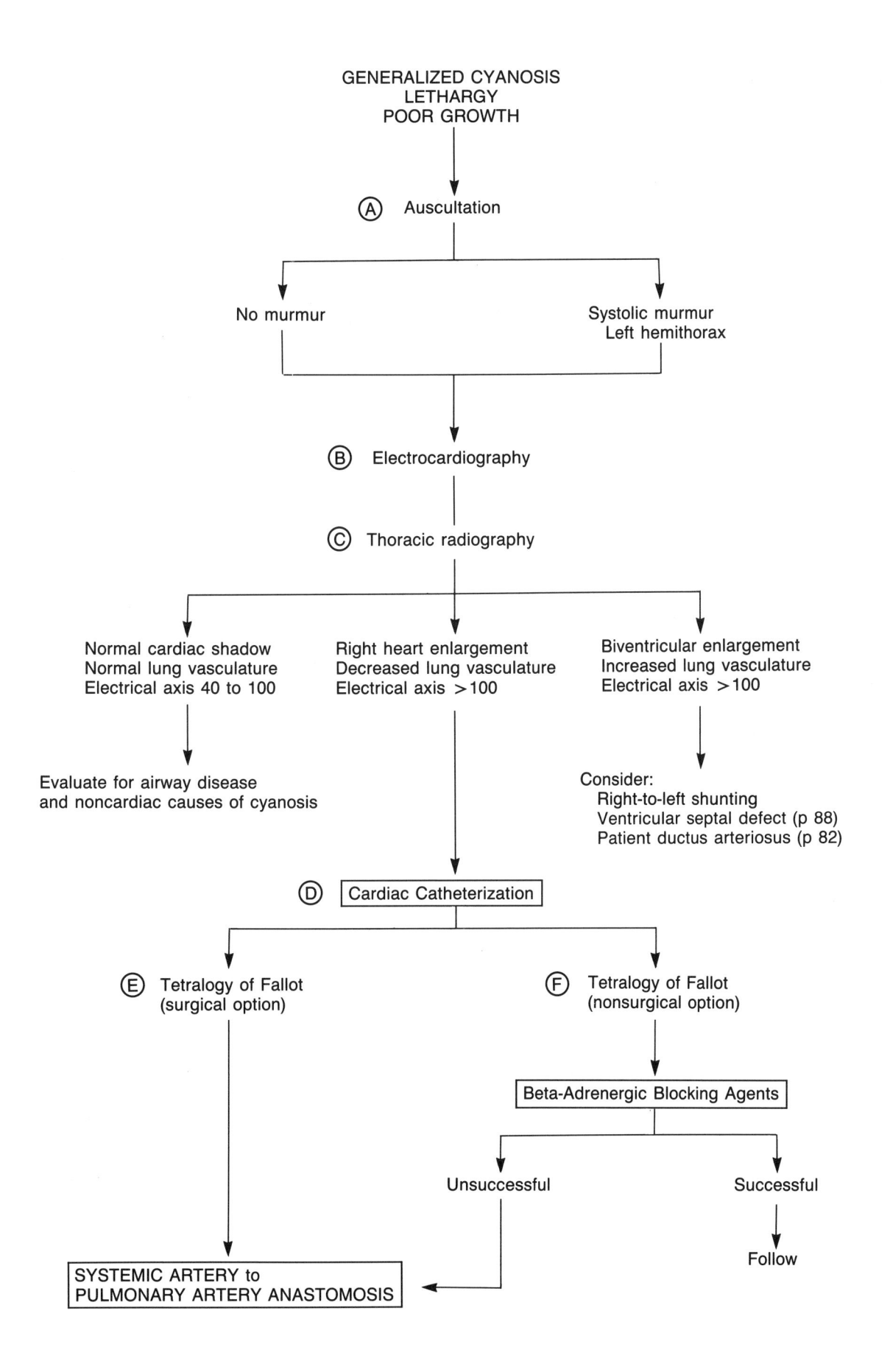

(A) Auscultation

- No murmur
- Systolic murmur Left hemithorax

(B) Electrocardiography

(C) Thoracic radiography

- Normal cardiac shadow
  Normal lung vasculature
  Electrical axis 40 to 100
  → Evaluate for airway disease and noncardiac causes of cyanosis

- Right heart enlargement
  Decreased lung vasculature
  Electrical axis >100

- Biventricular enlargement
  Increased lung vasculature
  Electrical axis >100
  → Consider:
    Right-to-left shunting
    Ventricular septal defect (p 88)
    Patient ductus arteriosus (p 82)

(D) Cardiac Catheterization

- (E) Tetralogy of Fallot (surgical option)
  → SYSTEMIC ARTERY to PULMONARY ARTERY ANASTOMOSIS

- (F) Tetralogy of Fallot (nonsurgical option)
  → Beta-Adrenergic Blocking Agents
    - Unsuccessful → SYSTEMIC ARTERY to PULMONARY ARTERY ANASTOMOSIS
    - Successful → Follow

VASCULAR RING ANOMALY

David L. Holmberg

Vascular ring anomalies (VRA) have many variations based on the degree of patency and association with other cardiac anomalies. Five main types are of concern: persistant right aortic arch with a left ligamentum arteriosum (Fig. 1); left aortic arch with a right ligamentum arteriosum; double aortic arch; and aberrant right or left subclavian arteries. Clinical signs associated with VRA are caused by the adjacent esophagus and trachea being trapped within a ring formed by these structures and the base of the heart.

A. Patients with VRA usually present soon after weaning; however, mature dogs have also been diagnosed with this condition. Regurgitation soon after eating solid food and poor weight gain are common owner complaints. Physical examination may be unrewarding other than showing generalized malnutrition. Nasal discharge, harsh lung sounds, and a palpable dilation of the cervical esophagus are occasionally seen secondary to chronic retention and aspiration of food.

B. Test feedings of solid dog food may be helpful in determining the level of the obstruction. Cricopharyngeal achalasia causes difficulty in swallowing, but with persistant mastication and repeated attempts, the food is passed normally to the stomach. Animals with VRA have no trouble swallowing food, but regurgitate within several minutes of consuming a moderate-sized meal. Older patients may have prolonged retention of food within the esophagus before regurgitation. Vomition of stomach contents is not typical of animals with VRA and may be suggestive of gastric or upper intestinal disease.

C. Survey thoracic radiographs are either normal or show a dilated esophagus filled with air or food. Contrast studies are usually required for diagnosis. Feeding a paste of barium sulfate mixed with soft dog food often facilitates the procedure.

D. Retention of the contrast media in a dilated pouch cranial to the base of the heart is diagnostic for the lesion. Some cases of VRA have dilatation of the esophagus caudal as well as cranial to the base of the heart. Dilatation of the entire thoracic esophagus is indicative of megaesophagus (e.g., idiopathic achalasia, myasthenia gravis), with or without a VRA. Differentiation can be made by serial radiographs and demonstration of a persistant narrowing of the esophagus at the heart base. Dilatation of the esophagus caudal to the heart significantly worsens the prognosis. Function of the lower esophageal sphincter must be evaluated in order to accurately determine the course of therapy.

E. Thoracotomy and isolation in combination with ligation and transection of the vascular ring and its associated scar tissue is therapeutic for an uncomplicated VRA. Resection or plication of the dilated pouch is usually not necessary as this improves clinically with time. If the thoracic esophagus is dilated throughout its length, but has a normally functioning lower sphincter, feeding the dog a gruel with its forequarters elevated assists in the normal passage of food. Some of these patients regain normal function of their esophagus by 1 year of age.

F. Abnormal function of the lower sphincter probably represents a generalized esophageal neuromuscular problem and has a poorer prognosis. Treatment of these animals must include an esophagomyotomy through the lower sphincter.

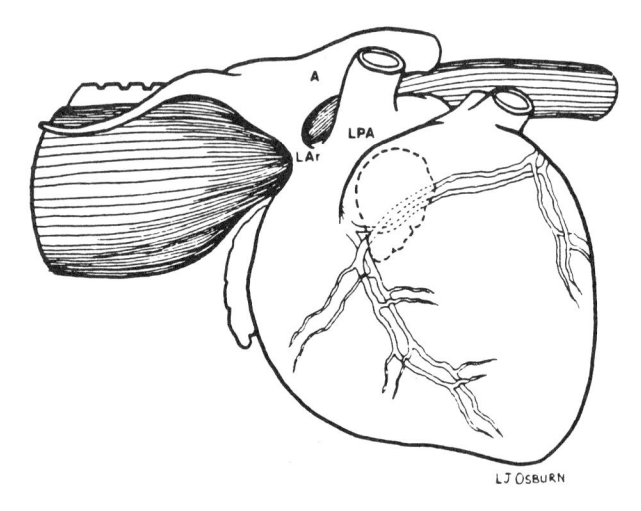

Figure 1 View of the heart from the left side showing a stricture of the esophagus due to a persistent right aortic arch. Aorta (A); ligamentum arteriosum (LAr); and left pulmonary artery (LPA).

References

Holmberg DL, Presnell KR. Vascular ring anomalies: case report and brief review. Can Vet J 1979; 20:78.

Shires PK, Liu W. Persistent right aortic arch in dogs: a long term follow-up after surgical correction. JAAHA 1981; 17:773.

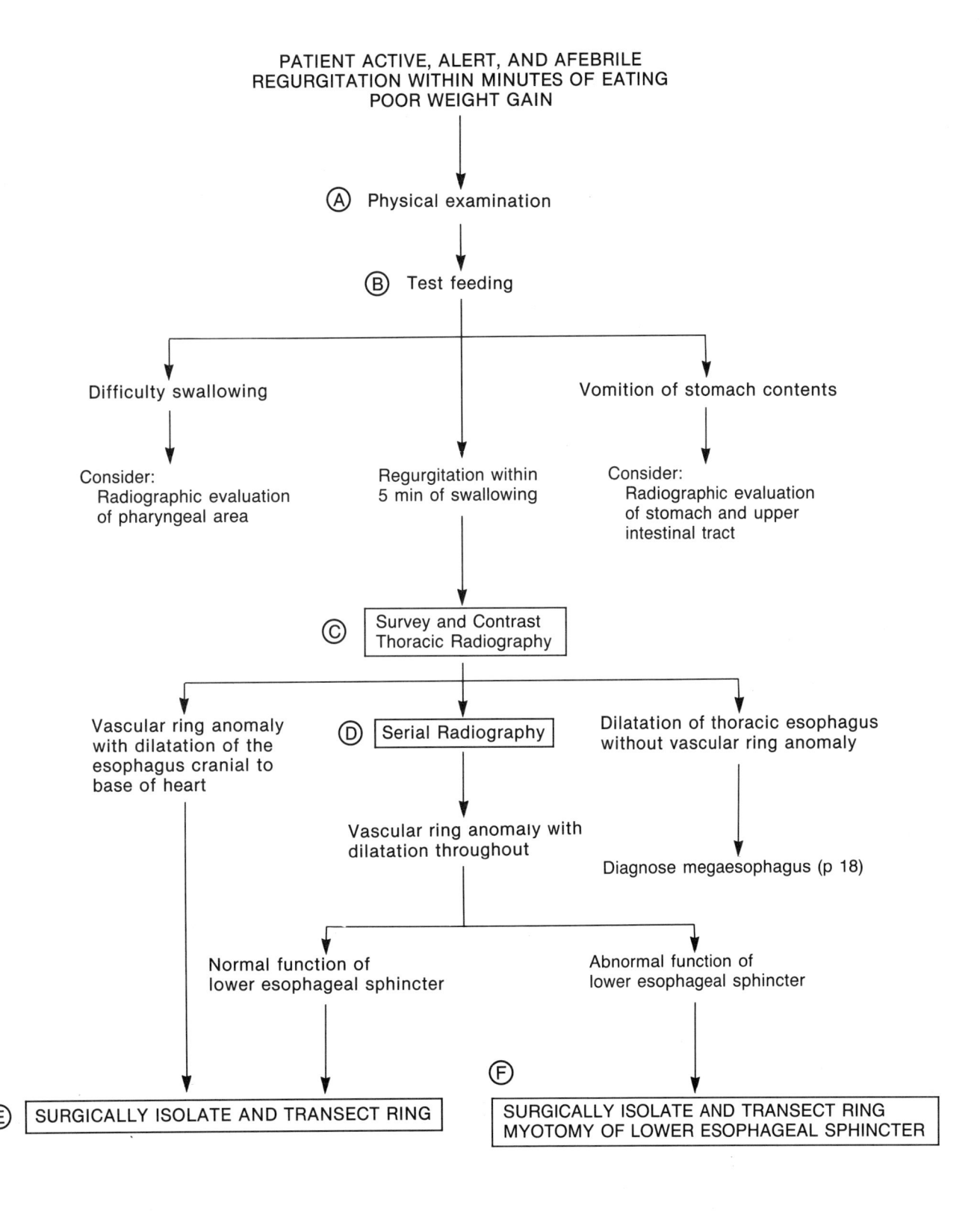

PATIENT ACTIVE, ALERT, AND AFEBRILE
REGURGITATION WITHIN MINUTES OF EATING
POOR WEIGHT GAIN
↓
Ⓐ Physical examination
↓
Ⓑ Test feeding

- Difficulty swallowing
  → Consider: Radiographic evaluation of pharyngeal area
- Regurgitation within 5 min of swallowing
  → Ⓒ Survey and Contrast Thoracic Radiography
- Vomition of stomach contents
  → Consider: Radiographic evaluation of stomach and upper intestinal tract

From Ⓒ Survey and Contrast Thoracic Radiography:
- Vascular ring anomaly with dilatation of the esophagus cranial to base of heart
- Ⓓ Serial Radiography
- Dilatation of thoracic esophagus without vascular ring anomaly → Diagnose megaesophagus (p 18)

From Ⓓ Serial Radiography:
- Vascular ring anomaly with dilatation throughout
  - Normal function of lower esophageal sphincter → Ⓔ SURGICALLY ISOLATE AND TRANSECT RING
  - Abnormal function of lower esophageal sphincter → Ⓕ SURGICALLY ISOLATE AND TRANSECT RING; MYOTOMY OF LOWER ESOPHAGEAL SPHINCTER

ARTIFICIAL CARDIAC PACEMAKER

David L. Holmberg

Implantation of an electric cardiac pacemaker (ECP) is performed on dogs that have a pathologically slow heart rate. Clinical signs of this problem are syncope, lethargy, and exercise intolerance. Some cases may also have signs of congestive heart failure superimposed on those of bradycardia. Although all breeds are susceptible, the miniature Schnauzer is affected most frequently.

A. Physical examination reveals whether an abnormal heart rate is present. Tachycardia is suggestive of heart failure or many tachyarrhythmias; a normal heart rate may indicate a noncardiac basis for the presenting complaint. Murmurs are not uncommon in dogs with bradycardia.

B. Differentiating the causes of bradycardia requires electrocardiographic evaluation. Atrial standstill or third-degree heart block with a slow ventricular response are obvious abnormalities. Marked sinus arrhythmia or temporary sinus arrest may occur only sporadically and often may progress to the more easily recognizable disturbances. These electrical conduction problems are generally referred to as part of the "sick sinus syndrome."

C. Thoracic radiographs are of little value in determining the need for an ECP. Significant signs of pulmonary edema may, however, suggest the early use of diuretics, sodium restriction, and cage rest. Various degrees of cardiomegaly are usually present.

D. Clinical pathologic results for a dog with a primary myocardial conduction disturbance are usually normal unless the animal is in congestive heart failure. However, laboratory evaluation is useful in identifying some noncardiac causes of bradycardia such as hypothyroidism or hyperkalemia.

E. The use of systemic atropine or isoproterenol may increase the ventricular rate in dogs with slow sinus rhythms or prolonged atrioventricular (A–V) conduction times.

F. Transvenous cardiac pacing can be used to increase the ventricular rate in dogs that are unresponsive to medical management. This treatment permits easier preoperative stabilization of the patient and safer anesthesia if a permanent ECP is later implanted. Placement of the transvenous pacemaker lead may be done with sedation and local anesthesia and is usually performed via the jugular vein, with the electrode coming to rest within the right ventricle. Dogs that fail to respond to medical management or temporary pacemaker implantation are unlikely to benefit from a permanent ECP and have a poor prognosis. These animals should be treated conservatively with rest; dietary salt restriction and diuretics are indicated if the animal is in heart failure.

G. Implantation of a permanent ECP requires a lateral thoracotomy or ventral midline laparotomy. The electrode is screwed and/or sutured into the apex of the heart. The lead cable is exited from the chest and tunneled subcutaneously towards the abdomen. The pulse generator is placed in a subcutaneous pocket in medium and large dogs and within the abdomen of small patients.

References

Bonagura JD, Helphrey ML, Muir WW. Complications associated with permanent pacemaker implantation in the dog. JAVMA 1983; 182:149.

Lombard CW, Tilley LP, Yoshioka M. Pacemaker implantation in the dog: survey and literature review. JAAHA 1981; 17:751.

Yoshioka MM, Tilley LP, Harvey HJ, et al. Permanent pacemaker implantation in the dog. JAAHA 1981; 17:746.

LETHARGY
SYNCOPE
EXERCISE INTOLERANCE

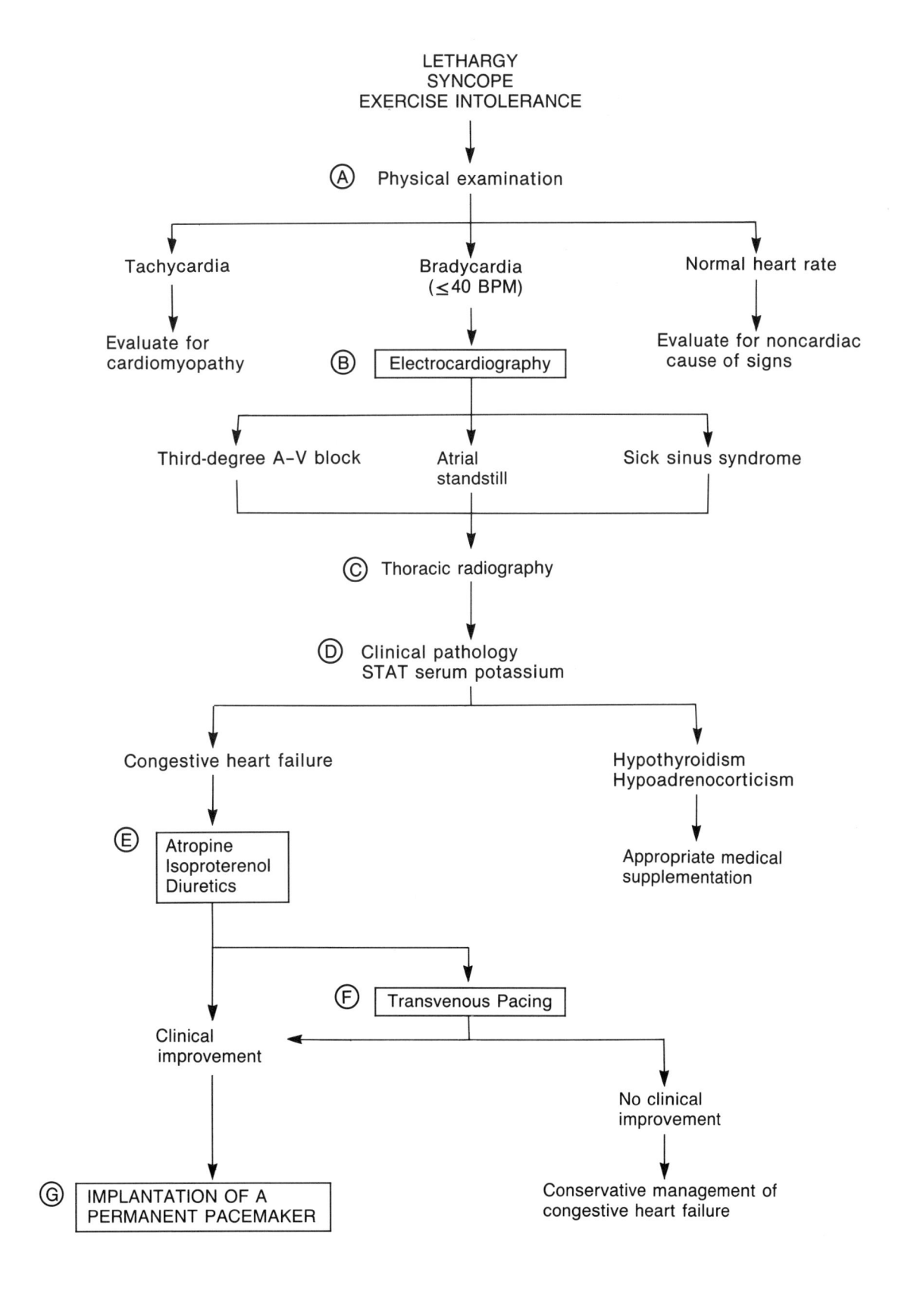

↓

Ⓐ Physical examination

- Tachycardia → Evaluate for cardiomyopathy
- Bradycardia (≤40 BPM) → Ⓑ Electrocardiography
- Normal heart rate → Evaluate for noncardiac cause of signs

Ⓑ Electrocardiography
- Third-degree A–V block
- Atrial standstill
- Sick sinus syndrome

↓

Ⓒ Thoracic radiography

↓

Ⓓ Clinical pathology
STAT serum potassium

- Congestive heart failure → Ⓔ Atropine / Isoproterenol / Diuretics
- Hypothyroidism / Hypoadrenocorticism → Appropriate medical supplementation

Ⓔ → Clinical improvement → Ⓖ IMPLANTATION OF A PERMANENT PACEMAKER

Ⓔ → Ⓕ Transvenous Pacing → No clinical improvement → Conservative management of congestive heart failure

PERICARDIAL EFFUSION TAMPONADE

David L. Holmberg

A. There is no age or breed predilection for this condition. Larger dogs over 8 years of age may present more frequently because of their higher incidence of cardiac tumors. Pericardial effusion tamponade (PET) inhibits diastolic filling of the heart and results in poor ventricular stroke volumes. Distended veins, poor peripheral pulse, and muffled heart sounds are classic signs of PET. Depending on the rate of fluid accumulation, animals may present with histories ranging from lethargy to acute collapse. Because PET is usually secondary to other diseases, diagnostic testing should be directed at determining the underlying condition.

B. Electrocardiography is useful in ruling out congestive cardiomyopathies that can cause signs and radiographic findings similar to PET. Increased amounts of fluid within the pericardial sac may decrease the amplitude of the QRS complex; however, experimental trials have not shown this to be consistent. Electrical alternans can be seen with PET, but most cases have normal electrocardiograms.

C. Typical PET survey radiographs are described as having a large globoid cardiac shadow. However, this requires that the fluid accumulation has been chronic enough to allow significant stretching of the pericardial sac. Relatively small amounts of fluid can cause acute clinical signs without creating obvious changes on the survey radiographs.

D. Contrast radiography can be used to determine the presence of PET as well as its etiology. Upper gastrointestinal studies may demonstrate pericardiodiaphragmatic hernias in younger animals. Angiocardiography and/or contrast studies of the pericardial sac itself help to determine the actual heart size and can assist in the visualization of cardiac neoplasms. Positive or negative contrast studies of the pericardium are usually performed at the time of pericardiocentesis for cytologic purposes. Although not currently available at most veterinary clinics, echocardiography is probably the most sensitive method of detecting PET. False-negative studies are possible with any of the aforementioned techniques.

E. Cytologic examination of fluid removed by pericardiocentesis may be helpful in determining the etiology of the PET. Transudative effusions are usually associated with congestive heart failure or hernias. Exudative effusions occur uncommonly and are secondary to foreign body penetration. Nonclotting bloody effusions suggest slowly bleeding neoplasms, whereas blood that clots after removal occurs with rapid bleeding such as that caused by left atrial rupture or iatrogenic puncture of a coronary vessel. Although a nonclotting serosanguinous effusion is suggestive of benign idiopathic pericardial effusion, this type of sample may be seen with any of the previously mentioned conditions. Treatment of PET is directed at the underlying cause of the fluid accumulation. Medical management of congestive heart failure may be indicated. Exploration of the pericardial sac for removal of a foreign body or evaluation and/or excision of a cardiac neoplasm is usually approached through a lateral thoracotomy. Idiopathic effusions may be controlled by repeated pericardiocentesis; however, subphrenic pericardectomy is curative.

References

Berg RJ, Wingfield W. Pericardial effusion in the dog: a review of 42 cases. JAAHA 1984; 20:721.

Bolton GR. Pericardial diseases. In: Ettinger SJ, ed. Textbook of veterinary internal medicine. 1st ed. Toronto: WB Saunders, 1975:1039.

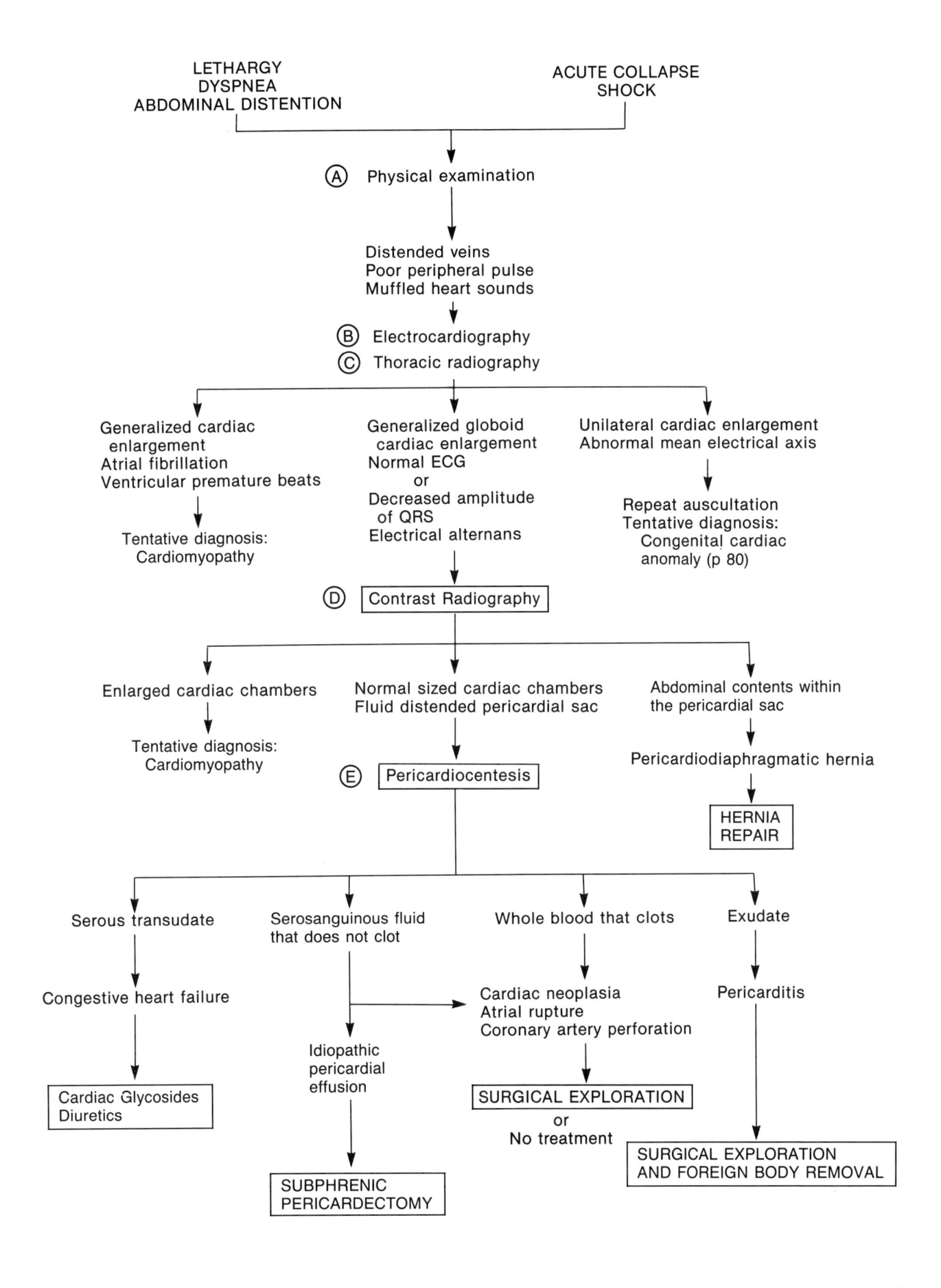

```
                    LETHARGY                          ACUTE COLLAPSE
                    DYSPNEA                               SHOCK
              ABDOMINAL DISTENTION
                          │                                │
                          └────────────────┬───────────────┘
                                           ▼
                                    Ⓐ Physical examination
                                           │
                                           ▼
                                    Distended veins
                                    Poor peripheral pulse
                                    Muffled heart sounds
                                           │
                                           ▼
                                    Ⓑ Electrocardiography
                                    Ⓒ Thoracic radiography
                                           │
            ┌──────────────────────────────┼──────────────────────────────┐
            ▼                              ▼                              ▼
   Generalized cardiac          Generalized globoid           Unilateral cardiac enlargement
       enlargement              cardiac enlargement           Abnormal mean electrical axis
   Atrial fibrillation              Normal ECG                            │
   Ventricular premature beats          or                                ▼
            │                  Decreased amplitude            Repeat auscultation
            ▼                         of QRS                  Tentative diagnosis:
    Tentative diagnosis:         Electrical alternans             Congenital cardiac
      Cardiomyopathy                    │                          anomaly (p 80)
                                        ▼
                               Ⓓ Contrast Radiography
                                        │
            ┌───────────────────────────┼───────────────────────────┐
            ▼                           ▼                           ▼
   Enlarged cardiac chambers   Normal sized cardiac chambers   Abdominal contents within
            │                  Fluid distended pericardial sac    the pericardial sac
            ▼                           │                           │
    Tentative diagnosis:                ▼                           ▼
      Cardiomyopathy           Ⓔ Pericardiocentesis       Pericardiodiaphragmatic hernia
                                        │                           │
                                        │                           ▼
                                        │                      ┌─────────┐
                                        │                      │ HERNIA  │
                                        │                      │ REPAIR  │
                                        │                      └─────────┘
   ┌────────────────┬────────────────┬──────────────────┐
   ▼                ▼                ▼                  ▼
Serous        Serosanguinous    Whole blood that     Exudate
transudate    fluid that        clots                   │
   │          does not clot        │                    ▼
   ▼                │              ▼                Pericarditis
Congestive          │         Cardiac neoplasia         │
heart failure       │         Atrial rupture            │
   │                │         Coronary artery perforation
   ▼                ▼              │                    ▼
┌──────────┐    Idiopathic         ▼           ┌──────────────────────┐
│ Cardiac  │    pericardial   ┌──────────────┐ │ SURGICAL EXPLORATION │
│Glycosides│    effusion      │   SURGICAL   │ │ AND FOREIGN BODY     │
│Diuretics │        │         │  EXPLORATION │ │      REMOVAL         │
└──────────┘        ▼         └──────────────┘ └──────────────────────┘
             ┌──────────────┐       or
             │  SUBPHRENIC  │   No treatment
             │PERICARDECTOMY│
             └──────────────┘
```

ARTERIOVENOUS FISTULA

David L. Holmberg

An arteriovenous fistula (AVF) may be congenital or acquired, multiple or single, central or peripheral. The most common examples of congenital AVF are single and central (patent ductus arteriosus or ventricular septal defect). Congenital AVFs can also be peripheral and multiple, but are rarely treated surgically. Acquired peripheral AVFs are the result of abnormal healing of ruptured adjacent arteries and veins. Rather than reestablishing normal circulation, a direct arteriovenous shunt is formed as the hematoma is resolved. The increased pressure in the venous system obstructs blood flow through the veins distal to the shunt and results in dilatation and valvular incompetence within the veins. The body responds by increasing the collateral blood supply to the area, but as the intravascular pressure exceeds the venous oncotic pressure, edema of the limb distal to the AVF occurs. Acquired peripheral AVF is the form of the disease dealt with in this chapter.

A. Although most AVFs are secondary to local trauma, the animals are usually presented weeks to months after the injury. Small painless swellings may be overlooked by owners until the condition progresses to lameness with generalized limb edema. Poor circulation may lead to ulceration, infection, and, in severe cases, gangrene of the limb distal to the AVF. Physical examination and palpation are extremely important in early differentiation of AVF from other diseases.

B. Because the pressure difference between the artery and vein results in continuous shunting of blood, turbulence can be detected as a palpable thrill or auscultated as a continuous murmur. Small AVFs may occur in the pinna of dogs secondary to ear scratching. These dogs may be presented for chronic shaking of their heads, or the owners may complain of an insect-like buzzing sound. Careful listening by the examiner in a quiet room is required to confirm this finding. Pressure on the affected artery may reduce the shunt and stop the characteristic murmur and thrill. If the volume of blood being shunted is large, the immediate decrease in venous return to the heart causes a reflex bradycardia called Branham's sign. This is a common finding when dealing with large central AVF, but is unusual with peripheral lesions.

C. Clinicopathologic findings are normal with uncomplicated AVF. However, secondary infection or vascular impairment of an organ may lead to changes characteristic of the area.

D. Survey radiographs are usually normal with small or early AVF. Large, long-standing AVF causes increased vascularity to an area and results in bone demineralization or periosteal proliferation. Destruction of normal bone structure is not seen with AVF and is considered more characteristic of neoplasia or infection.

E. Contrast radiography is necessary for the accurate diagnosis and treatment of AVF. Direct injection of iodinated dye into the proximal artery that supplies the shunt is acceptable when dealing with lesions in the distal two-thirds of the leg. When the AVF is within the body or proximal on a limb, catheterization of the aorta, passage of the catheter into the affected vessel, or flooding the aortic branching with dye is preferred. Premature venous filling and tortuous varicose vessels are diagnostic for AVF. Blood gas analysis shows the venous oxygen content of the limb to be highest proximal to the shunt.

F. The surgical correction of AVF is difficult and is aimed at the elimination of the shunt. Careful dissection, good hemostasis, and removal of all abnormal vessels are required for a cure. Ligation of the artery proximal to the shunt does not stop the AVF and may lead to ischemia of the distal portion of the limb. In chronic, recurring or infected cases, amputation of the limb may be the only effective treatment.

References

Litwak P. Peripheral vascular disorders. In: Slatter DH, ed. Textbook of small animal surgery. Toronto: WB Saunders, 1985:1151.

Olivier NB. Pathophysiology of arteriovenous fistulae. In: Slatter DH, ed. Textbook of small animal surgery. Toronto: WB Saunders, 1985:1051.

Suter PF. Diseases of the peripheral vessels. In: Ettinger SJ, ed. Textbook of veterinary internal medicine. 1st ed. Toronto: WB Saunders, 1975:1003.

Thompson JE, Garrett MD. Peripheral-arterial surgery. N Engl J Med 1980; 302:491.

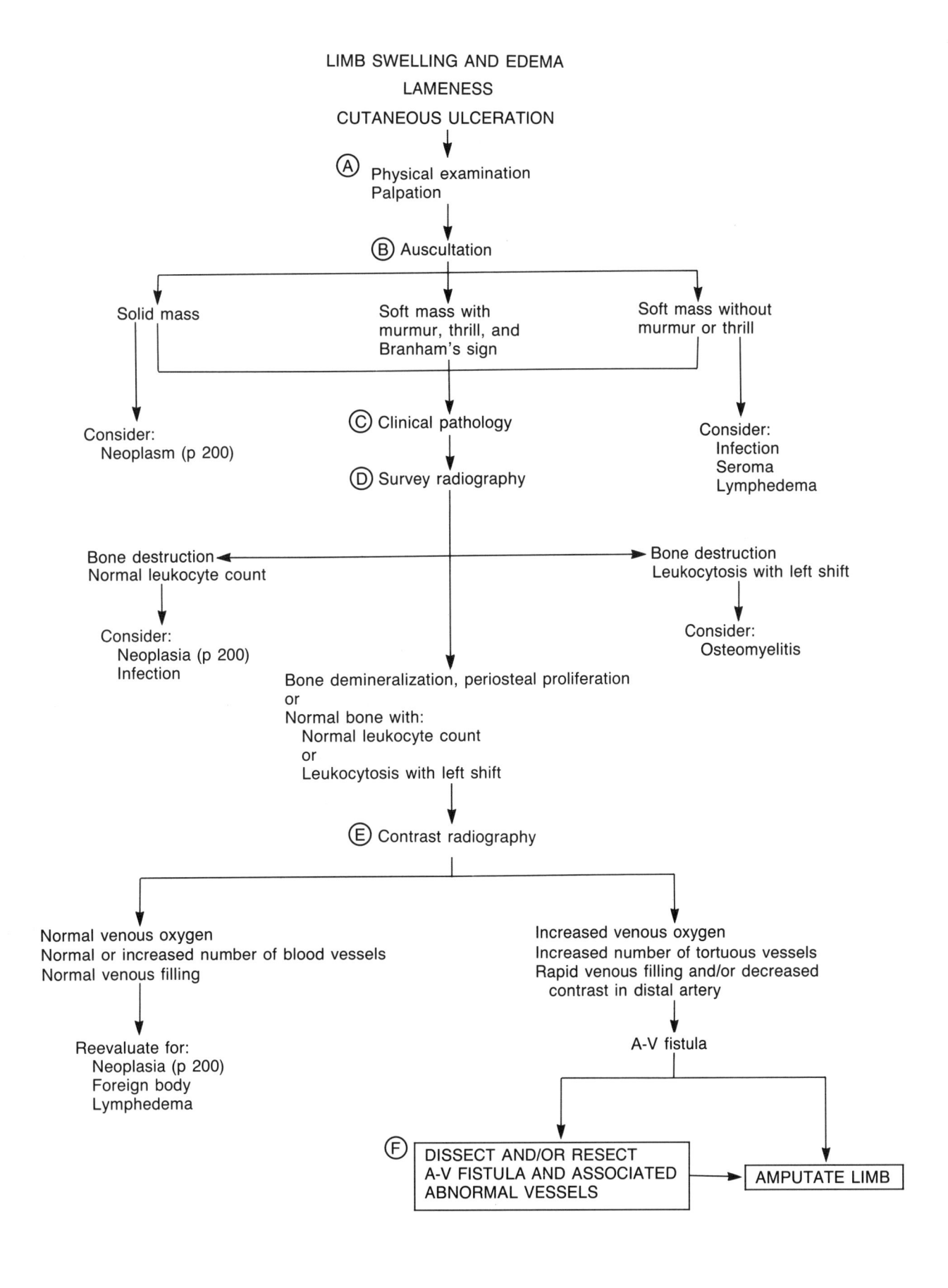

LIMB SWELLING AND EDEMA
LAMENESS
CUTANEOUS ULCERATION

(A) Physical examination
Palpation

(B) Auscultation

- Solid mass
- Soft mass with murmur, thrill, and Branham's sign
- Soft mass without murmur or thrill

Solid mass →
Consider:
　Neoplasm (p 200)

Soft mass without murmur or thrill →
Consider:
　Infection
　Seroma
　Lymphedema

(C) Clinical pathology

(D) Survey radiography

Bone destruction
Normal leukocyte count →
Consider:
　Neoplasia (p 200)
　Infection

Bone destruction
Leukocytosis with left shift →
Consider:
　Osteomyelitis

Bone demineralization, periosteal proliferation
or
Normal bone with:
　Normal leukocyte count
　or
　Leukocytosis with left shift

(E) Contrast radiography

Normal venous oxygen
Normal or increased number of blood vessels
Normal venous filling →
Reevaluate for:
　Neoplasia (p 200)
　Foreign body
　Lymphedema

Increased venous oxygen
Increased number of tortuous vessels
Rapid venous filling and/or decreased contrast in distal artery →
A-V fistula

(F) DISSECT AND/OR RESECT A-V FISTULA AND ASSOCIATED ABNORMAL VESSELS → AMPUTATE LIMB

ACUTE VASCULAR EMBOLISM

David L. Holmberg

A. The signs of acute vascular embolism (AVE) are attributable to ischemia of the organ or body part supplied by its vessel. Because the causes of acute organ failure are numerous, only occlusion of the terminal aorta is considered in this chapter. Severe pain on palpation of the affected limb(s), lameness, and/or paresis are noted in most cases. These signs are similar to those of other unrelated conditions such as long bone fracture(s), infection, or spinal disease. The initial diagnosis of vascular occlusion can be based on lack of femoral pulse, slow capillary refill time, and decreased surface temperature of the leg.

B. Survey radiographs may be of use in order to determine the etiology of the disease, as well as the location of the vascular obstruction. *All animals presenting with AVE should be evaluated for heart disease.* The changes in the cardiac shadow associated with cardiomyopathy (the most common cause of aortic obstruction) have been well characterized. Radiodense foreign bodies such as airgun pellets or intravascular catheters can be accurately identified and located without using contrast agents. However, the damage these agents may have done to the heart wall or valve leaflets may not be obvious.

C. Electrocardiographic and laboratory evaluation of the patient should precede surgical intervention for AVE. Impaired renal function, electrolyte imbalance, and cardiac arrhythmias can have significant effects on the anesthetic management of these cases. The severity of these changes depends on the etiology and duration of the occlusion and should be minimized whenever possible. If no evidence of life-threatening damage to the cardiopulmonary system exists, patients with radiodense intravascular foreign bodies should be taken directly to surgery.

D. Contrast radiography helps determine the etiology and location of radiolucent vascular obstructions. Injection of iodinated contrast media directly into the heart has been used in the past but causes further myocardial damage. Placing a jugular catheter into the right atrium and allowing the dye to be pumped from the heart gives good visualization of the aorta to the affected site without the risk of percutaneous cardiac puncture. Obstruction proximal to the renal arteries is indication for emergency surgical intervention. Vascular embarrassment to the kidneys and/or the intestinal tract carries a poor prognosis and must be corrected within hours of onset.

E. Vascular obstruction distal to the renal arteries permits the option of medical rather than surgical intervention. Heparin (150 IU per kilogram) helps decrease further thrombus growth but requires additional care with hemostasis if surgery is performed later. Alpha-adrenergic blocking agents, such as acepromazine (0.2 mg per kilogram), can be effective in reducing arterial spasm and may improve blood flow distal to the obstruction. Propranolol should be used with caution for cardiac arrhythmias as this agent can enhance the existing vasoconstriction.

F. If surgical intervention is to be of maximal value, it should be performed within 6 hours after the onset of signs. However, if a significant paresis persists after medical stabilization or if the patient deteriorates while being treated, surgical intervention may be indicated. A ventral abdominal incision permits easy access to the terminal aorta. When the obstruction has been removed and blood flow reestablished, potassium, which has moved out of the cells during the period of anoxia, is flushed into the circulatory system. To minimize the effects of this flush on the heart, a 5 percent dextrose drip should be maintained during the surgery, and sodium bicarbonate (1 mEq per kilogram) should be infused intravenously several minutes before slowly returning normal blood flow to the hind limbs.

References

Robins GM, Wilkinson GT, Menrath VH, Atwell RB, Riesz G. Long-term survival following embolectomy in two cats with aortic embolism. J Small Anim Pract 1982; 23:165.

Thompson JE, Garrett WV. Peripheral-arterial surgery. N Engl J Med 1980; 302:491.

Van Vleet JF, Ferrans VJ, Weirich WE. Pathologic alterations in hypertrophic and congestive cardiomyopathy of cats. Am J Vet Res 1980; 41:2037.

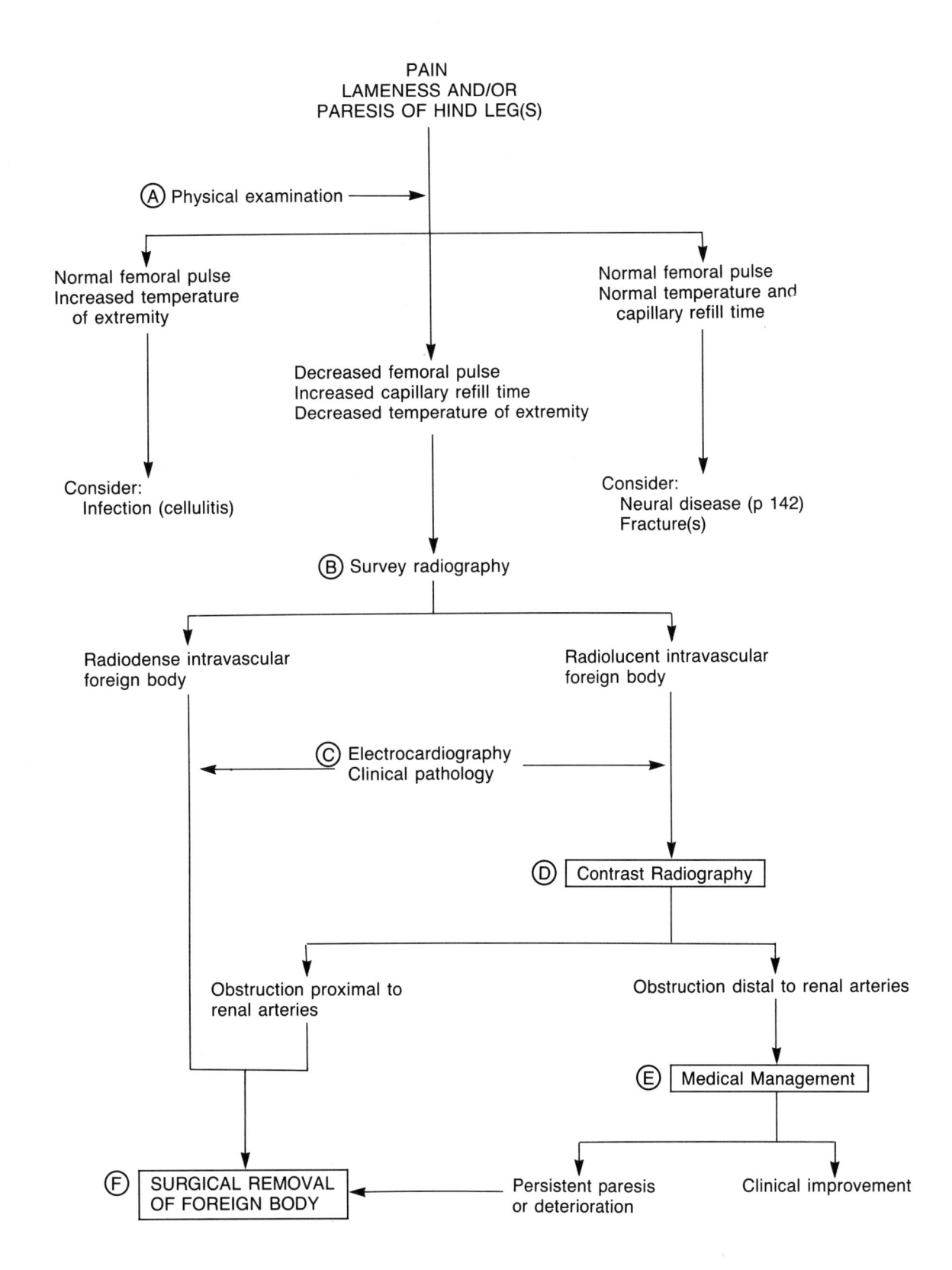

```
                    PAIN
                LAMENESS AND/OR
             PARESIS OF HIND LEG(S)
                         │
                         ▼
         (A) Physical examination ──────▶
          │              │                    │
          ▼              ▼                    ▼
  Normal femoral pulse   Decreased femoral pulse   Normal femoral pulse
  Increased temperature  Increased capillary       Normal temperature and
  of extremity           refill time               capillary refill time
                         Decreased temperature
                         of extremity
          │              │                    │
          ▼              ▼                    ▼
      Consider:                            Consider:
      Infection (cellulitis)               Neural disease (p 142)
                                           Fracture(s)
```

(B) Survey radiography

- Radiodense intravascular foreign body
- Radiolucent intravascular foreign body

(C) Electrocardiography / Clinical pathology

(D) Contrast Radiography
- Obstruction proximal to renal arteries
- Obstruction distal to renal arteries

(E) Medical Management
- Persistent paresis or deterioration
- Clinical improvement

(F) SURGICAL REMOVAL OF FOREIGN BODY

CANINE HEARTWORM

David L. Holmberg

A. Canine heartworm disease (CHD) is caused by infestation of the pulmonary and venous side of the cardiovascular system with *Dirofilaria immitis* (DI). Although most cases of CHD are found during routine laboratory screening of asymptomatic animals, clinical signs associated with the condition can be divided into two groups. Dogs that are moderately affected may present with coughing and exercise intolerance. If emptying of the right ventricle is delayed because of obstruction of the pulmonary artery by adult worms, a systolic murmur over the pulmonic valve and splitting of the second heart sound may be heard on auscultation. Hepatomegaly and ascites occur if the obstruction is adequate to cause right heart failure. The second group includes young dogs that are acutely exposed to a massive number of infective DI larvae. The simultaneous maturation and/or migration of a large number of worms can result in obstruction of the right atrium and posterior vena cava, causing severe liver destruction. Such dogs present in distress with distended jugular veins, decreased peripheral pulse, and, in some cases, shock (postcaval syndrome).

B. Thoracic radiographs are useful in differentiating CHD from other diseases such as mitral insufficiency or pericardial effusion, which may present with similar signs. Classically, dogs with long-standing CHD have enlargement of the right ventricle and main pulmonary artery. Embolism of the adult worms can result in acute termination or pruning of the peripheral pulmonary arteries. Dogs with acute obstruction of the vena cava may not have time to develop the typical changes and may have normal radiographs.

C. Electrocardiographic changes associated with CHD are those of right ventricular enlargement. Right deviation of the mean electrical axis and S-waves in leads I, II and III are often present but, like radiographic changes, require time for development.

D. Demonstration of DI microfilariae by one of the concentration techniques is diagnostic for the disease. The number of eosinophils circulating in the peripheral blood usually increases with CHD. An unexplained eosinophilia can be useful in diagnosing CHD in animals without circulating microfilariae. Dogs with severely hemolyzed blood samples, hemoglobinuria, and anemia should be considered to have the postcaval syndrome, and surgical treatment should begin as soon as possible. These dogs do not tolerate anesthesia well, and removal of the worms from the right atrium and posterior vena cava is carried out with long alligator forceps passed down the jugular vein (Fig. 1). If untreated, these animals may die within hours of presentation.

E. Dogs with CHD should be checked for adequate liver and kidney function. Because the compounds currently used to treat DI are nephrotoxic and hepatotoxic, preexisting disease of these organs may preclude medical treatment. Animals with significant impairment of renal or hepatic function may be better handled by surgical removal of the worms rather than treatment with arsenical drugs. The technique for removal of the DI is via a lateral thoracotomy and pulmonary arteriotomy following venous occlusion (see chapter on *Pulmonic Stenosis*, (p 84).

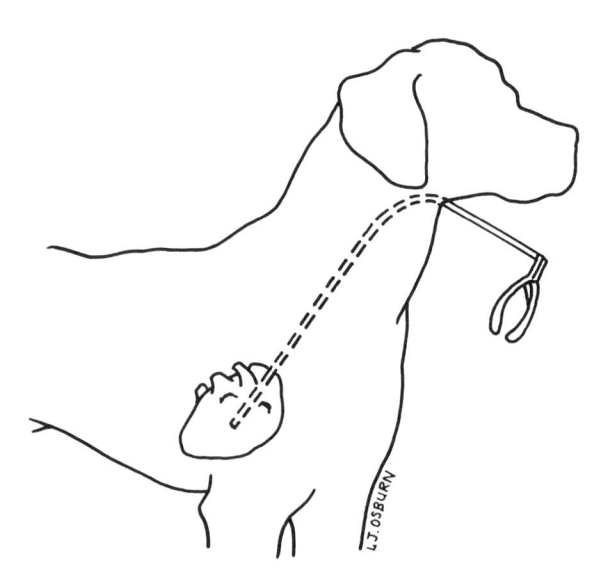

Figure 1 Heartworm removal from the heart using alligator forceps introduced into the jugular vein.

References

Jackson RF, Seymour WG, Growney PJ, Otto GF. Surgical treatment of the caval syndrome of canine heartworm disease. JAVMA 1977; 171:1065.

Rawlings CA, Lewis RE, McCall JW. Development and resolution of pulmonary arteriographic lesions in heartworm disease. JAAHA 1980; 16:17.

Special Report. Management of canine heartworm disease. JAVMA 1978; 173:1342.

```
                          CANINE HEARTWORM DISEASE Suspected
                                        |
                    ┌───────────────────┴───────────────────┐
                    ▼                                       ▼
        Middle age to older dogs                    Young dogs
        Exercise intolerance                        Acute collapse
        Coughing                                    Tachypnea
                    │       ◄──── Ⓐ Physical examination ────►
                    ▼                                       ▼
        Systolic murmur                             Systolic tricuspid murmur
          Split 2nd heart sound                     Distended veins
          Hepatomegaly (p 54)                       Poor peripheral pulse
          Ascites (p 204)
                            ◄──── Ⓑ Thoracic radiography ────►
                            ◄──── Ⓒ Electrocardiography ────►
```

┌────────────────────────┬──────────────────────────┬────────────────────────┐
▼   ▼   ▼

Left heart enlargement   Right heart enlargement   Biventricular enlargement
Normal or left axis   Pruning of pulmonary   Decreased amplitude QRS
  deviation   vessels   Normal pulmonary vessels
Normal pulmonary   Electrical axis >100
  vessels   S-waves in leads I, II, III
         │   │   │
         ▼   ▼   ▼
    Consider: Ⓓ Clinical pathology   Consider:
    Other causes   Possible
    of congestive   pericardial effusion
    heart failure   (p 96)

                  ┌──────────────┼──────────────┐
                  ▼   ▼   ▼
            Eosinophilia   Eosinophilia   Hemolysis
            No Microfilariae Microfilariae Hemoglobinuria
                             in blood   Anemia
                  │   │   │
                  ▼   ▼   ▼
         Occult dirofilariasis Dirofilariasis   Postcaval syndrome
                  │   │   │
                  ▼   ▼   ▼
         Recheck for   Ⓔ Assess renal   ┌─────────────────────────┐
         microfilariae   function   │ REMOVAL OF HEARTWORMS   │
         Treat as   │ WITH ALLIGATOR FORCEPS │
         dirofilariasis   │ AND LOCAL ANESTHETIC   │
                                                  │ VIA JUGULAR VEIN   │
                                                  └─────────────────────────┘

                  ┌──────────────────────┴──────────────────────┐
                  ▼   ▼
        Adequate renal and   Fixed specific gravity urine
        liver function   Increased serum urea
                                                   Increased alanine
                                                     aminotransferase
                  ▼   ▼
        ┌────────────────────────────┐   ┌─────────────────────────────┐
        │ Medical Treatment with   │   │ SURGICAL REMOVAL OF ADULT   │
        │ Arsenical Compound and   │   │ WORMS VIA PULMONARY   │
        │ Filaricide   │   │ ARTERIOTOMY   │
        └────────────────────────────┘   └─────────────────────────────┘

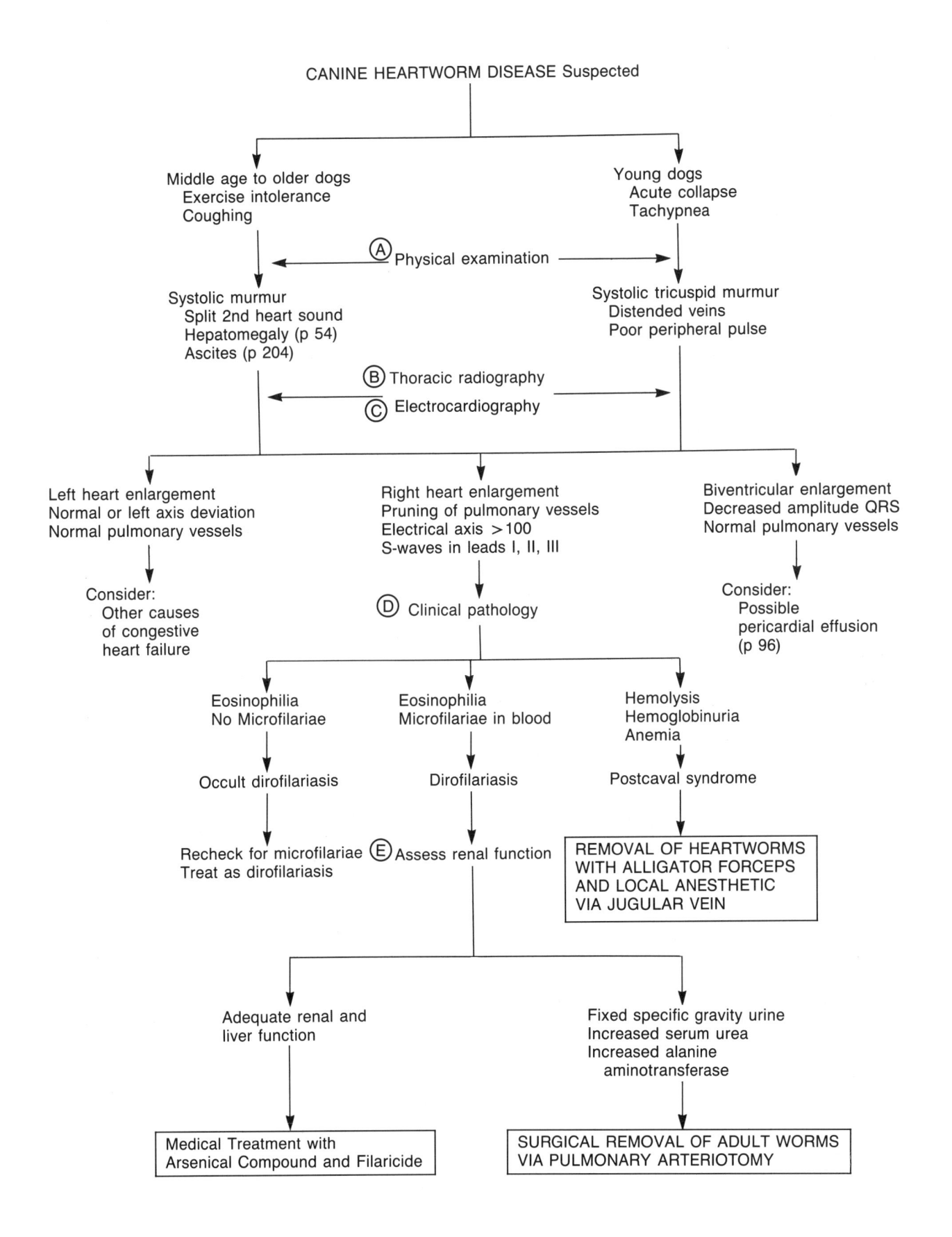

PORTOSYSTEMIC SHUNT

Karol A. Mathews

A. In the majority of cases, the history consists of a combination of both neurologic and nonneurologic signs. Neurologic signs include depression and apathy, stupor, coma, amaurotic blindness, head pressing, seizures, circling, pacing, and behavioral changes such as unprovoked aggression, timidity, and disobedience. Truncal ataxia and weakness may occur. Nonneurologic signs include anorexia, vomition, diarrhea, ptyalism, and, rarely, dysphagia. Stunted growth, poor hair coat, weight loss, and emaciation are also reported. Polyuria, polydipsia, stranguria, hematuria, and urethral obstruction may occur. Prolonged recovery from anesthesia or tranquilization may be the only historic abnormality in congenital portosystemic shunts.

B. Physical examination may reveal a thin, stunted animal with pale mucous membranes. Unless the dog is depressed or blind, the neurologic status may be normal except during a seizure episode. Cystic calculi may be palpated, or urethral calculi may obstruct urine flow. Ascites may be present in animals with advanced liver disease or atrophy but not in dogs with congenital shunts. In cases of arteriovenous (A-V) fistulas involving the liver, a heart murmur and vague gastrointestinal signs may be noted as well as ascites.

C. With portosystemic shunts, abdominal radiographs reveal a small liver and, occasionally, large kidneys. Similar findings may occur in patients with chronic primary liver disease. The liver may be normal or increased in size with active inflammation or neoplasia. There is usually poor abdominal detail caused by ascites or an absence of abdominal fat. Definitive diagnosis of portosystemic shunts may be made through transabdominal splenoportography, or, when an intrahepatic shunt is suspected (more common in the large breeds), cranial mesenteric angiography. With hepatic A-V fistulae, cardiomegally and increased pulmonary vasculature may be noted. Celiac angiography may identify the fistula.

D. Most patients with portosystemic shunts have a low erythrocyte mean corpuscula volume (MCV). The packed cell volume (PCV), hemoglobin, RBC count, and mean corpuscular hemoglobin (MCHC), may be reduced or normal. Coagulation studies are usually normal but may be abnormal in primary liver disease. Total serum protein, albumin, and urea are frequently significantly decreased. Serum alanine aminotransferase (ALT), serum aspartate aminotransferase (AST), and alkaline phosphatase are variably elevated in congenital and acquired portosystemic shunts, and may be significantly elevated in patients with acquired shunts secondary to liver disease. Total bilirubin may be elevated in patients, with liver disease but rarely in those with congenital shunts. Resting serum ammonia may or may not be elevated, but is frequently increased by more than 100 percent following ammonia tolerance tests. Postprandial serum bile acids are elevated and bromsulphalein retention is frequently prolonged. Ammonium biurate crystals or calculi are present in fewer than 50 percent of patients with congenital portosystemic shunts.

E. Exploratory laparotomy allows direct visualization of the liver and abdominal vasculature. In most instances, identification of single or multiple extrahepatic shunts can be made.

F. Because of the variable location, congenital portosystemic shunts, especially intrahepatic, may be difficult to locate. Perform intraoperative mesenteric portography and portal pressure measurements if necessary.

G. Jejunal or mesenteric vein catheterization facilitates portal pressure measurements and mesenteric portography. Normal portal pressures are reported to be 8 to 15 cmH_2O; lower pressures are associated with single congenital shunts; higher pressures are usually associated with post, intra, and prehepatic portal hypertension. Portal pressure measurements are also of value when attenuating portosystemic shunts.

H. Multiple extrahepatic shunts are frequently associated with primary liver disease, intrahepatic A-V fistulae and portal venous obstruction. Fremitus and blood filled cavities are present within the liver. Fistula removal is facilitated by lobectomy or selective dearterialization. An abdominal mass or constrictive lesion may cause portal venous obstruction. An attempt should be made to correct this. Blood flow through the shunt frequently persists even following correction of the initiating cause. Banding of the posterior vena cava at the hiatus, to raise the vena cava pressure above the portal pressure, can reverse the hepatofugal splanchnic blood flow forcing it into the portal vein and through the liver.

I. If primary liver pathology is suspected, obtain a liver biopsy. Hepatic insufficiency may be caused by a urea enzyme deficiency; submit the liver biopsy for quantitiative argino succinate synthetase analysis.

J. The prognosis in portal vein agenesis is poor. Medical management is palliative.

K. Single intrahepatic portocaval shunts usually occur in large breeds of dogs. The shunt may be completely or partially surrounded by hepatic parenchyma and, therefore, may be difficult to identify and correct.

L. Single extrahepatic shunts generally occur in small breeds of dogs and can be identified without intraoperative mesenteric portography. These shunts commonly originate from the gastrosplenic or splenic vein and usually terminate in the caudal vena cava proximal to the phrenicoabdominal vein. The decision to partially or totally occlude the shunt is based on bowel appearance and portal pressures.

M. A low protein diet is recommended for 3 weeks after shunt attenuation, with gradual introduction of normal diet, in order to avoid precipitating signs of hepatic en-

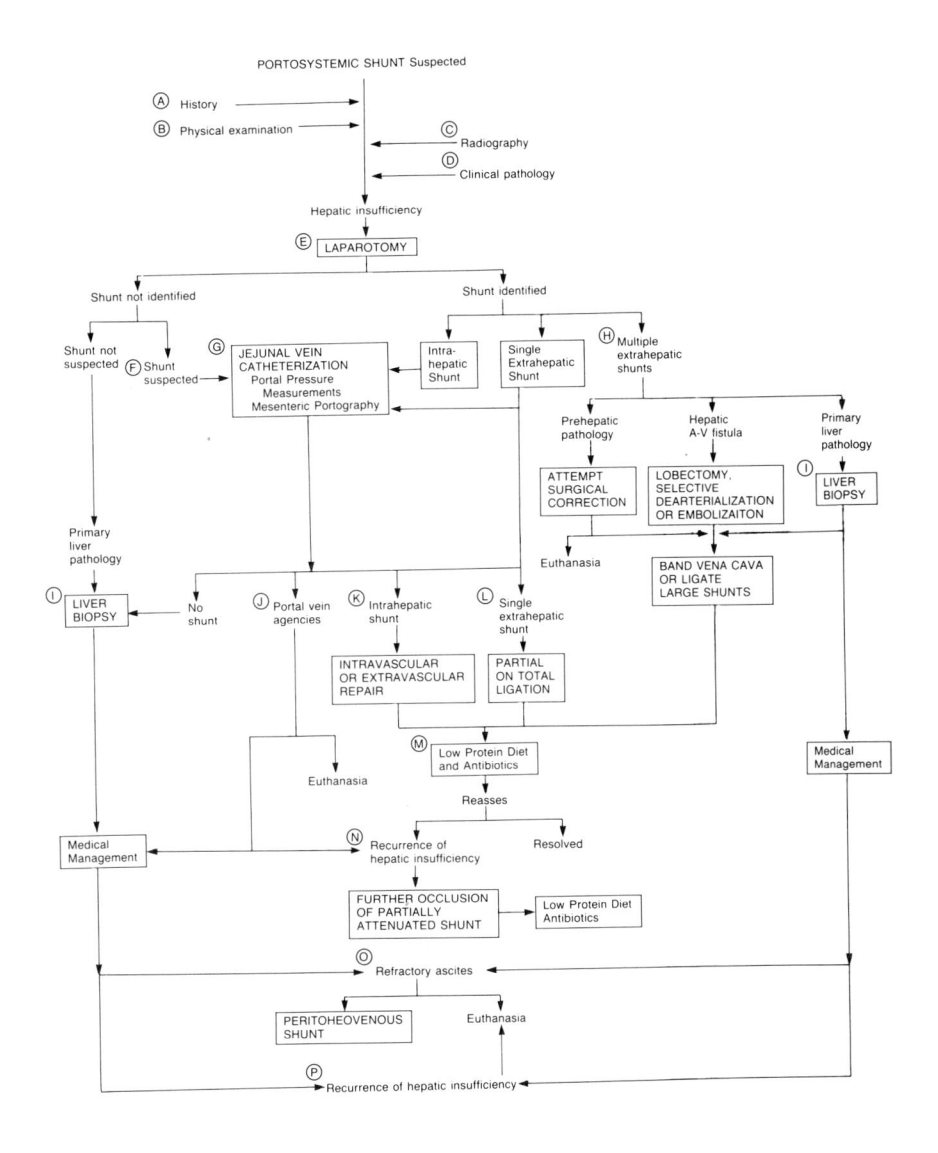

```
                    PORTOSYSTEMIC SHUNT Suspected
         Ⓐ History          →
         Ⓑ Physical examination →   ← Ⓒ Radiography
                                  ← Ⓓ Clinical pathology
                           ↓
                    Hepatic insufficiency
                      Ⓔ ┌─────────────┐
                        │  LAPAROTOMY │
                        └─────────────┘
              ┌──────────────┴──────────────┐
         Shunt not identified          Shunt identified
         ┌──────┴──────┐          ┌─────────┼─────────────┐
    Shunt not    Ⓕ Shunt       Intra-    Single      Ⓗ Multiple
    suspected    suspected →   hepatic  Extrahepatic  extrahepatic
                              Shunt     Shunt         shunts
              Ⓖ ┌──────────────────┐
                │ JEJUNAL VEIN     │
                │ CATHETERIZATION  │
                │ Portal Pressure  │
                │ Measurements     │
                │ Mesenteric       │
                │ Portography      │
                └──────────────────┘
                                    Prehepatic  Hepatic    Primary
                                    pathology   A-V        liver
                                                fistula    pathology
                                    ┌────────┐ ┌──────────┐  Ⓘ ┌────────┐
                                    │ATTEMPT │ │LOBECTOMY,│    │ LIVER  │
                                    │SURGICAL│ │SELECTIVE │    │ BIOPSY │
                                    │CORRECT.│ │DEARTERIAL│    └────────┘
                                    └────────┘ │IZATION OR│
                                               │EMBOLIZAIT│
                                               └──────────┘
                                    Euthanasia  ┌──────────┐
                                                │BAND VENA │
                                                │CAVA OR   │
                                                │LIGATE    │
                                                │LARGE     │
                                                │SHUNTS    │
                                                └──────────┘
      Primary       Ⓙ       Ⓚ           Ⓛ Single
      liver        Portal  Intrahepatic  extrahepatic
      pathology    vein    shunt         shunt
     Ⓘ┌──────┐    agencies
       │LIVER │ No   ┌──────────┐  ┌─────────┐
       │BIOPSY│ shunt│INTRAVASC.│  │PARTIAL  │
       └──────┘      │OR EXTRA- │  │ON TOTAL │
                     │VASCULAR  │  │LIGATION │
                     │REPAIR    │  └─────────┘
                     └──────────┘
                            Ⓜ ┌──────────────┐
                              │Low Protein   │           Medical
                              │Diet and      │           Management
                              │Antibiotics   │
                              └──────────────┘
   Medical              Reasses
   Management        Ⓝ    ↓
                      Recurrence of      Resolved
                      hepatic insufficiency
                      ┌──────────────┐
                      │FURTHER OCCLUS│→ Low Protein Diet
                      │OF PARTIALLY  │  Antibiotics
                      │ATTENUATED    │
                      │SHUNT         │
                      └──────────────┘
              Ⓞ → Refractory ascites ←
                ┌──────────────┐
                │PERITOHEOVENOUS│  Euthanasia
                │SHUNT         │
                └──────────────┘
              Ⓟ
              ← Recurrence of hepatic insufficiency ←
```

cephalopathy. Ampicillin should be given for 3 postoperative days.

N. The prognosis following surgical attenuation of a congenital portosystemic shunt is good to excellent. Hepatic insufficiency may recur if only partial attenuation was achieved, therefore, perform complete attenuation of the shunt, if possible. Recurrence of clinical signs, when associated with multiple extrahepatic shunts, should be managed medically.

O. Primary liver disease may result in ascites. If medical control fails, a peritoneovenous shunt may be palliative. The prognosis is poor.

P. Persistence or recurrence of hepatic insufficiency following thorough surgical and/or medical management indicates a poor prognosis.

References

Breznock EM, Whiting PG. Portacaval shunts and anomalies. In: Slatter DH, ed. Textbook of small animal surgery, Vol I. Philadelphia: WB Saunders, 1985:1156.

Ewing GO, Suter PF, Bailey CS. Hepatic insufficiency associated with congenital anomalies of the portal vein in dogs. JAAHA Sept/Oct 1974; 10:463.

Griffiths GI, Lumsden JH, Valli VEO. Hematologic and biochemical changes in dogs with portosystemic shunts. JAAHA Sept/Oct 1981; 17:205.

Mathews K, Gofton N. Congenital extrahepatic portosystemic shunt occlusion in the dog: the importance of gross observations during surgical correction. JAAHA 1986.

Meyer DJ. Liver function tests in dogs with portosystemic shunts: measurement of serum bile acid concentration. JAVMA 1986; 188(2):168.

Meyer DJ, Strombeck DR, Stone EA, Zenoble RD, Buss DD. Ammonia tolerance test in clinically normal dogs and in dogs with portosystemic shunts. JAVMA 1978; 173(4):377.

URINARY TRACT INFECTION

Elizabeth A. Stone

A. A dog with urinary tract infection (UTI) may present with dysuria, hematuria, or may have no symptoms. Risk factors to be considered when planning surgical treatment include urine retention, urethral catheterization, and indwelling urinary catheters.

B. The urine sample should be obtained by cystocentesis in cats and dogs or by aseptic catheterization in male dogs (Fig. 1).

C. Acute, uncomplicated, urinary tract infections (UTI) in female dogs are usually caused by bacterial cystitis.

D. A urine culture from a cystocentesis sample is considered positive when there are greater than 10^2 organisms on quantitative culture. In a catheterized sample, 10^5 organisms are considered positive.

E. Acute, uncomplicated infections may be treated with a 7-day course of a penicillin derivative, (ampicillin or amoxicillin), or a trimethoprim-sulphonamide. Chronic infections and infections that are associated with risk factors are treated with an antibiotic determined by the culture and sensitivity result.

F. A urine culture should be done on a urine specimen collected 2 to 4 days after completion of the antibiotic regimen.

G. Use double-contrast cystography in order to diagnose cystic calculi, bladder diverticula, and bladder masses.

H. Urinary tract calculi continue to be nidi for infection and may make it impossible to control UTI. After removal, calculi should be analyzed for mineral content. A *quantitative* mineral analysis is indicated for recurrent calculi, radiolucent calculi, and following ambiguous *qualitative* analysis results. Medical management is necessary to prevent recurrence of calculi. The therapy used depends on the type of calculus and UTI present.

I. Complete surgical excision is curative for benign bladder masses. Transitional cell carcinoma (TCCa) is the most frequent bladder neoplasia. Effective treatments for TCCa in dogs have not been determined.

J. The most frequent causes of chronic UTI in a male dog are chronic prostatitis and pyelonephritis. Chronic bacterial prostatitis is diagnosed by cytologic examination, culture of prostatic fluid, and culture and examination of a prostatic biopsy (p 134).

K. Renoliths are removed because they predispose the kidney to infection and may prevent elimination of the infection.

L. Choice of an antibiotic is based on sensitivity results, the activity in acid or alkaline urine, and the penetration into the renal medulla. A urine culture is done on the fourth day of therapy to determine the effectiveness of the chosen antibiotic. If it is effective, the antibiotic is continued for 4 weeks. A repeat culture is done 1 week after completion of the antibiotics. If still effective, the antibiotic is continued for another 4 weeks and another culture is taken. Once the urine is sterile, cultures are repeated monthly for 3 months to diagnose reinfection.

M. When one kidney has severe architectural changes and the other is normal, a unilateral nephroureterectomy is performed to remove the source of infection and prevent spread of infection to the healthy kidney.

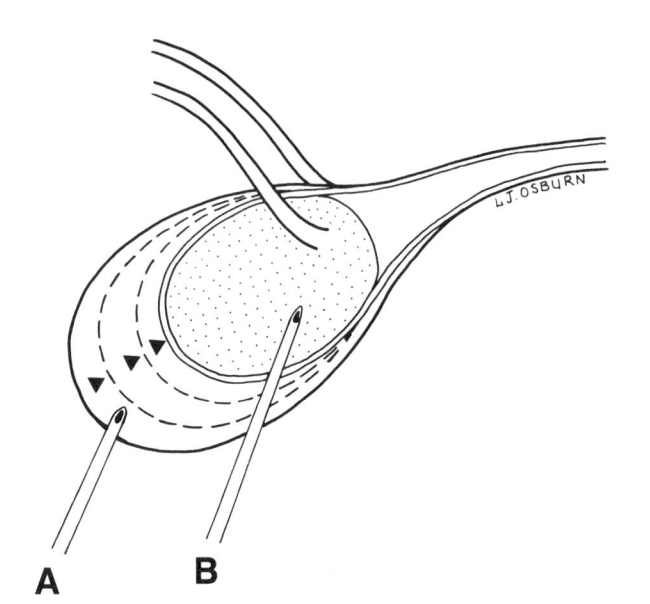

Figure 1 Needle placement for obtaining urine sample by cystocentesis *A*, is incorrect; *B*, is correct.

References

Klausner JS, Osborne CA. Urinary tract infection and urolithiasis. Vet Clin North Am 1979; 9:701.

Ling GV. Treatment of urinary tract infections with antimicrobial agents. In: Kirk RW, ed. Current veterinary therapy VIII. Philadelphia: WB Saunders, 1983:1051.

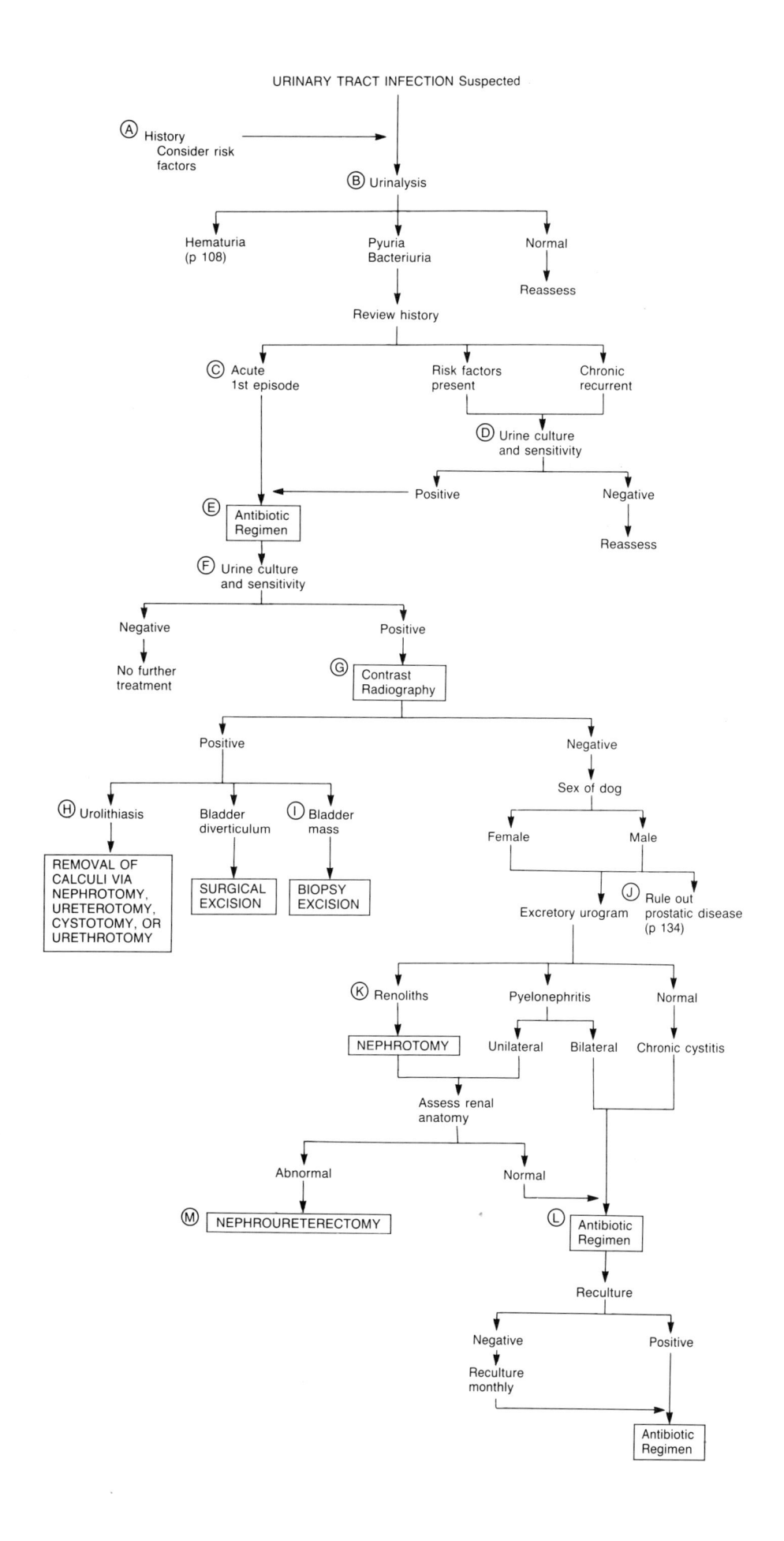

URINARY TRACT INFECTION Suspected

Ⓐ History
Consider risk factors

Ⓑ Urinalysis
- Hematuria (p 108)
- Pyuria / Bacteriuria → Review history
- Normal → Reassess

Review history:
- Ⓒ Acute 1st episode
- Risk factors present
- Chronic recurrent

Ⓓ Urine culture and sensitivity
- Positive
- Negative → Reassess

Ⓔ Antibiotic Regimen

Ⓕ Urine culture and sensitivity
- Negative → No further treatment
- Positive → Ⓖ Contrast Radiography
  - Positive:
    - Ⓗ Urolithiasis → REMOVAL OF CALCULI VIA NEPHROTOMY, URETEROTOMY, CYSTOTOMY, OR URETHROTOMY
    - Bladder diverticulum → SURGICAL EXCISION
    - Ⓘ Bladder mass → BIOPSY EXCISION
  - Negative → Sex of dog
    - Female → Excretory urogram
    - Male → Ⓙ Rule out prostatic disease (p 134) → Excretory urogram

Excretory urogram:
- Ⓚ Renoliths → NEPHROTOMY
- Pyelonephritis
  - Unilateral → Assess renal anatomy
    - Abnormal → Ⓜ NEPHROURETERECTOMY
    - Normal → Ⓛ Antibiotic Regimen
  - Bilateral → Ⓛ Antibiotic Regimen
- Normal → Chronic cystitis → Ⓛ Antibiotic Regimen

Ⓛ Antibiotic Regimen → Reculture
- Negative → Reculture monthly
- Positive → Antibiotic Regimen

HEMATURIA

Elizabeth A. Stone

A. The owner should be questioned carefully about the onset and duration of the hematuria, the possibility of it being trauma-induced, and the presence of any other clinical signs.

B. Screening tests for renal dysfunction and urinary tract infection (UTI) may demonstrate concurrent problems.

C. The presence of red cell casts indicates that the hematuria originated from the kidney rather than from the lower urinary tract.

D. Renal biopsy can be done with a keyhole percutaneous technique or by exploratory laparotomy. Glomerular diseases such as glomerulonephritis or amyloidosis rarely cause hematuria; proteinuria is the predominant sign.

E. The reproductive and estrus history helps to rule out uterine diseases and estrual bleeding. Subinvolution of placental sites (SIPS) occurs after whelping; pyometra is a post-estral disease. Vaginal masses may be noted on palpation or directly visualized with an otoscope or vaginal speculum (p 128).

F. Prostatic disease is diagnosed by examination of prostatic cytology from ejaculate, massage, or aspirate and histopathologic examination of a biopsy sample (p 134).

G. A positive-contrast urethrogram reveals space-occupying masses within the urethra.

H. A double-contrast cystogram is useful to evaluate the luminal surface of the urinary bladder.

I. An excretory urogram is used to detect abnormalities in the renal parenchyma, renal pelvis, and ureter.

J. Coagulopathies, which can cause hematuria, include thrombocytopenia, factor deficiencies, von Willebrand's disease, coumarin poisoning, and disseminated intravascular coagulation.

K. If only one kidney is grossly abnormal, a nephroureterectomy can be done. If both kidneys are abnormal, biopsies are taken.

L. If no abnormalities are apparent, a ventral cystotomy is made, and the ureteral openings are catheterized. Urine from each ureter is examined to determine which kidney is the source of hemorrhage.

M. If the source of bleeding can be identified and controlled, the kidney is not removed. Otherwise a nephroureterectomy is done.

N. Massive hematuria of nontraumatic renal origin without an obvious source or mechanism of hemorrhage has been reported in dogs (also called idiopathic hematuria or benign essential hematuria). There is no history of renal surgery, radiation therapy, or trauma. Renal function and urinalysis are normal except for red blood cells in the urine.

References

Crow SE. Hematuria: an algorithm for differential diagnosis. Comp Cont Ed 1980; 2:941.

Stone EA, DeNovo RC, Rawlings CA. Massive hematuria of nontraumatic renal origin in dogs. JAVMA 1983; 183:868.

Stone EA. Renal hematuria in dogs. In: Kirk RW, ed. Current veterinary therapy IX. Philadelphia: WB Saunders, 1986:1130.

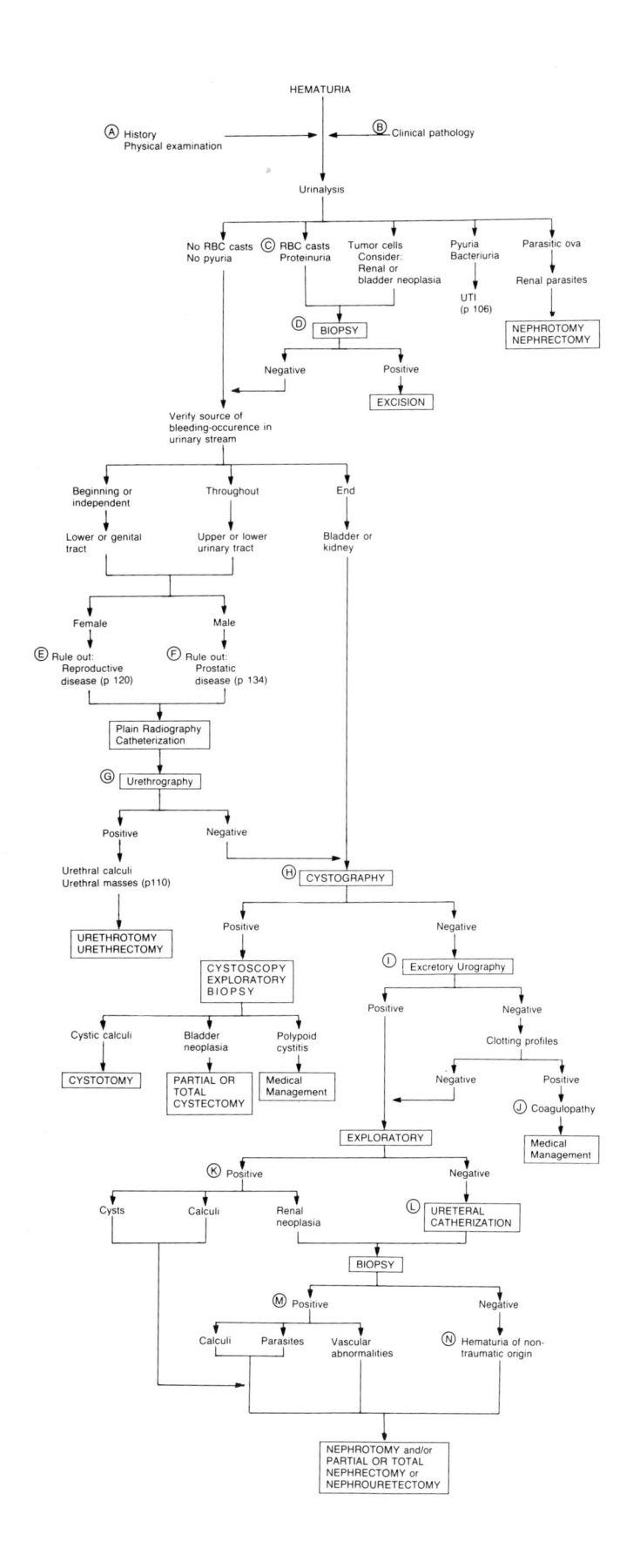

HEMATURIA

- (A) History, Physical examination
- (B) Clinical pathology

Urinalysis

- No RBC casts, No pyuria
- (C) RBC casts, Proteinuria
- Tumor cells — Consider: Renal or bladder neoplasia
- Pyuria, Bacteriuria → UTI (p 106)
- Parasitic ova → Renal parasites → NEPHROTOMY NEPHRECTOMY

(D) BIOPSY
- Negative → Verify source of bleeding-occurence in urinary stream
- Positive → EXCISION

Verify source of bleeding:
- Beginning or independent → Lower or genital tract
  - Female → (E) Rule out: Reproductive disease (p 120)
  - Male → (F) Rule out: Prostatic disease (p 134)
- Throughout → Upper or lower urinary tract
- End → Bladder or kidney

Plain Radiography, Catheterization

(G) Urethrography
- Positive → Urethral calculi, Urethral masses (p110) → URETHROTOMY URETHRECTOMY
- Negative → (H) CYSTOGRAPHY

(H) CYSTOGRAPHY
- Positive → CYSTOSCOPY EXPLORATORY BIOPSY
  - Cystic calculi → CYSTOTOMY
  - Bladder neoplasia → PARTIAL OR TOTAL CYSTECTOMY
  - Polypoid cystitis → Medical Management
- Negative → (I) Excretory Urography
  - Positive → EXPLORATORY
  - Negative → Clotting profiles
    - Negative → EXPLORATORY
    - Positive → (J) Coagulopathy → Medical Management

EXPLORATORY
- (K) Positive: Cysts, Calculi, Renal neoplasia
- Negative → (L) URETERAL CATHERIZATION → BIOPSY
  - (M) Positive: Calculi, Parasites, Vascular abnormalities
  - Negative → (N) Hematuria of non-traumatic origin

→ NEPHROTOMY and/or PARTIAL OR TOTAL NEPHRECTOMY or NEPHROURETECTOMY

CANINE URETHRAL OBSTRUCTION

Elizabeth A. Stone

A. The presenting complaint is frequently stranguria or anuria, but the owners may present the dog for vomiting or weakness not realizing that the dog has urethral obstruction. A distended bladder may be noted on examination.

B. Renal function is assessed by serum creatinine and serum urea nitrogen (BUN) levels. If the dog shows signs of uremia (weakness, depression, vomiting, dehydration), a complete blood count (CBC), electrolytes, and blood gas levels help to determine fluid therapy requirements.

C. The bladder is initially decompressed by cystocentesis with a syringe, a 3-way stopcock, and a 22-gauge needle. The dog must be adequately restrained to prevent movement during penetration of the bladder. Decompression may dislodge an obstructing calculus and allow urination or catheterization.

D. A specific gravity value of less than 1.035 in a dehydrated dog suggests primary renal failure in addition to probable prerenal and postrenal causes of azotemia. The urine sediment is examined for evidence of urinary tract infection (UTI) or neoplasia.

E. Appropriate fluid therapy is administered to correct the water, electrolyte, and acid-base imbalances. An azotemic dog may require osmotic diuresis to decrease the serum urea and creatinine levels after rehydration. An obligatory postobstructive diuresis with inappropriate water, sodium, and potassium losses may occur following relief of the obstruction. Fluid intake, urine output, packed cell volume, serum electrolytes, and hydration status should be monitored and replacement therapy administered as needed.

F. An attempt is made to pass a small-gauge, soft rubber catheter beyond the obstruction and into the bladder. Hydropulsion may dislodge calculi and allow passage of the catheter.

G. A severely uremic dog is not a good candidate for anesthesia. If a catheter cannot be passed, it may be necessary to place a temporary cystostomy catheter to drain the urine (Fig. 1). After rehydration and diuresis, further diagnostic tests and definitive treatment can be done.

H. The radiographs should be carefully examined for radiopaque calculi in other parts of the urinary tract.

I. If a dog has a fractured os penis, an attempt is made to pass a urethral catheter in order to decompress the bladder. A temporary prescrotal urethrotomy is performed to divert urine from the healing fracture. If a urethral stricture forms, a permanent scrotal urethrostomy may be performed.

J. A positive-contrast retrograde urethrogram is used in order to delineate urethral lesions. The technique is straightforward except that injected air bubbles may be mistaken for calculi or masses.

K. A double-contrast cystogram outlines radiolucent calculi in the bladder. The kidneys should also be evaluated for calculi with an excretory urogram.

L. The dog's clinical signs should correlate with the radiographic findings since a radiographic stricture may not be clinically significant. A short stricture can be excised and a urethral anastomosis performed. The urine is diverted from the healing urethra by a cystostomy catheter. Longer strictures must be bypassed by a prescrotal, scrotal, or perineal urethrostomy (Fig. 2). An intrapelvic urethral stricture may necessitate an antepubic urethrostomy.

M. In an uremic dog, the prescrotal urethrotomy procedure can be done with local anesthesia alone or in combination with a narcotic analgesic. It enables removal of calculi and placement of a catheter into the bladder. A

Figure 1 Cystostomy drainage of bladder using a Foley catheter. The catheter is passed through a layer of omentum to help prevent leakage of urine around the catheter.

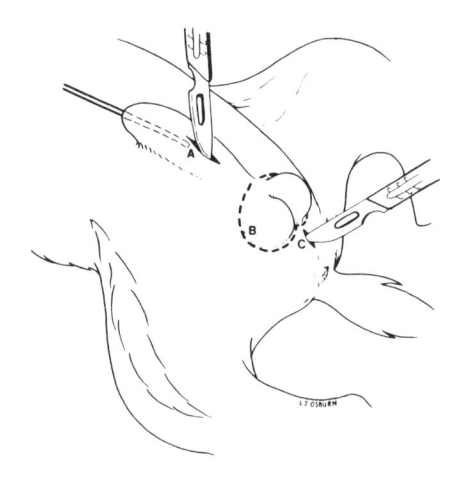

Figure 2 Urethrostomy sites in the male dog: A, prescrotal; B, scrotal; and C, perineal.

CANINE URETHRAL OBSTRUCTION Suspected

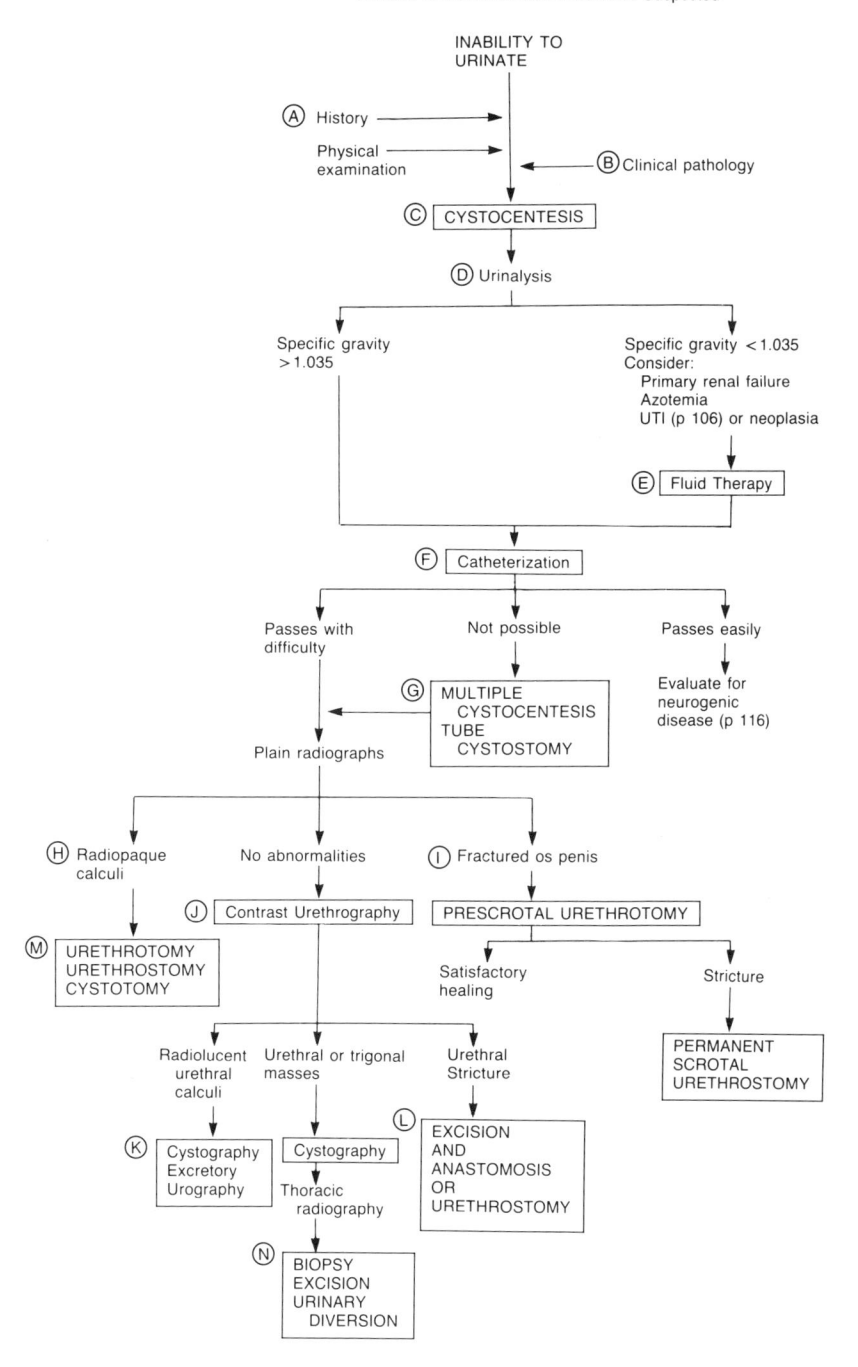

```
                    INABILITY TO
                     URINATE
    Ⓐ History ─────────→ ↑
       Physical ────────→ ←─── Ⓑ Clinical pathology
       examination
                         ↓
                    Ⓒ [CYSTOCENTESIS]
                         ↓
                    Ⓓ Urinalysis
                    ↙           ↘
         Specific gravity     Specific gravity <1.035
            >1.035            Consider:
                                Primary renal failure
                                Azotemia
                                UTI (p 106) or neoplasia
                                       ↓
                                Ⓔ [Fluid Therapy]
                    ↓           ↓
                    Ⓕ [Catheterization]
              ↙         ↓          ↘
       Passes with   Not possible   Passes easily
       difficulty        ↓              ↓
          ↓       Ⓖ MULTIPLE         Evaluate for
          ↓         CYSTOCENTESIS    neurogenic
          ↓         TUBE             disease (p 116)
          ↓         CYSTOSTOMY
       Plain radiographs
       ↙       ↓          ↘
    Ⓗ Radiopaque  No abnormalities  Ⓘ Fractured os penis
       calculi         ↓                    ↓
          ↓       Ⓙ [Contrast Urethrography]  PRESCROTAL URETHROTOMY
     Ⓜ URETHROTOMY                          ↙         ↘
       URETHROSTOMY                  Satisfactory   Stricture
       CYSTOTOMY                     healing           ↓
                                                  PERMANENT
              ↙       ↓        ↘                  SCROTAL
       Radiolucent  Urethral or  Urethral         URETHROSTOMY
       urethral    trigonal     Stricture
       calculi     masses          ↓
         ↓           ↓        Ⓛ EXCISION
       Ⓚ Cystography  Cystography    AND
         Excretory     ↓            ANASTOMOSIS
         Urography   Thoracic       OR
                     radiography    URETHROSTOMY
                       ↓
                     Ⓝ BIOPSY
                       EXCISION
                       URINARY
                       DIVERSION
```

permanent scrotal urethrostomy is indicated when the prescrotal urethra is damaged or irreparably strictured or when the dog is a recurrent stone former. Cystic calculi are removed by cystotomy.

N. A biopsy for cytologic and histopathologic examination is essential for formulating a treatment plan for urethral or trigonal masses. Excision and anastomosis of the urethra with maintenance of urinary continence is seldom possible. Urinary diversion procedures require careful patient selection and owner cooperation in order to limit postoperative complications and management problems. The prognosis for resection of urethral tumors is guarded because the full extent of the tumor is usually not known. Chemotherapy may improve patency of the urinary outflow tract.

References

Osborne CA, Klausner JS. War on canine urolithiosis: problems and solutions. Proceedings 45th Annual Meeting of the AAHA 1978:569.

Stone EA. Surgical therapy for urolithiasis. Vet Clin North Am 1984; 14:77.

FELINE URETHRAL OBSTRUCTION

Elizabeth A. Stone

A. A male cat may be presented for persistent straining. The owners may think the cat is constipated. If signs of renal failure have developed, the cat may be depressed, anorectic, and vomiting.

B. Abdominal palpation should be done gently to prevent rupture of a tense, distended bladder.

C. Determine whether the cat is showing signs of uremia that is secondary to urethral obstruction.

D. Depending on the duration of obstruction, serum creatinine, postassium, magnesium, and phosphorus may be elevated. The cat may have metabolic acidosis, hyponatremia, and hypocalcemia. Hyperkalemia is life-threatening and increases the risk of use of general anesthesia.

E. Electrocardiographic changes occur secondary to hyperkalemia and include increased T-wave, ST-depression, sinoatrial arrest, and widening of the QRS complex.

F. The type and amount of intravenous fluids depends on the degree of acidosis, hyperkalemia, and dehydration. Usually sodium chloride is given at the outset (p 190).

G. If the cat is very depressed, it may be possible to pass a urethral catheter without anesthesia. A low dose of an ultrashort-acting barbiturate preceded by atropine can be used in a normokalemic cat. If the cat is hyperkalemic or has electrocardiographic changes, an inhalant anesthetic combined with nitrous oxide may be administered by means of a face mask or induction chamber. Intravenous ketamine is less arrhythmogenic than barbiturates but must be used with caution and in very low doses (2 to 3 mg per kilogram) since it is excreted by the kidneys. Calculi most commonly lodge in the penile urethra (Fig. 1). Hydropulsion, combined with massage of the penis may disloge calculi and permit catheterization.

H. Infrequently the urethra cannot be unblocked by back flushing and catheterization because of obstructing material or urethral stenosis. Urethral stenosis may occur in previously traumatized urethras or following unsuccessful perineal urethrostomosis. In a healthy cat, a perineal urethrostomy (PU) is done to unblock the urethra and create a wider urethral opening. If the cat is not a good anesthetic risk for the length of time required to do a PU, or if the clinician is unfamiliar with the PU technique, a cystostomy catheter is placed into the bladder using local anesthetic. Bladder distension is relieved and the urine drained, simultaneously, the uremia and hyperkalemia are treated by diuresis. A PU is done after the cat's condition has improved.

I. Following relief of urethral obstruction, an obligatory diuresis may occur. It is managed by matching fluid intake to urine output. A cat that is drinking may be supplemented with subcutaneous fluids. Alternatively, a multiple electrolyte solution may be given intravenously. The BUN or serum creatinine and electrolytes (especially potassium) should be monitored to assess effectiveness of fluid therapy.

J. There is a high rate of recurrence of feline urologic syndrome (FUS) and urethral obstruction. Salting the food to induce polydypsia has been suggested in order to dilute the urine and help prevent recurrence. The etiology of FUS is unknown, and the efficacy of many recommendations to prevent recurrence have not been proven. A calculolytic diet may be beneficial.

K. If the cat reobstructs, a perineal urethrostomy is recommended. However, the owners should be warned that the PU procedure only prevents recurrence of urethral obstruction; therefore the signs of FUS (dysuria, hematuria, pollakiuria) may still occur. An increased incidence of urinary tract infection (UTI) has been reported to occur following PU procedures. Cats with a PU and signs of UTI should have a urinalysis and urine bacterial culture and sensitivity (p 106).

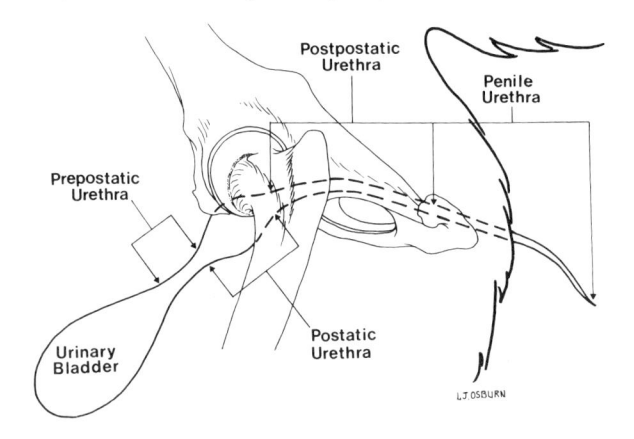

Figure 1 Normal urethra and urinary bladder in male cat.

References

Finco DR, Barsanti JA. Obstructive uropathies. In: Kirk RW, ed. Current veterinary therapy—small animal practice. Philadelphia: WB Saunders, 1986:1164.

Polzin DJ, Osborne CA. Feline urologic syndrome. In: Slatter DH, ed. Textbook of small animal surgery. Philadelphia: WB Saunders, 1985:1827.

INABILITY TO VOID

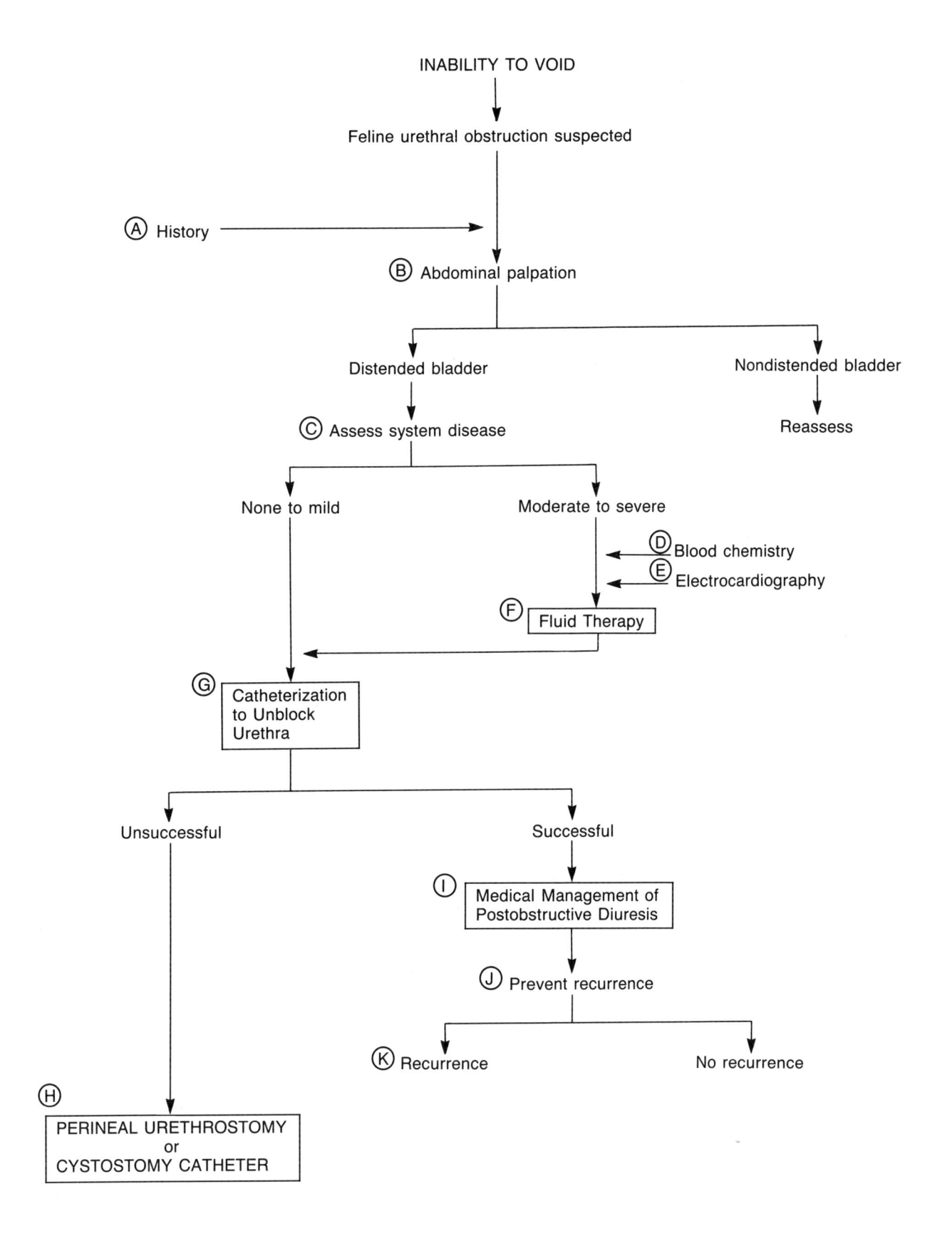

↓

Feline urethral obstruction suspected

(A) History →

↓

(B) Abdominal palpation

↙ ↘

Distended bladder   Nondistended bladder

↓   ↓

(C) Assess system disease   Reassess

↙ ↘

None to mild   Moderate to severe

                    ← (D) Blood chemistry
                    ← (E) Electrocardiography

                    (F) Fluid Therapy

↓

(G) Catheterization to Unblock Urethra

↙ ↘

Unsuccessful   Successful

                     ↓

                     (I) Medical Management of Postobstructive Diuresis

                     ↓

                     (J) Prevent recurrence

                     ↙ ↘

                     (K) Recurrence   No recurrence

(H) PERINEAL URETHROSTOMY or CYSTOSTOMY CATHETER

UROPERITONEUM

Elizabeth A. Stone

A. Usually there is a history of trauma (blunt trauma, e.g., automobile accident; penetrating trauma, e.g., gunshot wound; or iatrogenic trauma, e.g., urethral catheterization).

B. A distended abdomen may be the only sign, or the animal may show signs of uremia (anorexia, dehydration, vomiting) or shock. If there is a slow leak from the urinary tract, abdominal distention and uremia may not develop until several days after the initial trauma.

C. The serum creatinine may be elevated because of post-renal kidney failure effects with possible pre-renal failure contributions (e.g., dehydration, shock).

D. Abdominocentesis is done using aseptic technique with a needle or peritoneal catheter. Fluid is obtained for creatinine analysis, and the sediment is examined microscopically.

E. Findings of free and intracellular bacteria and numerous toxic and degenerated neutrophils suggest bacterial peritonitis.

F. Serial packed blood cell volumes (PCV) can be used to identify persistent hemorrhage. However, a decrease in the PCV may not be seen for several hours following acute hemorrhage.

G. The creatinine of the abdominal fluid is compared to the serum creatinine*. If the serum creatinine is equal to or less than the abdominal fluid creatinine, other causes of ascites should be evaluated. If the fluid creatinine is greater than the serum creatinine, there is urine leakage into the abdomen. There may also be concomitant peritonitis or other organ damage.

H. Positive-contrast cystography is more reliable than negative-contrast cystography in the identification of bladder leaks.

I. Cystography is not diagnostic of ureteral rupture or avulsion from the bladder unless there is ureteral reflux.

J. If the contrast cystogram and excretory urogram are negative, the leak may have sealed, and further diagnostics may not be needed. If the animal remains uremic, a peritoneal catheter is placed to drain the urine from the abdomen and monitor urine reaccumulation.

K. A uremic animal that is dehydrated, hyperkalemic, and acidotic is a poor anesthetic risk. Anesthesia should be delayed until the metabolic problems are at least partially reversed.

L. After placement of peritoneal and urethral catheters, the animal is rehydrated, and diuresis is performed. The catheters are connected to a sterile collection set, and urine output is monitored.

M. Once the animal is stabilized, an exploratory laparotomy is performed to examine the entire abdomen.

N. Traumatized bladder edges are excised, and the bladder is closed as a cystotomy incision.

O. The ureter is reimplanted more cranially in the bladder after a ventral cystotomy incision.

P. In medium- to large-sized dogs, the ureter is reanastomosed using 6-0 suture material. In small dogs and cats, it is easier to remove the kidney and ureter provided that the other kidney is not damaged.

---

*Editor's note: Blood and abdominal fluid urea nitrogen levels can be used for patient evaluation if creatinine determinations are unavailable, but the former are less sensitive indicators of urine leakage.

Reference

Bjorling DE. Traumatic injuries of the urogenital system. Vet Clin North Am: Small Anim Pract 1984; 14:61.

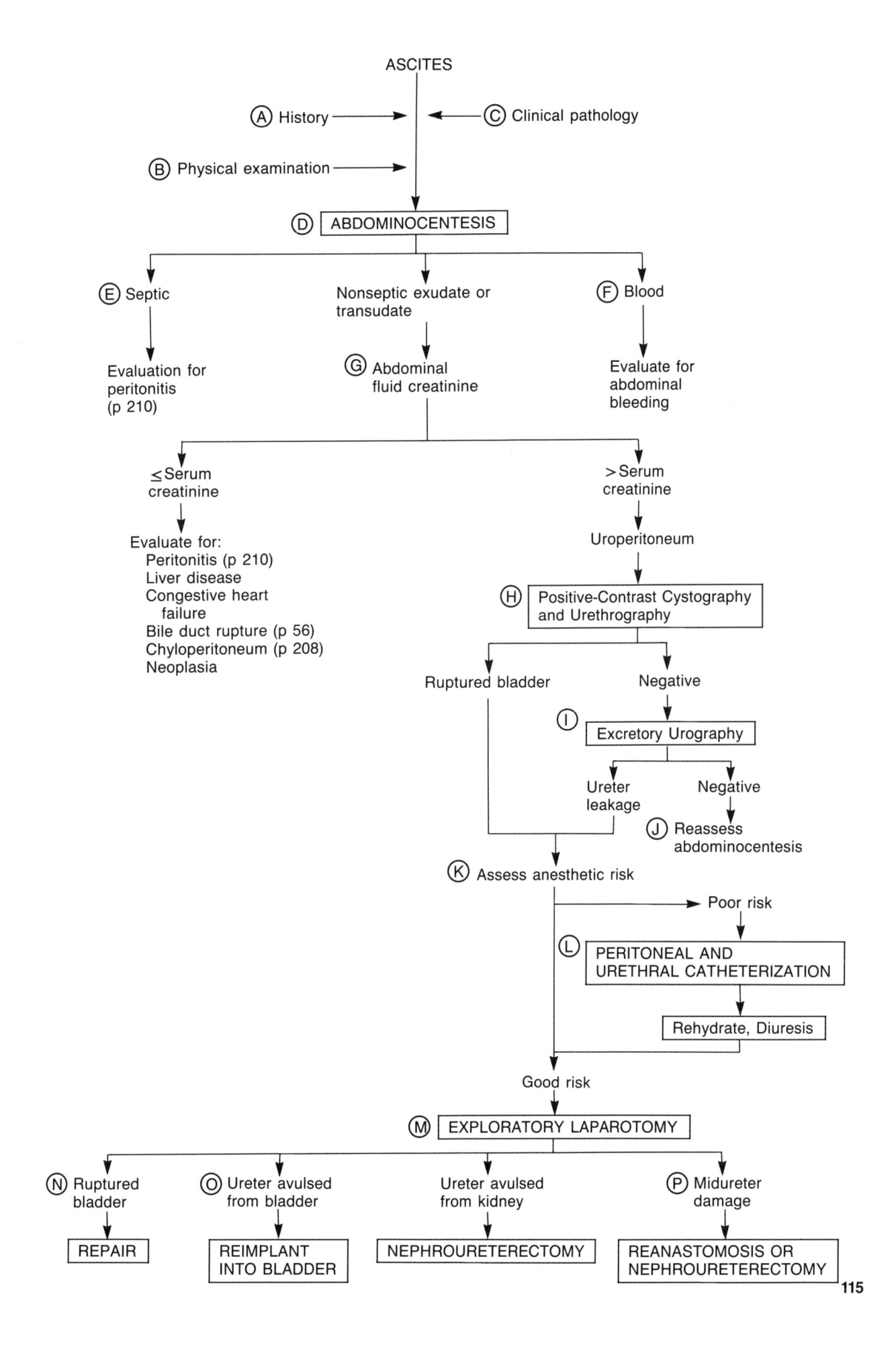

```
                              ASCITES
                                 │
         (A) History ─────────→  │  ←───────── (C) Clinical pathology
                                 │
         (B) Physical examination ─────→
                                 ↓
                         (D) ┌─────────────────┐
                             │ ABDOMINOCENTESIS │
                             └─────────────────┘
              ┌──────────────────┼──────────────────┐
              ↓                  ↓                  ↓
         (E) Septic      Nonseptic exudate      (F) Blood
              │           or transudate              │
              ↓                  ↓                   ↓
         Evaluation for    (G) Abdominal        Evaluate for
          peritonitis       fluid creatinine     abdominal
            (p 210)              │               bleeding
                      ┌──────────┴──────────┐
                      ↓                     ↓
                 ≤ Serum                > Serum
                 creatinine             creatinine
                      ↓                     ↓
              Evaluate for:             Uroperitoneum
                Peritonitis (p 210)         ↓
                Liver disease        (H) ┌──────────────────────────┐
                Congestive heart         │ Positive-Contrast Cystography │
                 failure                 │     and Urethrography       │
                Bile duct rupture (p 56) └──────────────────────────┘
                Chyloperitoneum (p 208)   ┌──────┴──────┐
                Neoplasia                 ↓             ↓
                                     Ruptured        Negative
                                      bladder           ↓
                                         │      (I) ┌──────────────────┐
                                         │          │ Excretory Urography │
                                         │          └──────────────────┘
                                         │           ┌────┴────┐
                                         │           ↓         ↓
                                         │        Ureter     Negative
                                         │        leakage      ↓
                                         │           │    (J) Reassess
                                         │           │        abdominocentesis
                                         └───────────┤
                                                     ↓
                                          (K) Assess anesthetic risk
                                                     │
                                                     ├──────→ Poor risk
                                                     │             ↓
                                                     │    (L) ┌────────────────────┐
                                                     │        │ PERITONEAL AND     │
                                                     │        │ URETHRAL CATHETERIZATION │
                                                     │        └────────────────────┘
                                                     │             ↓
                                                     │        Rehydrate, Diuresis
                                                     │
                                                Good risk
                                                     ↓
                                          (M) ┌──────────────────────┐
                                              │ EXPLORATORY LAPAROTOMY │
                                              └──────────────────────┘
              ┌──────────────┬──────────────────┬─────────────────┐
              ↓              ↓                  ↓                 ↓
         (N) Ruptured   (O) Ureter avulsed   Ureter avulsed  (P) Midureter
             bladder        from bladder     from kidney         damage
              ↓              ↓                  ↓                 ↓
         ┌────────┐   ┌──────────────┐   ┌──────────────────┐  ┌──────────────────┐
         │ REPAIR │   │ REIMPLANT    │   │ NEPHROURETERECTOMY │ │ REANASTOMOSIS OR │
         └────────┘   │ INTO BLADDER │   └──────────────────┘  │ NEPHROURETERECTOMY│
                      └──────────────┘                          └──────────────────┘
```

NEUROGENIC URINARY INCONTINENCE

Elizabeth A. Stone

A. Urinary incontinence is the inability to voluntarily control urination. The owner is questioned as to any incidents of trauma, duration of incontinence, ability to void normally, and frequency of voiding. The animal is observed voiding, and the volume, duration, and any stranguria are noted. The bladder is then palpated to assess distention, wall thickness, calculi, or masses. A complete neurologic examination is essential.

B. Concurrent urinary tract disease should be ruled out and infection treated, if present.

C. Voluntary control is determined from the history and from observation of voiding. A dog should be able to stop urination midstream if interrupted.

D. A urethral catheter is passed using aseptic technique. Urethral obstruction can be caused by uroliths, masses, or strictures (p 110).

E. Measure residual urine volume after voiding; a volume of less than 10 ml is normal.

F. An animal with detrusor dysfunction and normal urethral function dribbles urine, has a distended bladder, and does not voluntarily initiate urination. Cystometrography measures intravesical pressure during a detrusor reflex and assesses detrusor muscle function.

G. The urethral sphincter reflex is evaluated by observation and a urethral pressure profile (UPP). If the bladder is easily expressed and the dog dribbles urine, the urethral sphincter is incompetent.

H. A dog may be unwilling to urinate when it has severe pain from fractures or other causes, and may dribble because of overflow from the bladder, which must be kept decompressed to prevent primary detrusor dysfunction. Inappropriate urination (e.g., urinating on carpet) may be confused with incontinence.

I. Normal initiation of urination followed by sudden interruption of urine flow with continued straining suggests bladder-urethral incoordination, i.e., detrusor urethral reflex dyssynergia. The UPP may give a normal reading because this profile only measures resting pressure. Simultaneous bladder and urethral pressure measurements are necessary to demonstrate initiation of bladder contraction without relaxation of the urethral sphincter. Treatment for reflex dyssynergia is focused on relaxing the urethra without interfering with detrusor muscle contraction. An alpha-adrenergic blocking agent, phenoxybenzamine, is used to prevent smooth muscle contraction. Initially 5 to 10 mg once daily is given orally. The dose can be increased to up to 15 mg twice a day if needed. For striated muscle dyssynergia, dantrolene, 1 mg per kilogram three times a day is used to relax the striated muscle of the urethra. The dose can be increased to 5 mg per kilogram three times a day. Since it is difficult to determine if the problem is caused by smooth muscle or striated muscle, it is usually necessary to try both or a combination of the two drugs.

J. Damage to the sacral spinal cord or nerve roots may cause detrusor areflexia with or without sphincter areflexia. If the neurologic abnormality is reversible, the incontinence is managed medically in order to prevent irreversible changes in the urinary tract. The bladder is kept decompressed by intermittent aseptic catheterization performed every 8 hours. If the urethral sphincter is relaxed, manual expression of the bladder can be used; its effectiveness may be evaluated by periodic catheterization. Bethanechol, a cholinergic agent, is used to stimulate detrusor contraction in a neurogenic hypotonic bladder (5 to 10 mg orally three times a day). It should never be used in dogs with mechanical obstruction to voiding or defecation. Bethanechol may also cause increased urethral resistance. If the urethral sphincter reflex is present, administration of phenoxybenzamine may be necessary. Combined administration of bethanechol and phenoxybenzamine produces increased intravesical pressure and lowered urethral resistance.

K. Loss of pudendal nerve function causes striated muscle dysfunction in the urethra and external anal sphincter. In addition there is loss of the perineal and bulbocavernosus reflexes. Because there is continual urine leakage, the animal should be kept clean and water insoluble ointment should be applied to prevent urine scalds.

L. Upper motor neuron signs include hyperreflexia and loss of proprioception in the pelvic limbs. Immediately following trauma to the thoracolumbar spinal cord, the bladder is atonic and overfills. Early decompression of the spinal cord and/or stabilization of the vertebrae may contribute to return to function, as long as the bladder does not remain overdistended. One to 2 weeks after the injury, spinal reflexes initiate involuntary contraction and emptying of the spastic or "automatic" bladder. However, emptying is incomplete, resulting in residual urine retention.

M. Primary detrusor muscle dysfunction can result from

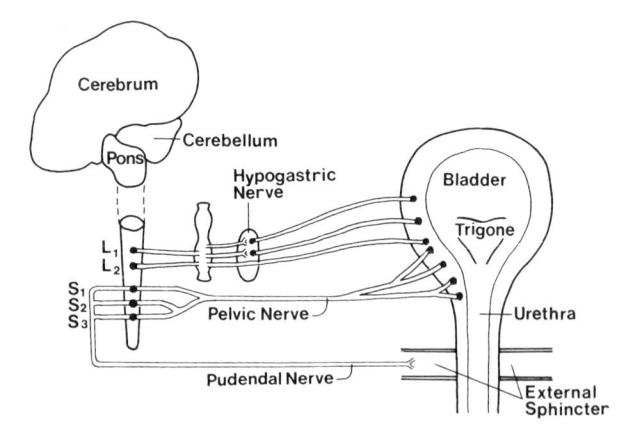

Figure 1 Simplified schematic illustration representing central control of micturition and peripheral innervation of bladder and urethra.

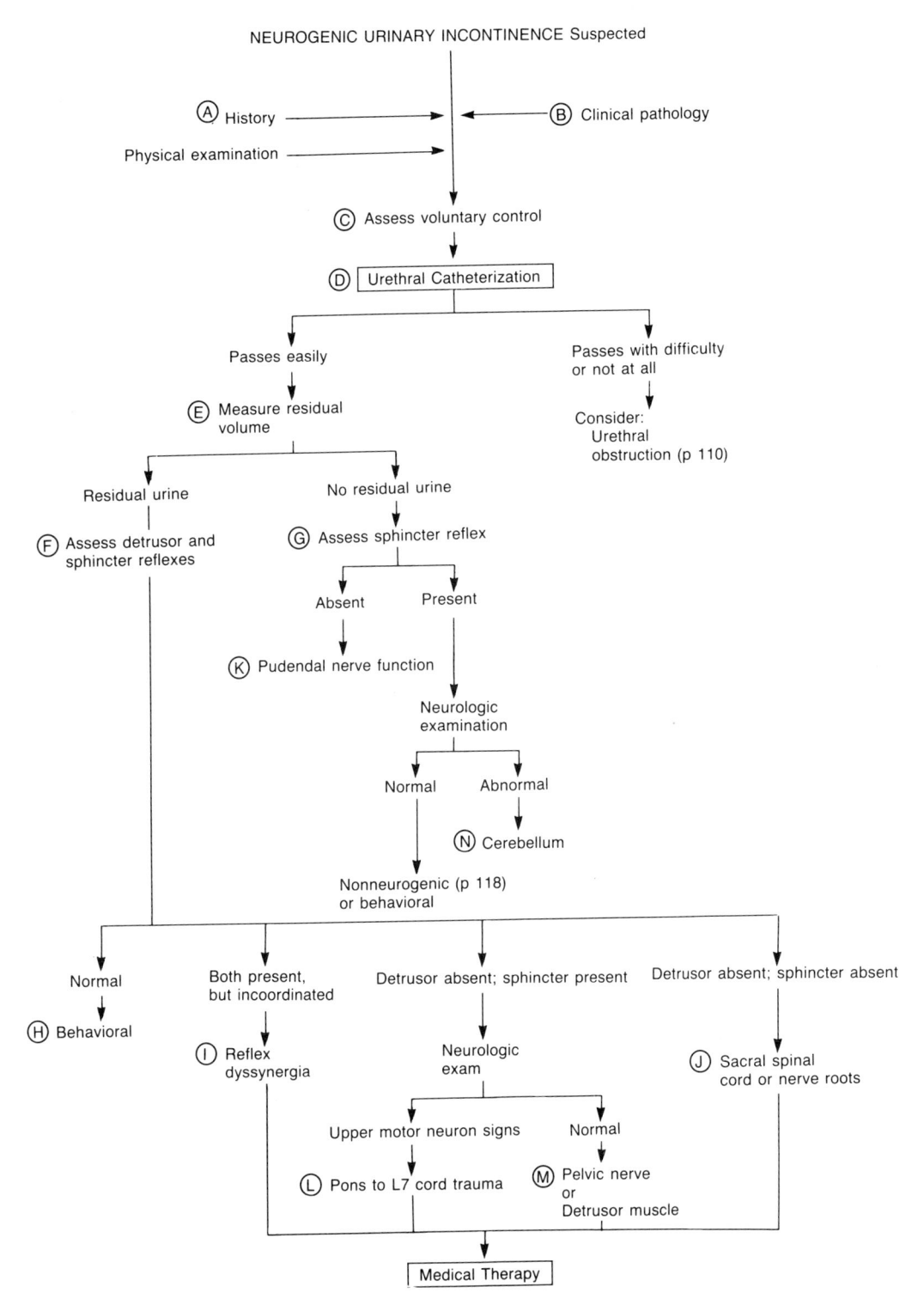

NEUROGENIC URINARY INCONTINENCE Suspected

```
                    NEUROGENIC URINARY INCONTINENCE Suspected
                                    │
      (A) History ──────────────────┼────────────── (B) Clinical pathology
      Physical examination ─────────┤
                                    ▼
                          (C) Assess voluntary control
                                    │
                                    ▼
                          (D) Urethral Catheterization
                           /                      \
                   Passes easily              Passes with difficulty
                          │                    or not at all
                          ▼                          │
                  (E) Measure residual               ▼
                      volume                    Consider:
                    /        \                  Urethral
          Residual urine    No residual urine   obstruction (p 110)
                │                │
     (F) Assess detrusor   (G) Assess sphincter reflex
         and sphincter         /         \
         reflexes         Absent       Present
                            │             │
                    (K) Pudendal nerve function
                                          │
                                          ▼
                                   Neurologic examination
                                     /          \
                                 Normal        Abnormal
                                                  │
                                            (N) Cerebellum
                                   │
                           Nonneurogenic (p 118)
                              or behavioral
```

Normal → (H) Behavioral

Both present, but incoordinated → (I) Reflex dyssynergia

Detrusor absent; sphincter present → Neurologic exam
 - Upper motor neuron signs → (L) Pons to L7 cord trauma
 - Normal → (M) Pelvic nerve or Detrusor muscle

Detrusor absent; sphincter absent → (J) Sacral spinal cord or nerve roots

→ **Medical Therapy**

prolonged distention of the urinary bladder. Treatment with bethanechol may be attempted.

N. Abnormalities of the cerebellum may result in detrusor hyperreflexia with little or no residual urine. Urination is frequent and inappropriate.

References

Moreau PM, Lees GE, Gross DR. Simultaneous cystometry and uroflowmetry (micturition study) for evaluation of the caudal part of the urinary tract in dogs: reference values for healthy animals sedated with xylazine. Am J Vet Res 1983; 44:1774.

Oliver JE. Dysuria caused by reflex dyssynergia. In: Kirk RW, ed. Current veterinary therapy VIII. Philadelphia: WB Saunders, 1983: 1088.

Oliver JE, Osborne CA. Neurogenic urinary incontinence. In: Kirk RW, ed. Current veterinary therapy VII. Philadelphia: WB Saunders, 1980: 1122.

Rosin AH, Ross L. Diagnosis and pharmacological management of disorders of urinary continence in the dog. Comp Cont Ed Pract Vet 1981; 3:601–612.

NONNEUROGENIC URINARY INCONTINENCE

Elizabeth A. Stone

A. The owner should be questioned regarding the dog's age at the onset of incontinence, its reproductive status, and the duration of incontinence.

B. Voluntary control is determined from the history and from observation. Loss of voluntary control must be differentiated from polyuria. Determine if the dog dribbles urine while sleeping. It may be impossible to assess voluntary control by observation in some instances, e.g., a dog with severe pelvic fractures or with bilateral ectopic ureters which bypass the bladder. Examination of the neurologic system that controls micturition should reveal no abnormalities (p 116). Urethral or prostatic masses may be palpable per rectum.

C. Concurrent urinary tract disease should be diagnosed and treated.

D. Owners may first notice continuous incontinence during housebreaking even though the animal has always been incontinent.

E. The abdominal wall is examined for moisture and abnormal openings. It may be necessary to shave a long-haired dog to facilitate examination.

F. A nondistended bladder should be carefully palpated for wall thickness, calculi, or masses.

G. The presence of a persistent urachus is confirmed by contrast cystography. For correction, a midline abdominal incision is made to locate the bladder and the urachus. The bladder wall around the urachal attachment is excised, and the bladder defect is closed. The distal end of the urachus is severed from the abdominal wall, and the abdominal incision is closed. Hypospadia repair may require a scrotal urethrostomy and excision of the exposed penis and prepuce. A perineal urethrostomy may be necessary with severe hypospadia.

H. Partial urethral obstruction can cause "paradoxical" incontinence. Resistance to urine flow is increased by the obstruction. The bladder distends until intravesical pressure exceeds urethral resistance, thereby permitting urine to dribble out. Detrusor dysfunction can be prevented by intermittent catheterization in order to keep the bladder compressed.

I. A combination of excretory urography and pneumocystography helps to identify ectopic ureters (Fig. 1). Some dogs have incompetent urethral sphincters and remain incontinent following surgical correction of the ectopic ureters. Urethral pressure profilometry may help identify these before surgery. Phenylpropanolamine (12.5 to 50 mg orally three times a day) may increase urethral sphincter competence.

J. Where an ectopic ureter travels in the bladder wall, a stoma is created into the bladder lumen and the ureter ligated distally. A ureter that bypasses the bladder is severed as distally as possible and implanted into the bladder. If neither of the above is possible, a unilateral nephroureterectomy can be performed.

K. The urethral pressure profile (UPP) measures intraluminal urethral pressure and allows the effective closure pressure of the resting urethra to be determined.

L. Hormone-responsive incontinence occurs in older bitches that were neutered at a young age or older dogs neutered for prostatic disease. The treatment is diethylstilbestrol (0.1 to 1.0 mg daily for 3 to 5 days). Thereafter it is administered as needed, and the minimum effective dosage should be used. Side effects include signs of estrus and bone marrow toxicity.

M. Severe chronic cystitis or neoplastic infiltration of the bladder can produce a small nondistensible bladder with limited capacity.

N. Urethral incompetence can occur following cystitis, urethritis, or chronic prostatic disease. It may respond to phenylpropanolamine at 12.5 mg to 50 mg orally three times a day.

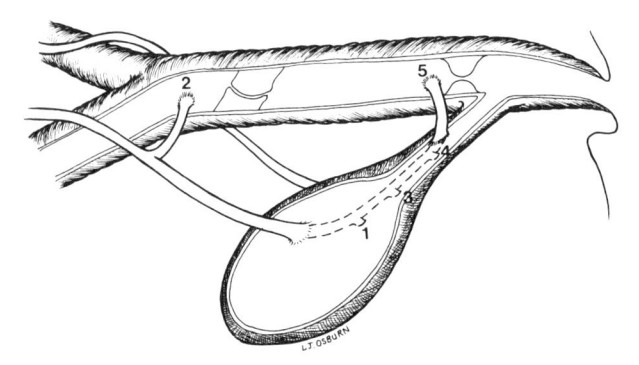

Figure 1 Ureteral ectopia: 1, normal opening into the urinary bladder. Abnormal openings into: 2, body of uterus; 3, bladder neck; 4, urethra; and 5, vagina.

References

Barsanti JA, Finco DR. Hormonal responses to urinary incontinence. In: Kirk RW ed. Current veterinary therapy VIII. Philadelphia: WB Saunders, 1983: 1086.

Rosin AE, Barsanti JA. Diagnosis of urinary incontinence in dogs: role of the urethral pressure profile. JAVMA 1981; 178:814.

Rosin AH, Ross L. Diagnosis and pharmacologic management of disorders of urinary continence in the dog. Comp Cont Ed 1981; 3:601.

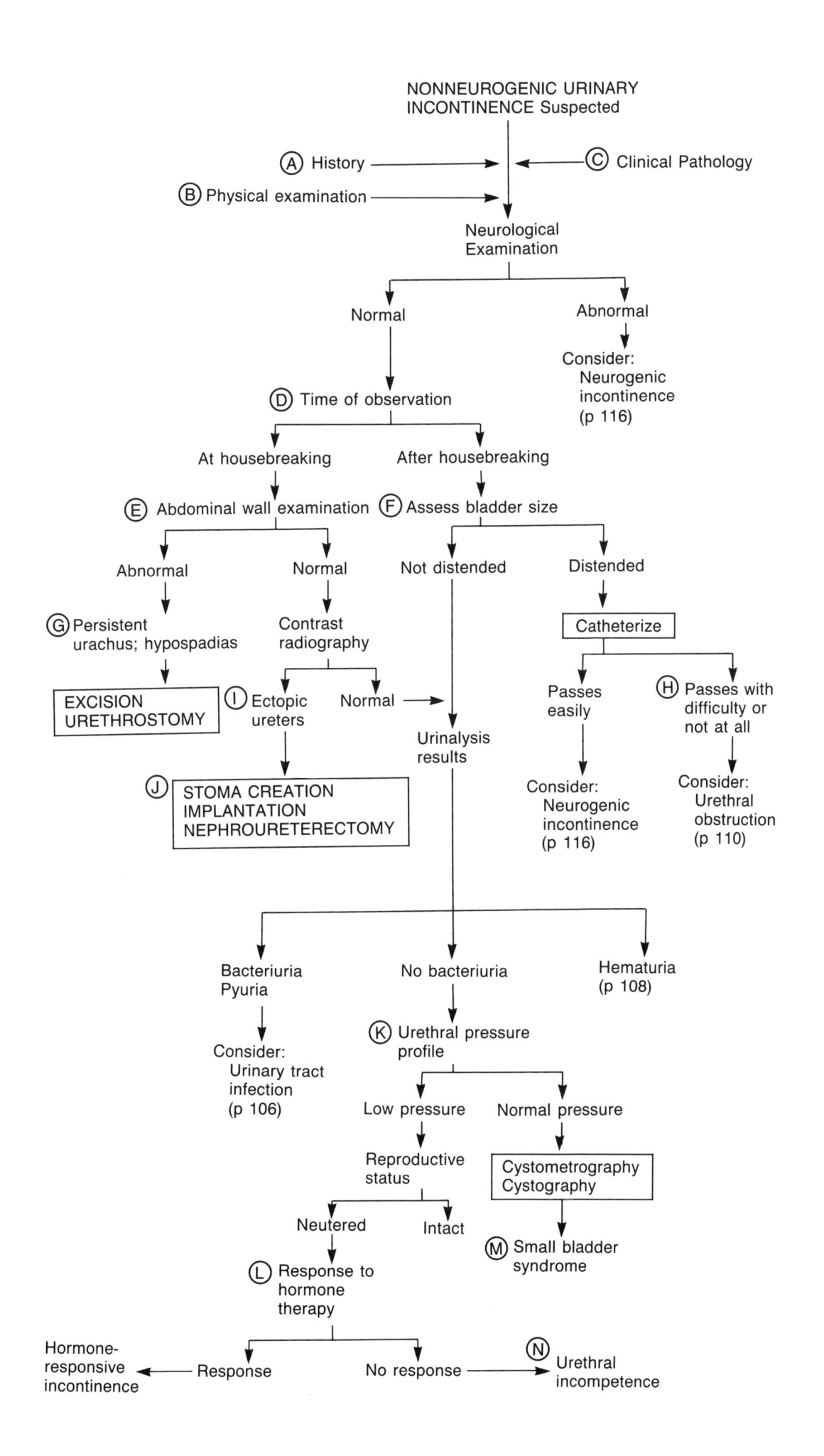

NONNEUROGENIC URINARY INCONTINENCE Suspected

- (A) History
- (B) Physical examination
- (C) Clinical Pathology

↓

Neurological Examination

- **Abnormal** → Consider: Neurogenic incontinence (p 116)
- **Normal** ↓

(D) **Time of observation**

- **At housebreaking** → (E) Abdominal wall examination
  - **Abnormal** → (G) Persistent urachus; hypospadias → **EXCISION URETHROSTOMY**
  - **Normal** → Contrast radiography
    - (I) Ectopic ureters → (J) **STOMA CREATION / IMPLANTATION / NEPHROURETERECTOMY**
    - Normal → Urinalysis results
- **After housebreaking** → (F) Assess bladder size
  - **Distended** → Catheterize
    - Passes easily → Consider: Neurogenic incontinence (p 116)
    - (H) Passes with difficulty or not at all → Consider: Urethral obstruction (p 110)
  - **Not distended** → Urinalysis results

Urinalysis results:

- **Bacteriuria Pyuria** → Consider: Urinary tract infection (p 106)
- **No bacteriuria** → (K) Urethral pressure profile
  - **Low pressure** → Reproductive status
    - **Neutered** → (L) Response to hormone therapy
      - Response → Hormone-responsive incontinence
      - No response → (N) Urethral incompetence
    - **Intact** → (N) Urethral incompetence
  - **Normal pressure** → Cystometrography / Cystography → (M) Small bladder syndrome
- **Hematuria** (p 108)

119

INFERTILITY IN THE CYCLIC BITCH

Brian C. Buckrell
Walter H. Johnson

A. A detailed description of breeding management, reproductive history, previous illness, hormone and drug use is required in all cases.

B. A complete physical examination is also required. Signs of endocrine imbalance (thyroid, adrenal) are particularly important.

C. Vulvar and perineal conformation are assessed. Evidence of vulvar irritation and vaginal discharge may indicate infection. Vaginal examination (digitally and using an otoscope or pediatric proctoscope) may identify anomalies.

D. Close scrutiny of the stages of the estrus cycle, by the use of vaginal cytology and teaser males, is often required. Breeding should occur every third day during the entire period of psychic and cytologic estrus and should continue to day one of diestrus. Behavioral problems or refusal to accept the male commonly occur. Artificial insemination (AI) may be required. AI yields normal conception rates if semen handling and insemination technique are correct. Insemination must be repeated throughout estrus.

E. Complete blood count and urinalysis should be performed. A biochemical profile may detect extrareproductive disease. Serology for *Brucella canis* should be included. Hypothyroidism is associated with a variety of reproductive disorders; infertility may resolve after thyroxine replacement therapy.

F. In cases of nonpregnancy at 30-days postbreeding, a diestrus progesterone level is taken (normal level is greater than 20 mg per milliliter) to confirm ovulation. When anovulation is diagnosed, human chorionic gonadotropin (hCG, 500 IU) given on day one of estrus may assist normal ovulation and corpus luteum formation in subsequent breedings.

G. It is important to take advantage of all available information. Whether or not the bitch is bred, vaginal cytology, taken at regular 2-day intervals up to day one of diestrus (D_1), pinpoints the day of ovulation (D_1 minus 6 days), which can be used during the next estrus cycle. Because of the great variability in the events of the estrus cycles of normal dogs, it is often difficult to differentiate between abnormal and normal, but unusual, cycles. An accurate reproductive history and monitoring of previous cycles is essential. The luteal function of diestrus can be plotted by taking progesterone levels at 30- and 60-days post-estrus. Serum, luteinizing hormone (LH), follicle stimulating hormone (FSH), estradiol, and testosterone measurements may be useful. Neutrophils that are present in vaginal cytology taken during estrus often indicate endometritis.

H. An interestrus period of less than 5 months may suggest inadequate luteal functions (use hCG, 500 IU, on day one of next estrus) or shortened anestrus, which reduces time for follicular development for the next estrus cycle. Mibolerone at the specified breed dose or megestrol acetate at 0.5 mg per kilogram per day for 2 to 3 weeks are unproven, but are suggested. Low dose diethylstilbestrol (0.05 to 0.1 mg, day one to three of proestrus) may improve physical acceptance of the male during estrus without reducing fertility.

I. Long-term antibiotic therapy (4 to 6 weeks) is followed by antibiotic administration during the next proestrus up to the point of breeding.

J. A hysterosalpingogram, which is useful in diagnosing uterine anomalies, may be performed by infusing non-irritating radiographic contrast material into the vagina through a Foley catheter. During estrus, the contrast should pass under light pressure through the cervix and enter the uterus.

K. Oviduct patency is assessed during anestrus by gently forcing saline, introduced at the uterotubular junction, retrograde out via the infundibulum. Laparotomy for ovarian and endometrial biopsy are indicated if the oviducts are patent. Samples may be taken from the uterus for culture and sensitivity and cytology.

L. Many cases of infertility remain undiagnosed. Early embryonic death (infectious, cytogenetic), antisperm antibodies, and implantation failures cannot always be readily confirmed.

M. Anatomic defects of the reproductive tract are uncommon. Most are diagnosed only by laparotomy.

References

Johnston SD. An algorithm for clinical approach to infertility in the bitch. Proc Soc Theriogen 1985: 25.

Lein DH. Reproductive disorders. In: Kirk RW, ed. Current veterinary therapy VIII. Philadelphia: WB Saunders, 1983: 885.

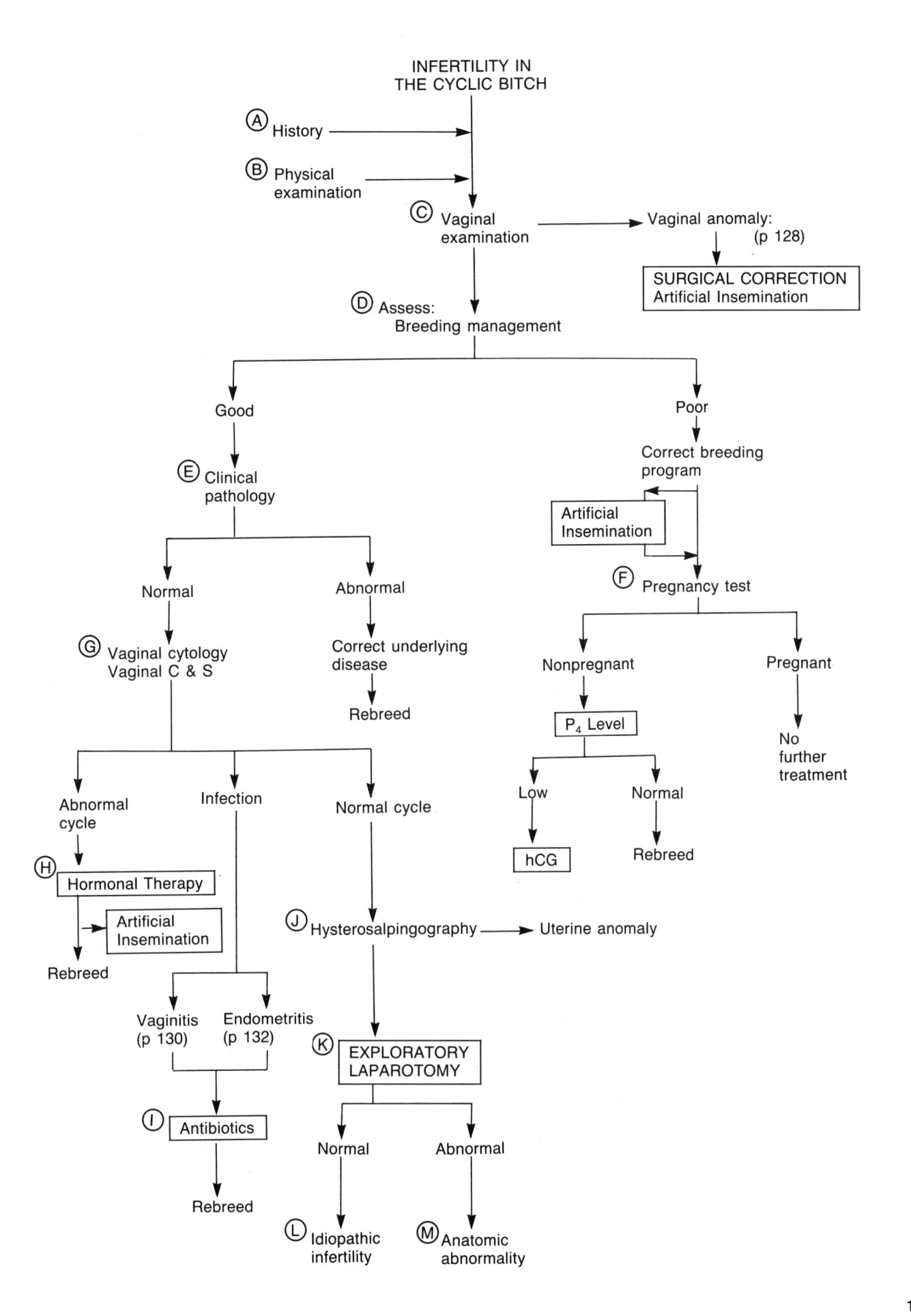

INFERTILITY IN THE CYCLIC BITCH

- A. History
- B. Physical examination
- C. Vaginal examination
  - → Vaginal anomaly: (p 128) → **SURGICAL CORRECTION** / Artificial Insemination
- D. Assess: Breeding management
  - **Good** → E. Clinical pathology
    - Normal → G. Vaginal cytology / Vaginal C & S
      - Abnormal cycle → H. Hormonal Therapy → Artificial Insemination → Rebreed
      - Infection → Vaginitis (p 130) / Endometritis (p 132) → I. Antibiotics → Rebreed
      - Normal cycle → J. Hysterosalpingography → Uterine anomaly
        - → K. **EXPLORATORY LAPAROTOMY**
          - Normal → L. Idiopathic infertility
          - Abnormal → M. Anatomic abnormality
    - Abnormal → Correct underlying disease → Rebreed
  - **Poor** → Correct breeding program → Artificial Insemination → F. Pregnancy test
    - Nonpregnant → P_4 Level
      - Low → hCG
      - Normal → Rebreed
    - Pregnant → No further treatment

121

INFERTILITY IN THE ACYCLIC BITCH

Brian C. Buckrell
Walter H. Johnson

A. A detailed history of prior illness, behavioral problems, reproductive function, and previous drug and hormone use is required. The owner's observation techniques and awareness of the signs of estrus are determined. Environmental factors, such as housing and the presence of other dogs, should be noted.

B. The bitch is examined for signs of hypothyroidism, hyperadrenalcorticalism, or systemic illness. Vaginal or clitoral anomalies and/or enlargement may indicate prenatal masculinization or inappropriate drug or hormone administration.

C. Heparinized blood and a skin biopsy are required by most laboratories for karyotyping to diagnose intersex conditions; XX males, X0 monosomy, XXX XXY trisomy, and mosaic chimeras XX/XY are some anomalies reported in the dog.

D. Complete blood count, blood chemistry, T_4, and serum cortisol levels are examined. A series of four progesterone assays, taken at 6-week intervals, indicates that ovulation has occurred during silent estrus if values greater than 2 mg per milliliter are obtained. Serum testosterone may be elevated in adrenal disease and with cystic ovaries.

E. Ovarian responsiveness to gonadotropin stimulation is determined by attempting to induce estrus. One regimen is to administer 200 IU of pregnant mare serum gonadotropin every 48 hours for five treatments. Most bitches respond since many cases of acyclicity are actually silent estrus cycles, delayed puberty, or the result of owner inexperience in estrus observation.

F. Few cases of congenital acylicity have a treatable cause. Most cases of true, acquired acyclicity have diagnosable systemic causes. Most often endocrine (thyroid or adrenal) disease is responsible.

G. The induction of estrus is primarily a diagnostic aid. The bitch may be bred, but fertility is reduced. Vaginal cytology is examined to record the events of the cycle, and pregnancy testing is done at 30 days postbreeding. Nonpregnant bitches are tested for ovulation (progesterone > 5 mg per milliliter).

H. Gonadotropin assays for luteinizing hormone (LH) and follicle stimulating hormone (FSH) levels and the gonadotropin stimulation test (50 IU of gonadotropin releasing hormone retest in 1 hour) can be performed.

I. Ovarian biopsy may detect a normal primary follicular population or ovarian aplasia and/or hypoplasia.

J. Idiopathic normogonadal hypogonadotropism seldom responds to therapy. Clomiphene citrate is used in women to stimulate gonadotropin levels, but its value is uncertain in the bitch. Bitches may respond to gonadotropin stimulation with a fertile estrus.

References

Johnston SD. An algorithm for clinical approach to infertility in the bitch. Proc Soc Theriogen 1984: 25.

Renton JP, Munro CD, Heathcote RH, Carmichael S. Some aspects of the aetiology, diagnosis and treatment of infertility in the bitch. J Reprod Fertil 1981; 61:289.

Shille VM, Thatcher MJ, Simmons KJ. Efforts to induce estrus in the bitch, using pituitary gonadotropins. JAVMA 1984; 184:1469.

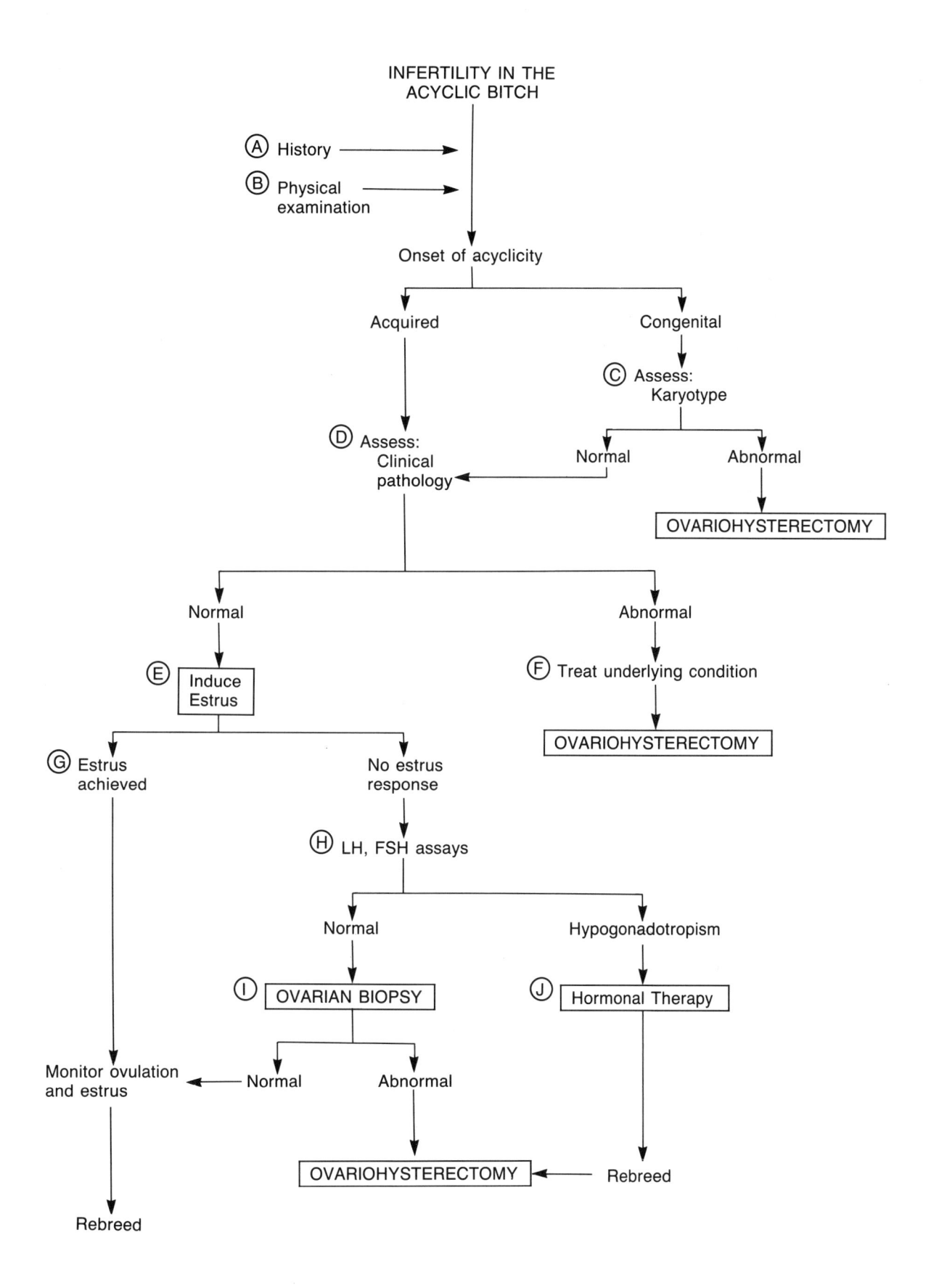

INFERTILITY IN THE ACYCLIC BITCH

- (A) History
- (B) Physical examination

↓

Onset of acyclicity
- Acquired
- Congenital

Congenital → (C) Assess: Karyotype
- Normal → (proceed to D)
- Abnormal → **OVARIOHYSTERECTOMY**

Acquired → (D) Assess: Clinical pathology
- Normal → (E) Induce Estrus
- Abnormal → (F) Treat underlying condition → **OVARIOHYSTERECTOMY**

Induce Estrus:
- (G) Estrus achieved → Monitor ovulation and estrus → Rebreed
- No estrus response → (H) LH, FSH assays
  - Normal → (I) OVARIAN BIOPSY
    - Normal → Monitor ovulation and estrus → Rebreed
    - Abnormal → **OVARIOHYSTERECTOMY**
  - Hypogonadotropism → (J) Hormonal Therapy → Rebreed → **OVARIOHYSTERECTOMY**

INFERTILITY IN THE DOG

Brian C. Buckrell

A. Obtain a detailed history of illness, breeding management, libido, mounting and behavioral problems, hormone and drug use. It is important to determine whether infertility is acquired or if the dog is unproven and has never been fertile. Consider breed predisposition to chromosomal anomalies (e.g., Cocker Spaniels).

B. Date signs of endocrine abnormalities such as thyroid and adrenal disease and feminization, and examine scrotal skin for trauma and irritation. Carefully palpate the testes and prostate for size, consistency, and lumps and the epididymides for enlargements. Examine the penis for anomalies or injury, and the prepuce for signs of balanoposthitis. Note and record body condition and evidence of locomotor dysfunction. Observation of the breeding technique is necessary.

C. Inexperienced or timid males may require assistance or bitch restraint to complete intromission. Environmental stress must be avoided. Artificial insemination (AI) may be required.

D. Semen is collected and evaluated for sperm concentration, motility, abnormalities, pH, presence of red blood cells, neutrophils, and epithelial cells.

E. Transient causes of reduced fertility (illness, drugs, scrotal irritation) may resolve spontaneously; fertility may return within a few months.

F. Azoospermia (complete lack of sperm) in palpably normal testicles suggests tubular blockage or hypogonadotropism. If sperm count can be obtained by epididymal aspiration, blockage of the duct system is presumed.

G. Oligospermia (low sperm count) without infection suggests a systemic disease, often endocrine, that is causing depression of the hypothalamic-pituitary-gonadal axis. Semen evaluation is repeated to confirm the low sperm count as repeatability between samples is low.

H. Indications of infection in semen (white blood count, altered pH, bacteria, sperm morphology, sperm agglutination) call for complete prostatic fluid analysis, *Brucella canis* serology, urinalysis, and complete blood count. Semen culture and sensitivity are done for anaerobes, aerobes, mycoplasma, and ureaplasma.

I. Infertile normaspermic dogs may have sperm or semen anomalies as yet undefined.

J. Gonadotropin profiles of luteinizing (LH) and follicle stimulating hormone (FSH) and serum testosterone (T) levels (2 samples at 2-hour intervals) are done. Human chorionic gonadotropin (hCG) stimulation test (100 IU - T levels prestimulation and at 4 hours) or gonadotropin releasing hormone GNRH (50 µg - preadministration and retest at 1 hour) for testosterone may be performed. Dogs with systemic disease may have low testosterone values.

K. Antibiotics are administered for 6 to 8 weeks, and the semen is recultured 1 week after therapy ends.

L. A scrotal exploratory allows detailed examination to confirm a blockage such as a sperm granuloma. Such blockages are not correctable.

M. Testicular biopsy provides information on spermatogenesis and aids prognostication. Tissues must be preserved in Bouin's fixative for 12 hours then transferred to formalin (10 percent).

N. Long-term testosterone therapy acts through negative feedback to cause a net reduction in testicular steroids and eventual reduced fertility. Gonadotropins have not been studied adequately in the dog to justify their use. Low libido may be helped clinically by 100 IU of hCG given once to raise both serum and testicular testosterone levels.

References

Hardie EM. Selected surgeries of the male and female reproductive tracts. Vet Clin North Am 1984; 1:109.

Olson PN. Clinical approach to infertility in the stud dog. Proc Soc Theriogen 1984:33.

Rosenthal RC. Infertility in the male dog. Comp Cont Ed 1983; 12:983.

INFERTILITY IN THE MALE DOG

- Ⓐ History
- Ⓑ Physical examination

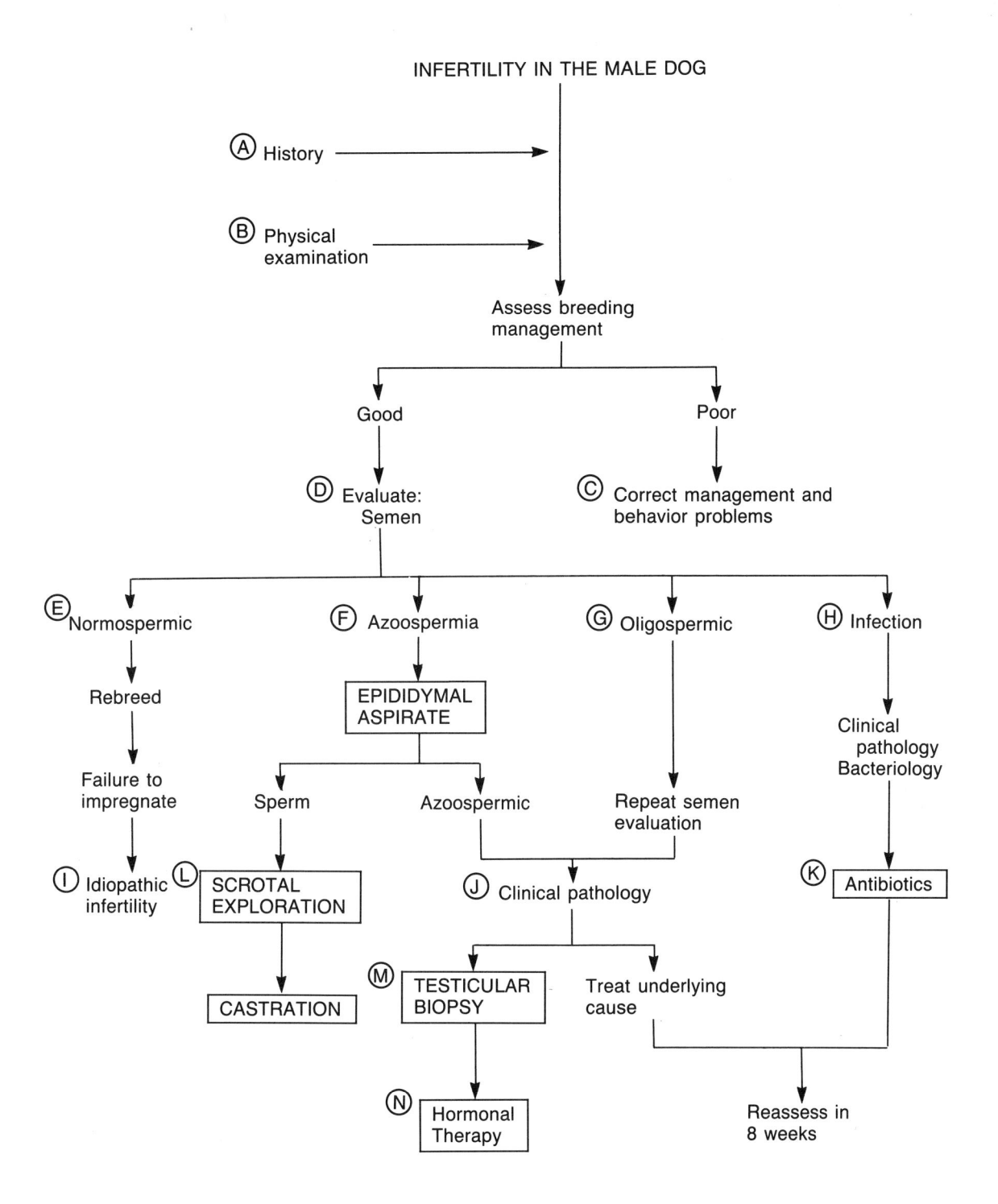

↓

Assess breeding management

- Good → Ⓓ Evaluate: Semen
- Poor → Ⓒ Correct management and behavior problems

Ⓓ Evaluate: Semen branches to:

- Ⓔ Normospermic → Rebreed → Failure to impregnate → Ⓘ Idiopathic infertility
- Ⓕ Azoospermia → **EPIDYMAL ASPIRATE**
  - Sperm → Ⓛ **SCROTAL EXPLORATION** → **CASTRATION**
  - Azoospermic → Ⓙ Clinical pathology
- Ⓖ Oligospermic → Repeat semen evaluation → Ⓙ Clinical pathology
- Ⓗ Infection → Clinical pathology / Bacteriology → Ⓚ **Antibiotics** → Reassess in 8 weeks

Ⓙ Clinical pathology:
- Ⓜ **TESTICULAR BIOPSY** → Ⓝ **Hormonal Therapy**
- Treat underlying cause

CANINE DYSTOCIA

Brian C. Buckrell

A. The normal variations observed in bitches at parturition make recognition of dystocia difficult. The following criteria assist in diagnosis:

 1. Prolonged gestation—based on previous whelping history, knowledge of breeding dates, and events of the estrus cycle (day 1 of diestrus), and drop in rectal temperature more than 24 hours previously;
 2. Pelvic obstruction—fetal presentation, breed predisposition, and anatomic problems such as pelvic fractures;
 3. Signs of maternal illness—toxemia, hypocalcemia;
 4. Unproductive, persistent straining for 30 minutes or more;
 5. Absence of straining for longer than 4 hours between pups;
 6. Evidence of fetal death in utero;
 7. Abnormal uterine discharge; and
 8. History of previous dystocias or cesareans.

B. Digital examination of the pelvic vagina confirms or rules out obstructive dystocia. Evidence of abnormal uterine discharge, vaginal dilation, and lubrication is noted. Mammary glands are examined for development and milk production.

C. Complete blood count, biochemical profile, and, if possible, blood calcium levels are assessed if signs of maternal illness are present. Fetal number and viability must be confirmed with the use of radiography or real-time ultrasonography.

D. It is not known if parturition is fetally initiated in the dog, but most cases of in utero litter deaths result in delayed parturition, dystocia and, eventually, maternal metritis and toxemia. Cesarean section, with supportive medical care, is indicated with dead litters.

E. A pup lodged in the pelvic canal will die unless freed immediately. Prolonged obstruction may lead to secondary uterine inertia.

F. Mild lubricants may assist delivery; an episiotomy aids visualization, but is rarely required. Instrument manipulation offers little advantage over digital manipulation and can damage the cervix and vagina. Oxytocin is contraindicated in obstructive cases. Fetotomy is a good alternative to prolonged manipulation if the pup is dead. Cesarean section is often required.

G. Oxytocin (5 to 10 IU, IM) injected at 30-minute intervals should cause fetal expulsion. When expulsion has not occurred 30 minutes after the second injection, an immediate cesarean section is done, since placental separation results in fetal death.

H. Cesarean section is an effective and safe alternative to manipulative and medical therapy, if undertaken prior to maternal fatigue and fetal death. In many cases of unresponsive uterine inertia, pelvic obstruction or fetal death, cesarean section is the only course to follow. In the event of uterine rupture or when there are dead or infected pups, an ovariohysterectomy may be performed instead. Oxytocin (5 to 10 IU, IM) is administered immediately following surgery to encourage involution, uterine evacuation, and milk let-down.

I. When obstructive causes are ruled out, uterine inertia is suspected. Oxytocin is administered. The bitch in primary inertia fails to respond to exogenous or endogenous oxytocin. Uterine contractions are inapparent or weak and unproductive. Primary inertia is most common in older, obese bitches (often with large litters). Heredity and neurogenic inhibition (i.e., fear) may play a role. Secondary uterine inertia attributable to maternal fatigue is responsive to oxytocin, but repeated injections may be required. Secondary inertia is the most common cause of dystocia in the bitch.

J. Calcium gluconate (5 to 10 ml of 10 percent solution, IV, slowly) and glucose (10 ml of 10 percent solution IV) are recommended. Promazine tranquilizers overcome voluntary inhibition of stage II labor in the nervous bitch. However, these sedatives cross the placenta and cause fetal depression.

K. Uterine torsion, rare in the dog, requires a cesarean section for correction. Ovariohysterectomy is often indicated if there is uterine damage.

L. A history of dystocia, breed disposition (e.g., some toy and brachycephalic breeds), previous pelvic fractures, or vaginal anomalies may indicate an elective cesarean section to prevent dystocia.

References

Christiansen IJ. Dystocia, obstetric and postparturient problems. In: Christiansen IJ, ed. Reproduction in the dog and cat. Toronto: Bailliere Tindall, 1984: 197.

Gaudet DA, Kitchell BE. Canine dystocia. Comp Cont Ed 1985; 5:406.

Hardie EM. Selective surgeries of the male and female reproductive tracts. Vet Clin North Am 1984; 1:109.

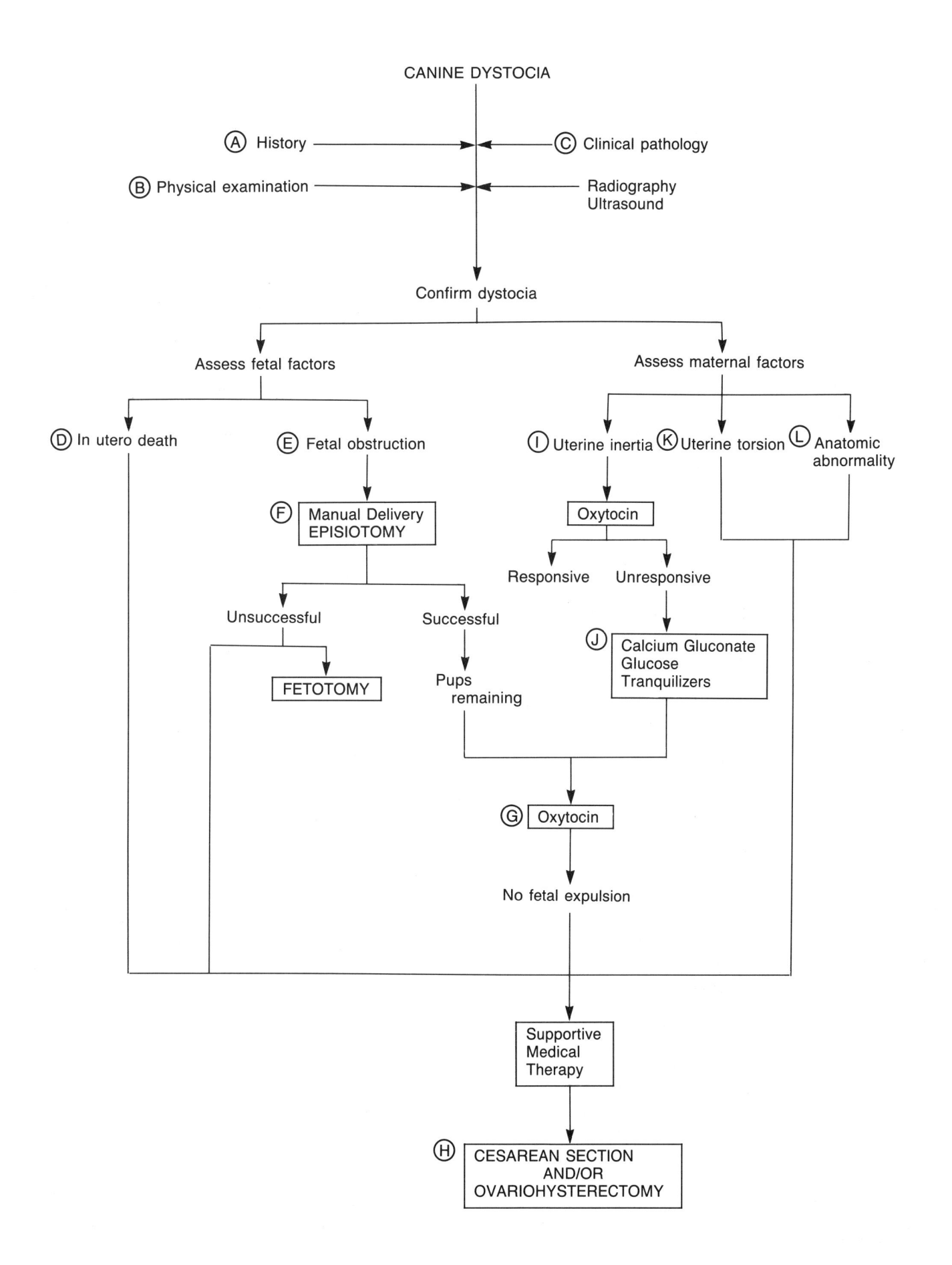

CANINE DYSTOCIA

- Ⓐ History
- Ⓑ Physical examination
- Ⓒ Clinical pathology
- Radiography Ultrasound

↓

Confirm dystocia

Assess fetal factors

- Ⓓ In utero death
- Ⓔ Fetal obstruction
  - Ⓕ Manual Delivery EPISIOTOMY
    - Unsuccessful → FETOTOMY
    - Successful → Pups remaining

Assess maternal factors

- Ⓘ Uterine inertia
  - Oxytocin
    - Responsive
    - Unresponsive → Ⓙ Calcium Gluconate / Glucose / Tranquilizers
- Ⓚ Uterine torsion
- Ⓛ Anatomic abnormality

↓

Ⓖ Oxytocin

↓

No fetal expulsion

↓

Supportive Medical Therapy

↓

Ⓗ CESAREAN SECTION AND/OR OVARIOHYSTERECTOMY

VAGINAL PROTRUSION

Brian C. Buckrell

A. A breeding history of nonpenetrance, pain, or bleeding may be presented. It is helpful to know the stage of the reproductive cycle to differentiate structures protruding from the vagina. Protrusions that occur during estrus are generally estrogen-induced tissue hyperplasia, whereas those that present postpartum are usually true prolapses. Tumors and polyps may be noticed at any time, usually in mature bitches. Breed predisposition to vaginal hyperplasia has been reported in Bull Mastiffs, Boxers, and Bulldogs.

B. Digital examination helps to differentiate vaginal polyps and tumors from vaginal hyperplasia or prolapse. Identifying the urethral opening may help orientation. Vaginal hyperplasia usually involves only the mucosa of the ventral floor, whereas a true prolapse involves the entire wall. The surfaces of protruding polyps and tumors usually remain intact; exposed mucosa of vaginal hyperplasia or prolapse becomes traumatized and ulcerated.

C. Vaginal polyps are common. They originate from mid vagina and have a narrow 3- or 4-inch long pedicle. Many enlarge or become visible only during estrus. Surgical excision with ligation near the base of the polyp(s) is readily accomplished. Leimyomas, leiomyosarcomas, lipomas, and transmissible venereal tumors may enlarge to the point of protruding from the vulva. A biopsy is necessary for confirmation, and surgical removal is required to reduce discomfort and pressure on the urethra. Chemotherapeutic agents such as vincristine or cyclophosphamide have proven useful in treating some vaginal tumors.

D. Uterine prolapse is rare in bitches and usually occurs immediately postparturition. Signs of hemorrhage and shock may be present. Exposed tissue is usually traumatized and bleeding.

E. A true vaginal prolapse is rare and involves the entire vaginal wall rather than just the mucosa.

F. Vaginal hyperplasia occurs in young bitches during proestrus or estrus in response to elevated serum estrogens. Hyperplasia usually regresses spontaneously once the bitch enters diestrus. In rare cases, hyperplasia recurs when estrogen levels rise prior to parturition.

G. Reduction of the prolapsed tissue is attempted following cleaning and lubrication with water-soluble gel. A vaginal tampon helps maintain the reduction of a prolapsed vagina. In the case of uterine prolapse, laparotomy may be required to align the uterine horns. The uterus may be sutured to the ventrolateral abdominal wall to prevent recurrence, or the bitch may be spayed. Oxytocin is administered (5 to 10 IU, IM) to encourage involution. Antibiotics and parenteral fluids are used to prevent infection and to treat shock.

H. Vaginal hyperplasia cannot be manually replaced. Urethral patency is established, and the mass is washed and treated topically with antibacterial creams.

I. Estrogen levels are reduced by inducing ovulation (500 IU of human chorionic gonadotropin IM) or suppressed with megestrol acetate (2 mg per kilogram once daily for 5 days).

J. In rare cases, even with the aid of a laparotomy, prolapsed vaginal or uterine tissues cannot be replaced, and amputation of protruding tissues is required.

K. If hyperplasia does not regress, or if a large amount of tissue is prolapsed or severely damaged, mucosal resection is indicated. Generally only mucosa of the ventral vagina need be removed. The urethra must be identified and preserved. An episiotomy aids exposure (Fig. 1).

L. Ovariohysterectomy results in a rapid reduction of vaginal hyperplasia and is also recommended when problems are likely to recur or future fertility is doubtful.

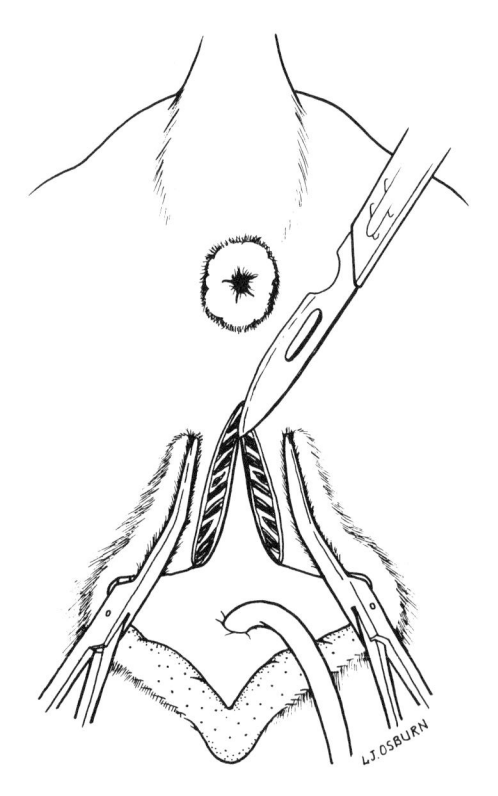

Figure 1 Episiotomy to increase exposure of vaginal vault. Urethra is catheterized for identification and to minimize danger of iatrogenic damage.

References

Hardie EM. Selective surgeries of the male and female reproductive tracts. Vet Clin North Am 1984; 14:109.

Herron MA. Tumors of the canine genital system. JAAHA 1983; 19:981.

VAGINAL PROTRUSION

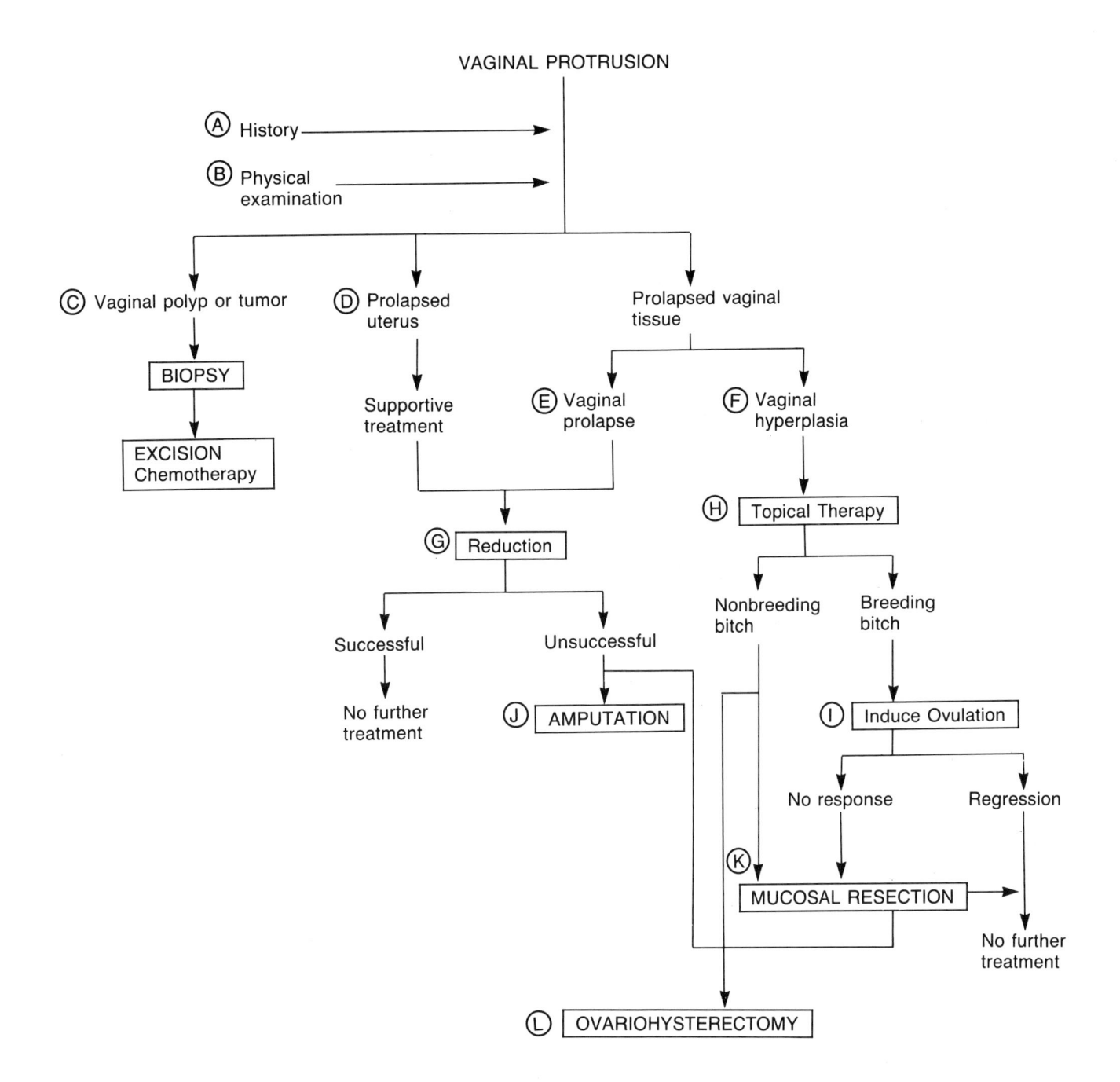

- Ⓐ History
- Ⓑ Physical examination

↓

- Ⓒ Vaginal polyp or tumor → **BIOPSY** → **EXCISION** Chemotherapy
- Ⓓ Prolapsed uterus → Supportive treatment
- Prolapsed vaginal tissue
  - Ⓔ Vaginal prolapse
  - Ⓕ Vaginal hyperplasia

Ⓖ Reduction
- Successful → No further treatment
- Unsuccessful → Ⓙ **AMPUTATION**

Ⓗ Topical Therapy
- Nonbreeding bitch → Ⓚ
- Breeding bitch → Ⓘ **Induce Ovulation**
  - No response → **MUCOSAL RESECTION**
  - Regression → No further treatment

Ⓛ **OVARIOHYSTERECTOMY**

VAGINITIS

Brian C. Buckrell

A. Prepuberal or puppy vaginitis occurs commonly. Pups display vaginal discharge and vulvar-perineal irritation accompanied by licking. Mature bitches with vaginitis have a variable amount of discharge and may attract males. Tenesmus and dysuria, associated with urinary infection, are commonly seen.

B. The degree of vulvar infolding and the presence of a prominent perineal fold are noted. Signs of skin irritation and infection may be present in the labial folds.

C. Prominent perineal folds or excessive perineal fat predispose to vulvar and vestibular infection. Infolding of the labia introduces hair and prevents a complete vulvar seal.

D. Prior to surgical repair, vigorous systemic and local antibiotic therapy and douching are used to reduce postsurgical complications.

E. Once the infection is controlled, episioplasty is performed to correct the vulvar-perineal anatomy. Antibiotics are continued for 3 weeks following surgery.

F. The vagina is examined digitally (sterile lubricated glove) for obstruction, foreign bodies, tumors, or conformational abnormalities. Visual examination using an otoscope or pediatric proctoscope with air insufflation is often needed to confirm the presence of an obstruction. The presence of lymphoid follicles, discharge, and inflammation are noted.

G. Vaginal anomalies are a common finding. Incomplete fusion of the müllerian ducts results in partitioning of the vagina. Annular strictures, dorsoventral septa, and stenoses occur in the region of the hymen. Each of these contributes to retention of vaginal secretions and thereby predisposes to infection.

H. Contrast material infused into the vagina may delineate strictures or other anomalies.

I. Minor strictures and vertical septa can be stretched or broken digitally, whereas more prominent strictures require intravaginal surgery. Examinations, manipulations, and surgery are more readily performed during proestrus or under the influence of estrogens (5 mg diethylstilbestrol daily for 3 days prior to surgery), but bleeding may be increased. Postsurgical care includes antibiotics and digital examination to avoid adhesions.

J. Most cases of puppy vaginitis resolve at puberty without treatment. Treatment is warranted for future breeding bitches. Systemic antibiotics are used for 3 weeks and mild disinfectant douches (e.g., povidone iodine) are used weekly. Reevaluation is made in 1 month.

K. Swabs are obtained aseptically from the anterior vagina for bacteria and mycoplasma culture. Commensal organisms include *Staphylococcus, Streptococcus, E. coli, Pasteurella, Proteus, Pseudomonas, Corynebacterium* and many *Mycoplasma* species. Their isolation is of significance only when present in large numbers or in pure cultures, or in association with clinical signs of vaginitis. Vaginal cytology is examined for bacteria and neutrophils. *Brucella canis* serology is taken from mature breeding bitches. A urinalysis should be included in the evaluation to rule out urinary tract disease.

L. Vaginitis is often refractory to therapy. Accurate microbial cultures are essential. In addition to parenteral antibiotics with weekly douches (e.g., povidone iodine), topical antibiotic-steroid ointments are used to reduce vulvar fold irritation. In recurring cases, especially in spayed females, estrogen supplementation may maintain vaginal health (diethylstilbesterol, 1 mg if bitch weighs more than 20 lb; 0.5 mg if less than 20 lbs, twice a day for 7 days; then every third day for 2 weeks; or topical stilbestrol ointment introduced into the vagina daily). It may be necessary to repeat periodically throughout the animal's life.

References

Barton CL. Canine vaginitis. Vet Clin North Am 1977; 7:711.

Olson PNS, Mather EC. Canine vaginal and uterine bacterial flora. JAVMA 1978; 172:708.

Osbaldiston GW. Bacteriological studies of reproductive disorders of bitches. JAAHA 1978; 14:363.

Wykes PM, Soderberg SF. Congenital abnormalities of the canine vagina and vulva. JAAHA 1983; 19:995.

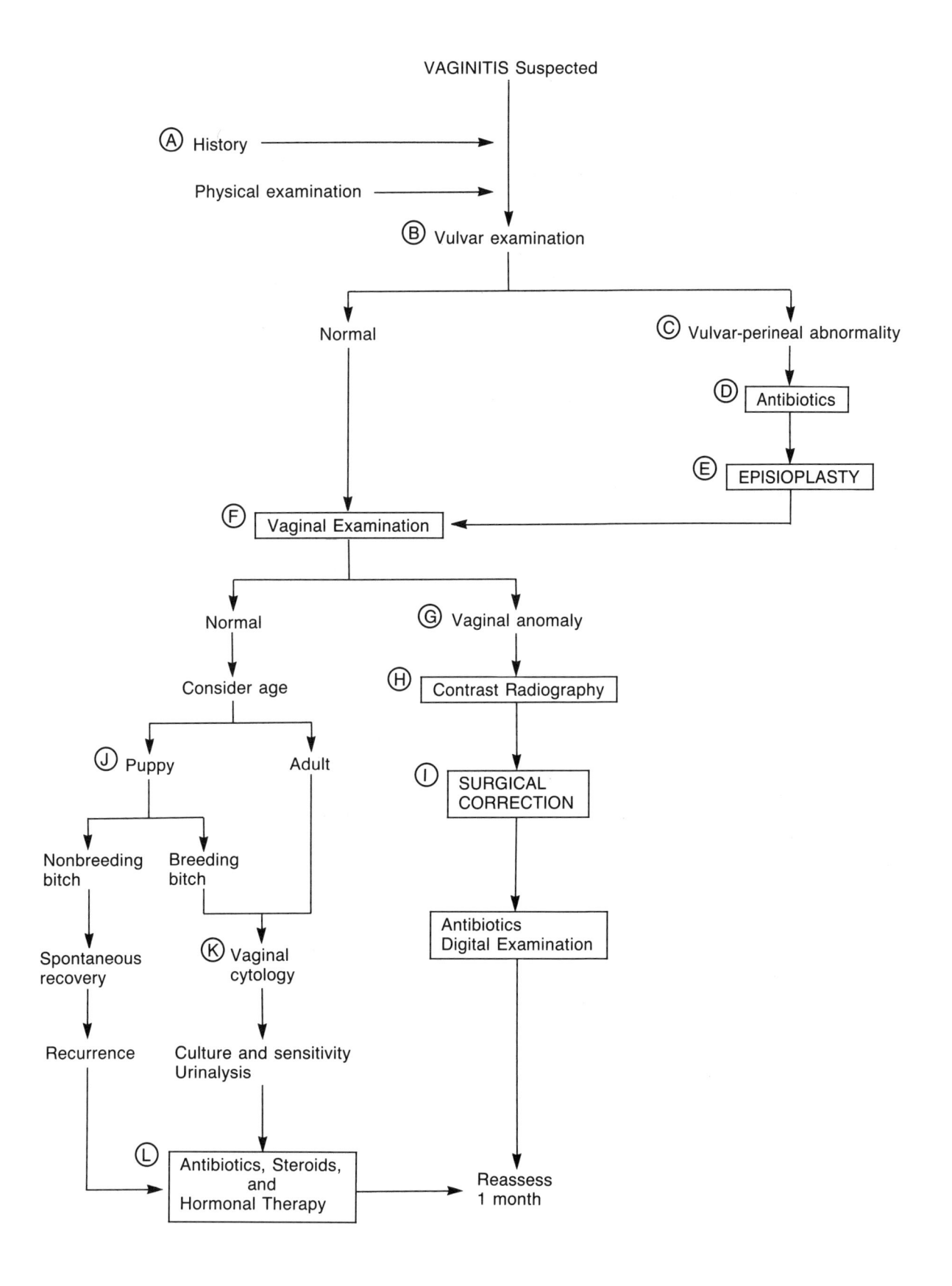

```
                        VAGINITIS Suspected
                                │
        Ⓐ History ──────────────▶│
                                │
        Physical examination ──▶│
                                ▼
                    Ⓑ Vulvar examination
                    ┌───────────┴───────────┐
                    ▼                       ▼
                  Normal         Ⓒ Vulvar-perineal abnormality
                    │                       │
                    │                       ▼
                    │                 Ⓓ ┌─────────────┐
                    │                   │ Antibiotics │
                    │                   └─────────────┘
                    │                       │
                    │                       ▼
                    │                 Ⓔ ┌─────────────┐
                    │                   │ EPISIOPLASTY│
                    │                   └─────────────┘
                    ▼                       │
        Ⓕ ┌─────────────────────┐◀──────────┘
          │ Vaginal Examination │
          └─────────────────────┘
                    │
        ┌───────────┴───────────┐
        ▼                       ▼
      Normal           Ⓖ Vaginal anomaly
        │                       │
   Consider age                 ▼
        │                 Ⓗ ┌─────────────────────┐
        │                   │ Contrast Radiography│
        │                   └─────────────────────┘
   ┌────┴────┐                  │
   ▼         ▼                  ▼
 Ⓙ Puppy   Adult          Ⓘ ┌─────────────┐
   │         │               │  SURGICAL   │
 ┌─┴──┐      │               │ CORRECTION  │
 ▼    ▼      │               └─────────────┘
Non-  Breeding                    │
breeding bitch                    ▼
bitch   │                  ┌─────────────┐
 │      │                  │ Antibiotics │
 ▼      ▼                  │ Digital     │
Spontaneous Ⓚ Vaginal      │ Examination │
recovery    cytology       └─────────────┘
 │          │                     │
 ▼          ▼                     │
Recurrence  Culture and sensitivity
 │          Urinalysis
 │          │
 │          ▼
 │    Ⓛ ┌──────────────────┐
 └───▶│ Antibiotics, Steroids,│
      │ and Hormonal Therapy  │────▶ Reassess
      └──────────────────────┘      1 month
```

PYOMETRA

Brian C. Buckrell

Cystic endometrial hyperplasia-pyometra complex in the bitch is a diestrual uterine disease in mature bitches that occurs 3 to 12 weeks post-estrus. It is a progressive, endometrial, glandular hyperplasia caused by progesterone stimulation of the estrogen-primed uterus over a series of reproductive cycles. The accumulation of glandular secretions provides an excellent environment for bacterial growth that is further enhanced by the inhibition of leukocytic response in the diestrual uterus. *Escherichia coli* is the most frequent bacteria recovered. Purulent material accumulates and produces systemic illness of varying severity. The severity depends on the duration of the illness and on whether or not the cervix is open to permit drainage. Cases with a closed cervix may be extremely ill, with symptoms that include polydypsia, polyuria, dehydration, depression, vomiting, and diarrhea. Bitches with open cervix pyometra generally have less severe systemic illness, but copious vaginal discharge.

A. A history of having received estrogens or progestational compounds during previous estrus cycles is not uncommon.

B. Physical examination includes palpation to detect the presence of an enlarged uterus. Body temperature is normal to subnormal. Presence of vaginal discharge is noted.

C. Complete blood count, blood chemistry, and urinalysis are required to rule out other causes of polyuria and polydypsia. Neutrophilia is usually marked (20,000 to 100,000 per cubic millimeter) and a normocytic, normochronic mild anemia is common. Cytology of vaginal discharge reveals toxic neutrophils and bacteria. Bacterial culture and antimicrobial sensitivity are performed. Radiography and ultrasonography help confirm the diagnosis of pyometra.

D. Dehydration and poor renal perfusion are corrected with fluid replacement (p 190). Antibiotics are given. If bacterial sensitivity results are not available, broad-spectrum antibiotics, such as a trimethoprim-sulphonamide or chloramphenicol, are suggested.

E. Prostaglandin (PGf2α) induces myometrial contraction, cervical dilatation, and luteolysis. Its effect is to evacuate uterine contents. PGf2α has not been thoroughly investigated in the dog. Dogs are kept under close observation for 30 minutes following treatment. In open pyometras, 0.25 mg per kilogram of the natural salt dinoprost is administered subcutaneously twice daily for 3 to 5 days. Closed pyometras are a greater risk and require a gradually increasing dosage: 0.175 mg per kilogram twice daily until uterine drainage begins (usually within 36 hours) followed by 0.25 mg twice daily for 2 more days.

F. Antibiotics are continued for 4 weeks, and used during the next proestrus until the bitch is bred. In spite of vigorous antibiotic therapy, fertility is poor and future reinfections should be anticipated.

References

Hardy RM, Osborne CA. Canine pyometra: pathophysiology, diagnosis and treatment of uterine and extra-uterine lesions. JAAHA 1974; 10:245.

Nelson RW, Feldman EC. Stabenfeldt GH. Treatment of canine pyometra and endometritis with prostaglandin $F_{2\alpha}$. JAVMA 1982; 181:899.

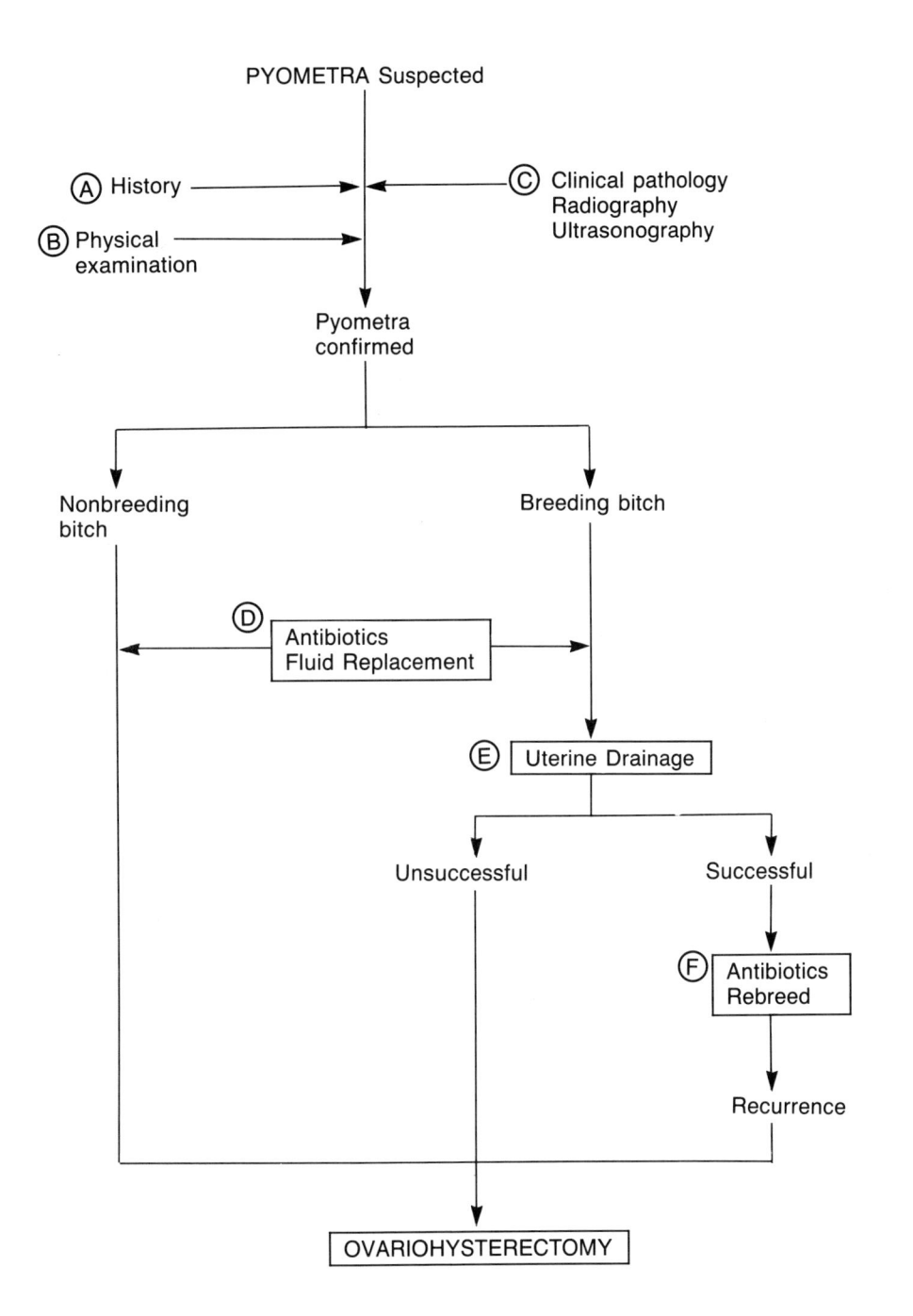

```
                    PYOMETRA Suspected
                             │
   Ⓐ History ─────────────→ │ ←───── Ⓒ Clinical pathology
                             │                Radiography
   Ⓑ Physical ─────────────→│                Ultrasonography
      examination            ↓
                         Pyometra
                         confirmed
                    ┌────────┴────────┐
                    ↓                 ↓
              Nonbreeding         Breeding bitch
                bitch                  │
                  │      Ⓓ  ┌──────────────────┐
                  │←────────│   Antibiotics    │────→
                  │         │ Fluid Replacement│
                  │         └──────────────────┘
                  │                    ↓
                  │         Ⓔ ┌─────────────────┐
                  │           │ Uterine Drainage │
                  │           └─────────────────┘
                  │            ↓              ↓
                  │      Unsuccessful      Successful
                  │            │              ↓
                  │            │       Ⓕ ┌────────────┐
                  │            │         │ Antibiotics│
                  │            │         │  Rebreed   │
                  │            │         └────────────┘
                  │            │              ↓
                  │            │          Recurrence
                  │            │              │
                  └────────────┼──────────────┘
                               ↓
                    ┌────────────────────┐
                    │ OVARIOHYSTERECTOMY │
                    └────────────────────┘
```

PROSTATIC DISEASE

Brian C. Buckrell

A. Prostatic disease is usually associated with symptoms of chronic disease, which include recurrent urinary tract disease, dysuria, difficulty in locomotion or defecation, bloody urethral discharge, and abdominal pain. Patients with acute disease may display pyrexia, anorexia, vomiting, and septicemia.

B. The prostate is palpated per rectum and abdominally for size, symmetry, location, surface texture, and pain. The testicles are examined for tumor development, and the prepuce is examined for balanoposthitis.

C. Plain and contrast radiography and real-time ultrasonography reveal prostatic size, location, and tissue density (e.g., cysts). Urine is obtained by cystocentesis to rule out urinary tract disease. Prostatic fluid is obtained by ejaculation or by urethral-prostatic wash. Prostatic fluid analysis is essential in order to establish a diagnosis and to provide a guide for therapy and prognosis. Consideration is given to color, volume, pH, epithelial cells, white blood count, red blood count, and bacteria (normal fluid contains fewer than 100 bacteria per milliliter). Bacterial and mycoplasma culture and sensitivity is performed on prostatic fluid or, in cases of acute prostatitis when prostatic fluid may be difficult to obtain, on urine. When prostatic enlargement is present, neutrophilia helps to differentiate acute disease and abscessation from prostatic cysts or neoplasia.

D. Benign prostatic hyperplasia (BPH) occurs in mature, intact dogs in response to estrogen and/or androgen stimulation. Although symptoms may be minor (mild discomfort, hematuria, hemospermia, urethral discharge), the condition is progressive, and treatment is advised. Castration is the preferred treatment, but hormonal therapy may be attempted in the valuable breeding dog.

E. Squamous metaplasia is an inflammatory change that results from estrogen stimulation (exogenous therapy or Sertoli cell tumors) in the intact dog. Large numbers of squamous epithelial cells are present in centrifuged prostatic fluid samples.

F. Fine-needle aspiration, rectally or transabdominally, may differentiate abscess formation from neoplasia, but there is a risk of producing iatrogenic peritonitis. Examination and biopsy during laparotomy may be more satisfactory.

G. Abscesses may be small and may be located in a slightly, or greatly, enlarged prostate gland. Initially prostatic abscesses are treated with antibiotics, but usually require surgical drainage.

H. With time, BPH alters the prostatic architecture, which results in cystic hyperplasia. These small multiple cysts contain blood or serosanguinous fluid and constantly discharge into the bladder and urethra. Hormonal therapy and castration are indicated for treatment of cystic hyperplasia. Cystic hyperplasia can be differentiated from noninflammatory prostatic retention cysts by evidence of inflammation in the prostatic fluid. Paraprostatic and prostatic retention cysts can enlarge to the point that surgical drainage is required.

I. Prostatic adenocarcinomas are androgen dependent and may be reduced in size by castration or by treatment with megestrol acetate (MA), thus providing temporary relief for the patient. Gonadotropin-releasing hormone agonists, presently on trial for human prostatic neoplasia, may be of help in the future. Prostatectomy, complete or partial, is difficult and may be attempted as a final solution. Most tumors have metastasized by the time diagnosis is made.

J. The prostate-blood barrier is disrupted in acute disease. Antibiotics are selected on the basis of prostatic or urine culture results. Megestrol acetate reduces prostatic inflammation. The patient should be castrated as soon as its condition is stabilized, as recurrences are common. Antibiotics are continued for 14 days, and the patient is reevaluated. In chronic prostatitis, the blood-prostate barrier remains intact. Antibiotics are selected based on prostatic fluid pH, antibiotic pKa, protein binding, lipid solubility, and the results of bacterial culture and sensitivity. Prostatic fluid usually remains acidic with chronic disease. Chloramphenicol, a trimethoprim-sulphonamide, and erythromycin are often the best choices. When pH is alkaline (for example, with Proteus infection), penicillin may be used. Antibiotics are continued for 4 weeks, and the dog is reevaluated. Further treatment is often required. Hormonal therapy reduces inflammation, but castration is suggested for long-term relief and to prevent recurrence. Fertility in most dogs is reduced by prostatitis.

K. Low dose oral diethylstilbestrol (DES) reduces androgen stimulation if used for short-term relief (0.5-1.0 mg once daily for 7 days). Prolonged low dose or high dose estrogen therapy acts synergistically with androgens to increase stromal hyperplasia and epithelial cell squamous metaplasia. Bone marrow depression is also of concern. An alternative is to use megestrol acetate at 0.5 mg per kilogram daily to effect (usually for 10 days), then once weekly. Studies on the long-term effects of MA in the dog have not been conducted.

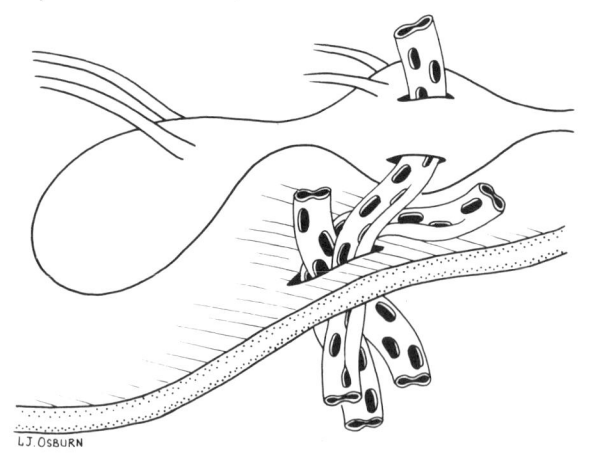

Figure 1 Drainage of prostatic abscess and periprostatic area using Penrose drains.

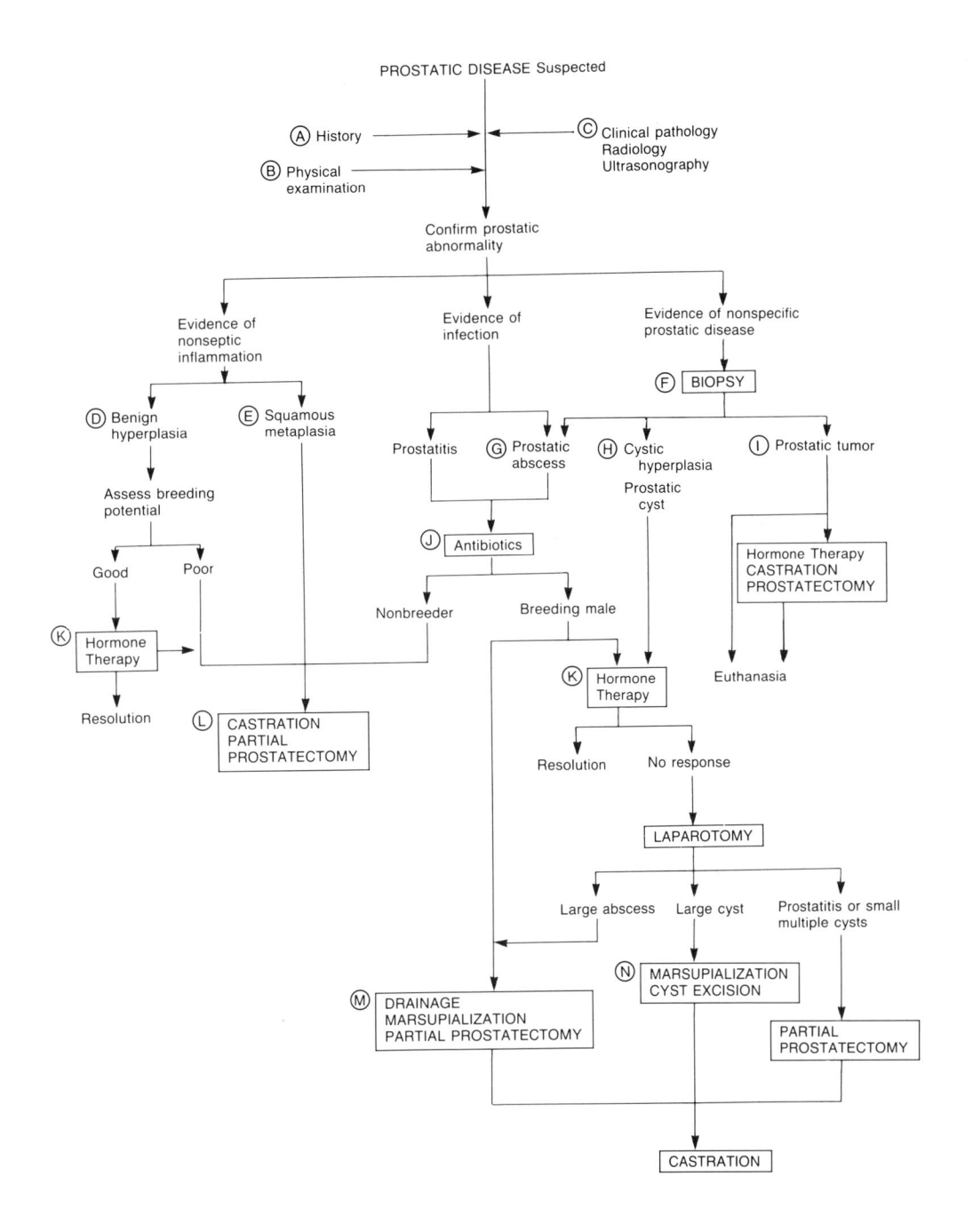

```
                    PROSTATIC DISEASE Suspected
                              │
    Ⓐ History ─────────────→  ←───────── Ⓒ Clinical pathology
                              │                 Radiology
    Ⓑ Physical ────────────→  │                 Ultrasonography
       examination            │
                              ▼
                    Confirm prostatic
                      abnormality
          ┌───────────────────┼───────────────────┐
          ▼                   ▼                   ▼
    Evidence of          Evidence of         Evidence of nonspecific
    nonseptic            infection           prostatic disease
    inflammation                                   │
       ┌──────┐                                    ▼
       ▼      ▼                              Ⓕ  BIOPSY
  Ⓓ Benign  Ⓔ Squamous    ┌──────┬─────┐    ┌──────┴──────┐
  hyperplasia metaplasia  ▼      ▼     ▼    ▼             ▼
       │                Prostatitis Ⓖ Prostatic  Ⓗ Cystic  Ⓘ Prostatic
       ▼                           abscess   hyperplasia    tumor
  Assess breeding                    │       Prostatic         │
    potential                        ▼       cyst              ▼
     ┌───┴───┐                  Ⓙ Antibiotics              Hormone Therapy
     ▼       ▼                       │                     CASTRATION
   Good     Poor                     ▼                     PROSTATECTOMY
     │       │              ┌────────┴─────────┐                │
     ▼       │              ▼                  ▼                ▼
  Ⓚ Hormone  │          Nonbreeder        Breeding male     Euthanasia
    Therapy │
     │      │                                  ▼
     ▼      ▼                              Ⓚ Hormone
  Resolution Ⓛ CASTRATION                    Therapy
            PARTIAL                         ┌────┴────┐
            PROSTATECTOMY                   ▼         ▼
                                        Resolution  No response
                                                      │
                                                      ▼
                                                  LAPAROTOMY
                                         ┌────────┬──────────┐
                                         ▼        ▼          ▼
                                    Large abscess Large cyst  Prostatitis or small
                                         │        │          multiple cysts
                                         ▼        ▼           │
                                      Ⓜ DRAINAGE  Ⓝ MARSUPIALIZATION
                                      MARSUPIALIZATION  CYST EXCISION
                                      PARTIAL PROSTATECTOMY   │
                                                              ▼
                                                         PARTIAL
                                                         PROSTATECTOMY
                                                              │
                                                              ▼
                                                         CASTRATION
```

L. Prostatic disease is androgen induced or androgen supported. Megestrol acetate and low dose estrogens are helpful for short-term therapy. However, fertility is impaired by these drugs, and as most prostatic disease recurs, castration is advised. Partial prostatectomy may be required for resolution of chronic prostatitis. Semen preservation may be offered in the case of a valuable breeding male.

M. Drainage is the preferred treatment for abscesses (Fig. 1). Very large abscesses may be amenable to marsupialization. Partial prostatectomy is indicated for chronic prostatitis or multiple small abscesses, but carries the risk of causing urinary incontinence.

N. Marsupialization is the recommended treatment for large cysts, and is less likely to result in cyst recurrence than simple drainage. Complete excision of the cyst may be possible, but this is contraindicated if extensive dissection is needed.

References

Hornbuckle WE, MacCoy DM, Allan GS, Gunther R. Prostatic disease in the dog. Cornell Vet 1978; 68:284.

Klausner JS, Osborne CA. Management of canine bacterial prostatitis. JAVMA 1983; 182:292.

McAnulty JF. Prostatic surgery in the dog. Vet Clin North Am 1984; 14:103.

Olsen PN. Disorders of the canine prostate gland. Proc Soc Theriogen 1984: 46.

LESION LOCALIZATION IN SPINAL CORD DISEASE

Joane Parent

A. Disc disease is unlikely in a dog less than 1 year of age. Consider atlantoaxial luxation in the miniature breed that suffers from a painful cervical disease. Neuroepithelioma is an occasional cause of thoracolumbar spinal compression in the young large breed dog (5 months to 3 years). Fibrocartilaginous embolic myelopathy also occurs most frequently in the young large dog.

B. Time of onset, progression, and clinical signs are important in diagnosis and prognostication. If compression occurs slowly, 50 percent of the spinal cord diameter can be lost without clinical evidence of neurologic deficit. If pain sensation is not lost, acute lesions generally have a good prognosis for return to normal function. Painful cord diseases include disc disease, vertebral fractures, discospondylitis, osteomyelitis, meningitis, atlantoaxial luxation, and, occasionally, vertebral tumor.

C. A thorough physical examination and basic laboratory data are required in order to rule out multisystemic disease. Specific abnormalities such as fever or pain should be noted.

D. A complete neurologic examination should always be performed, which includes evaluation of mental status, cranial nerves, gait and posture, postural reactions, spinal reflexes, and pain sensation.

E. There are three types of ataxia: vestibular, cerebellar, and spinal. Vestibular ataxia is characterized by head tilt, disequilibrium, and preservation of strength. In cerebellar ataxia, there is loss of coordination, but good purposeful movement and preservation of strength. With the more common spinal ataxia, there is a proprioceptive deficit and an inherent weakness. In mild spinal cord dysfunction, knuckling may not be present. Gait evaluation is most valuable in deciding if there is spinal ataxia. The single best question to answer is "Does the animal know where its feet are at all times?"

F. Neurologic abnormalities such as intention tremors, absence of menace response, opisthotonus, and increased extensor tone and reflexes may be solely caused by cerebellar disease.

G. Clinically, spinal cord disease implies the concomitant presence of weakness and a proprioceptive deficit.

H. If reflexes are normal, consider muscle or metabolic disease. In musculoskeletal disease, the gait appears stiff, choppy, and weak. Myasthenia gravis generally presents as episodic weakness. If the reflexes are decreased, peripheral neuropathy should be considered.

I. With lesions at L_{6-7} and L_7-S_1, only the spinal roots are affected; therefore, there is no ataxia, but there may be loss of flexor and pudendal reflexes and lack of tail function. In most cases, this syndrome is associated with hyperesthesia.

J. If only the white matter of the spinal cord is affected, diseases such as cervical vertebral instability in the Doberman ("Wobbler") and disc disease may demonstrate increased tone and reflexes in all four legs. If there is spinal root and/or nerve compression (C4 to C7), there can be forelimb lameness.

K. There may be Horner's syndrome (lesion T1 to T3) or forelimb lameness.

L. Hyperesthesia, line of anesthesia, or panniculus reflex can indicate more precisely the lesion location.

M. The spinal segments L5 to L7 are situated in the fourth lumbar vertebra; segments S1 to S3 lie in the fifth vertebra. In the dog, the spinal cord terminates in the cranial portion of the seventh lumbar vertebra (Fig. 1). Despite this disparity in spinal and vertebral numbering, each spinal nerve root at this level exits immediately caudal to the vertebra of the same number. This portion of the spinal cord is assessed using the patellar (femoral nerve, spinal segments L4 to L6) flexor (sciatic nerve, spinal segments L6 to S2); and perineal reflexes (pudendal nerve, S1 to S3). A vertebral lesion at L_{3-4} diminishes the patellar reflex; a vertebral lesion at L_{4-5} may decrease the patellar, flexor, and perineal reflexes; whereas a vertebral lesion at L_{5-6} may diminish the flexor and perineal reflexes.

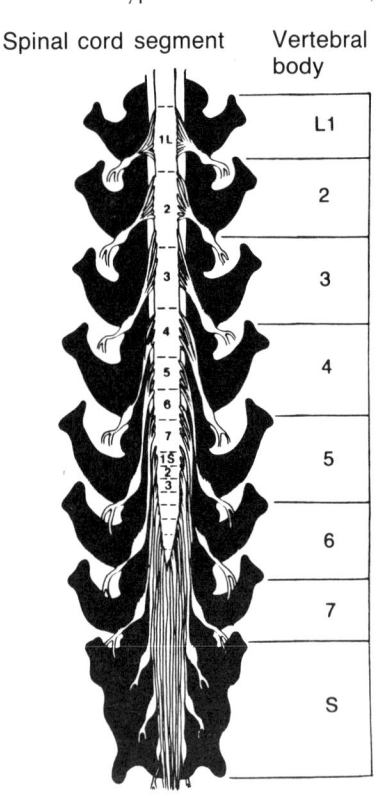

Figure 1 Relationship between spinal cord segments and vertebral bodies in the dog.

Reference

De Lahunta A. Veterinary neuroanatomy and clinical neurology. 2nd ed. Philadelpia: WB Saunders 1983:175.

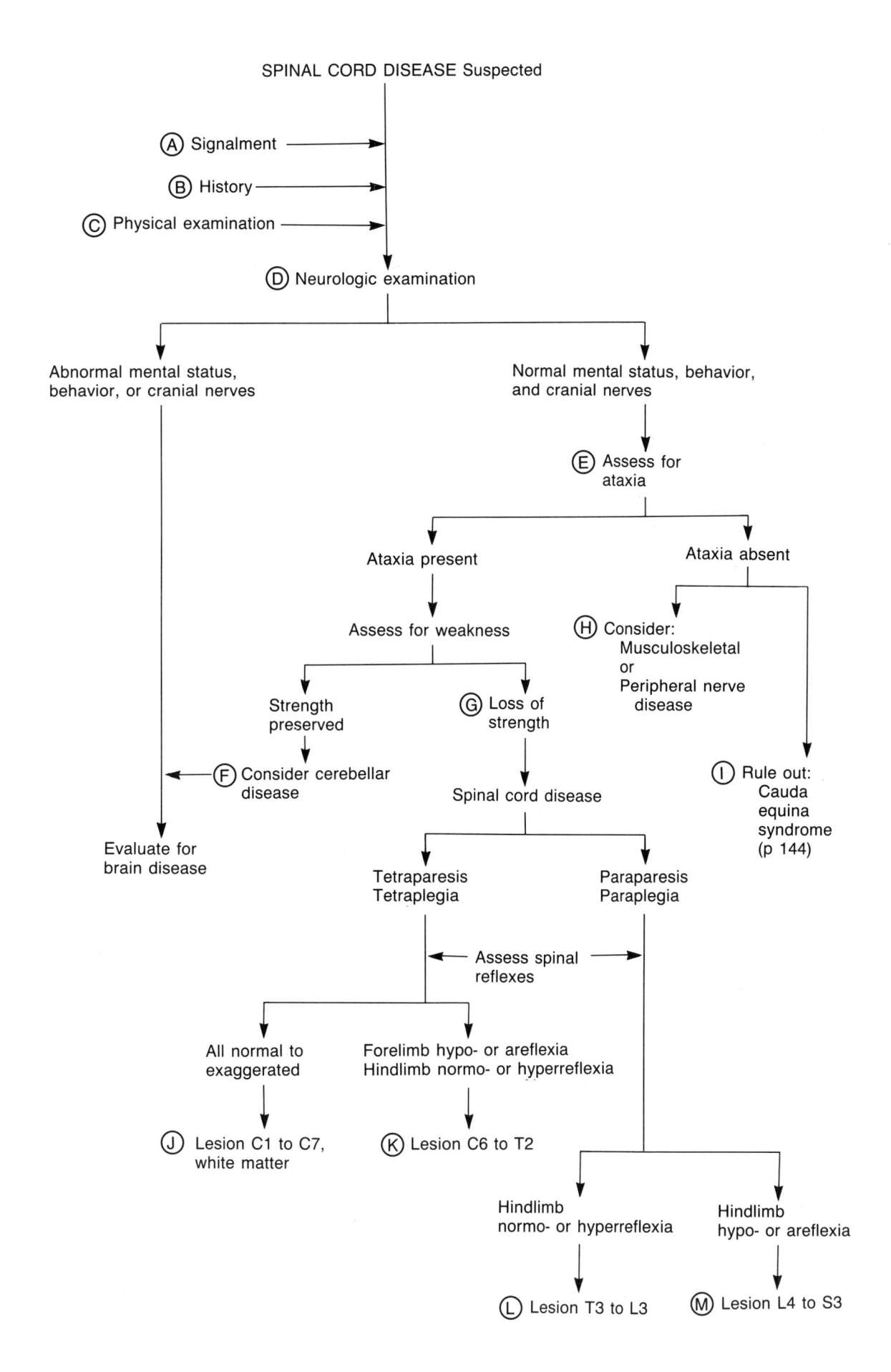

SPINAL CORD DISEASE Suspected

- (A) Signalment
- (B) History
- (C) Physical examination

→ (D) Neurologic examination

Abnormal mental status, behavior, or cranial nerves
→ Evaluate for brain disease

Normal mental status, behavior, and cranial nerves
→ (E) Assess for ataxia

Ataxia present
→ Assess for weakness

- **Strength preserved** → (F) Consider cerebellar disease
- **(G) Loss of strength** → Spinal cord disease

Ataxia absent
- (H) Consider: Musculoskeletal or Peripheral nerve disease
- (I) Rule out: Cauda equina syndrome (p 144)

Spinal cord disease

Tetraparesis / Tetraplegia
Assess spinal reflexes

- **All normal to exaggerated** → (J) Lesion C1 to C7, white matter
- **Forelimb hypo- or areflexia, Hindlimb normo- or hyperreflexia** → (K) Lesion C6 to T2

Paraparesis / Paraplegia
Assess spinal reflexes

- **Hindlimb normo- or hyperreflexia** → (L) Lesion T3 to L3
- **Hindlimb hypo- or areflexia** → (M) Lesion L4 to S3

137

NECK PAIN

Joane Parent
Susan M. Cochrane

A. Atlantoaxial luxation or subluxation is usually encountered in the young miniature breeds, whereas bacterial meningitis is usually seen in the young medium-sized dog. An animal less than a year old is unlikely to suffer from intervertebral disc disease (IVDD).

B. The animal may be presented with episodic or persistent neck pain. There may be restricted neck motion, reluctance to climb stairs, or arching of the back.

C. Pain associated with the neck region must be substantiated. Perform a thorough physical examination and a complete data base assessment (hematology, biochemical profile, and urinalysis). Fever may occur with meningitis or discospondylitis. An inflammatory hematologic response may be observed in the patient with an infectious disorder. Concurrent urinary tract infection may be seen in cases of discospondylitis.

D. A normal neurologic examination does not exclude spinal cord compression. In slowly progressive spinal cord disease, there is often tremendous compensation before clinical signs occur.

E. Use nonsteroidal anti-inflammatory drugs (NSAIDs) not only for treatment, but as an aid in diagnosis. In the older large dog, the discomfort of osteoarthritis may respond to NSAIDs. As a rule, it is unwise to use steroids or antibiotics without substantiating the cause of the cervical pain. Most spinal diseases that require steroid or antibiotic therapy need a minimum of 6 to 8 weeks of treatment.

F. Take spinal radiographs under general anesthesia unless a fracture or atlantoaxial luxation is suspected, in which case further spinal cord injury could occur during manipulation of the anesthetized patient. If chemical restraint must be used in these cases, careful handling is mandatory.

G. Discospondylitis, cervical vertebral instability (CVI), and vertebral tumors may be detected on survey radiographs, but myelography is necessary for full evaluation of the severity of the compression, especially if surgery is contemplated. Spondylosis and dural ossification are nonpainful and usually incidental findings. Vertebral malformation (e.g., hemivertebra) may be an incidental finding in breeds such as the English Bulldog and Boston Terrier.

H. Cervical vertebral instability is usually a nonpainful condition. However, in the Doberman Pinscher presented with neck pain, primary disc disease or disc disease secondary to CVI should be suspected. In CVI, stressed views should be done during myelography in order to document the dynamics of the compression. The Doberman breed has a high incidence of von Willebrand's disease, cardiomyopathy, and hypothyroidism. These factors, depending upon the severity and chronicity of the CVI, may be surgical deterrents.

I. In most cases, treatment is palliative. For benign tumors, resection may be possible.

J. Discospondylitis, in its early course, can be difficult to diagnose as the lesion may not be readily obvious on radiographs. Clinical signs such as recurrent fever, depression, and decreased appetite are suggestive. Perform blood and urine cultures.

K. Rule out inflammatory diseases by cerebrospinal fluid (CSF) analysis. If the cell count and cytology are normal, myelography can be performed safely. In cases of known trauma, myelography can be pursued even if the CSF is hemorrhagic. With extradural compression, the CSF analysis is usually normal. In neoplastic or degenerative intramedullary diseases, the CSF protein concentration may be increased, but the fluid is likely to be normal cytologically.

L. When the CSF analysis indicates the presence of inflammatory disease, surgical treatment is not indicated, and myelography can be detrimental. This category includes the meningeal infiltrations. It is essential to differentiate between infectious and noninfectious causes of inflammation. CSF analysis is essential for treatment selection (steroids versus antibiotics). CSF analysis should be repeated if no improvement has occurred after 3 to 5 days and before withdrawing or changing medication.

References

De Lahunta A. Veterinary neuroanatomy and clinical neurology. 2nd ed. Philadelphia: WB Saunders, 1983:195.

Oliver JE, Lorenz MD. Handbook of veterinary neurologic diagnosis. Philadelphia: WB Saunders, 1983:188.

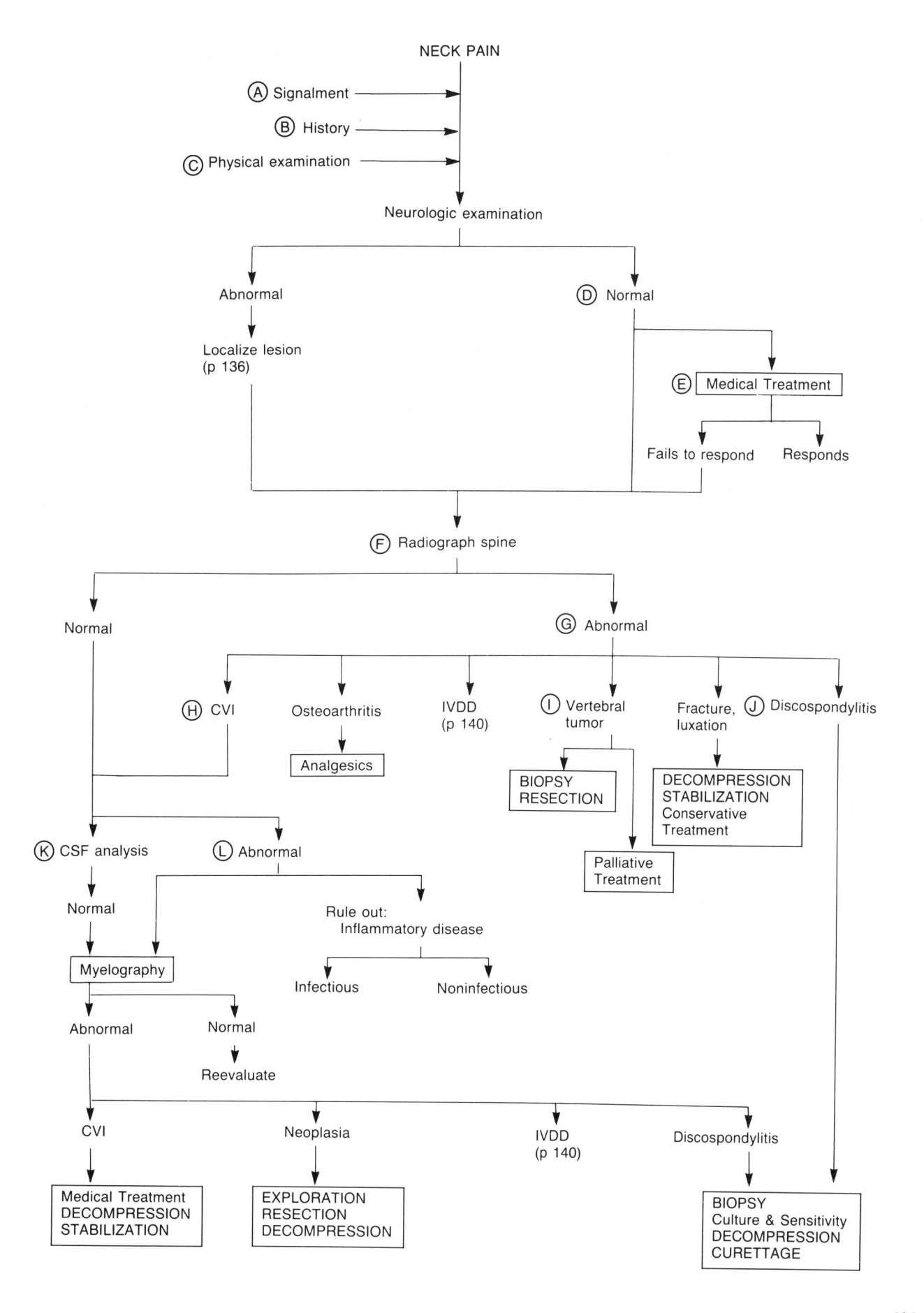

NECK PAIN

- (A) Signalment
- (B) History
- (C) Physical examination

↓

Neurologic examination

- Abnormal → Localize lesion (p 136)
- (D) Normal → (E) Medical Treatment
  - Fails to respond
  - Responds

↓

(F) **Radiograph spine**

- Normal
- (G) Abnormal
  - (H) CVI
  - Osteoarthritis → Analgesics
  - IVDD (p 140)
  - (I) Vertebral tumor → BIOPSY / RESECTION → Palliative Treatment
  - Fracture, luxation → DECOMPRESSION STABILIZATION Conservative Treatment
  - (J) Discospondylitis

From Normal / CVI:

- (K) CSF analysis
  - Normal → Myelography
  - (L) Abnormal → Myelography; Rule out: Inflammatory disease
    - Infectious
    - Noninfectious

Myelography
- Abnormal
  - CVI → Medical Treatment / DECOMPRESSION / STABILIZATION
  - Neoplasia → EXPLORATION / RESECTION / DECOMPRESSION
  - IVDD (p 140)
  - Discospondylitis → BIOPSY / Culture & Sensitivity / DECOMPRESSION / CURETTAGE
- Normal → Reevaluate

CERVICAL INTERVERTEBRAL DISC DISEASE

Joane Parent

A. Age and breed are important in the diagnosis of cervical intervertebral disc disease (CIVDD). Young to middle-aged Dachshunds, Cocker Spaniels, Poodles, and Beagles are at risk. The Doberman Pinscher is the most common large breed in which primary CIVDD is encountered; albeit in this breed it is more often secondary to cervical vertebral instability (CVI). The high incidence of atlantoaxial subluxation or luxation in the miniature breeds makes this an important differential diagnosis.

B. The history is usually one of acute and often recurrent symptoms. The owner may report neck pain, restricted neck motion, and yelping with abrupt movements. Muscle spasms may be observed and are sometimes interpreted by the owner as seizures.

C. The head may be held low with rigid neck extension. The patient may resist attempts to move the head and neck. Front leg lameness can be present as a result of spinal root compression by the abnormal disc between C4 to 5, C5 to 6 and C6 to 7. There may be neurogenic muscle atrophy as a consequence of this compression.

D. Medical treatment with steroids, muscle relaxants, or both is only palliative in CIVDD as the majority of patients relapse. This should be strongly stressed to the owner at the first presentation so that fenestration can be accomplished at this time or at the first recurrence. Long-term therapy with steroids or nonsteroidal anti-inflammatory drugs (NSAIDs) is not recommended.

E. The deficits vary from mild to severe tetraparesis with mild to severe front limb extension. The presence of spinal nerve signs (lameness, neurogenic atrophy) is indicative of lower cervical disc disease.

F. Take spinal radiographs under general anesthesia in order to obtain diagnostic films. Normal radiographs do not rule out disc disease. The most common sites involved are C2 to 3 and C3 to 4. Survey radiographs are often diagnostic; however, myelography is indicated in chronic cases or in cases with neurologic deficits so that spinal cord compression that requires decompression is not overlooked.

G. Cerebrospinal fluid (CSF) analysis should always be done before myelography, and before surgery (either decompression or fenestration), if the diagnosis is not clear cut. Meningomyelitis can present as neck pain with or without neurologic deficits.

H. The easiest and most common approach for removal of disc material in the cervical vertebral canal is ventral slotting. It should be combined with a prophylactic fenestration of the other cervical discs. Protrusion of a cervical disc with collapse of the intervertebral space or lateral protrusion of disc material may necessitate dorsal laminectomy. In rare cases of lateralization of clinical signs with nerve root entrapment, hemilaminectomy with foraminotomy may be necessary. If the patient has no neurologic deficits, the best treatment for cervical disc disease is fenestration.

Reference

Oliver JE, Lorenz MD. Handbook of veterinary neurologic diagnosis. Philadelphia: WB Saunders, 1983: 188.

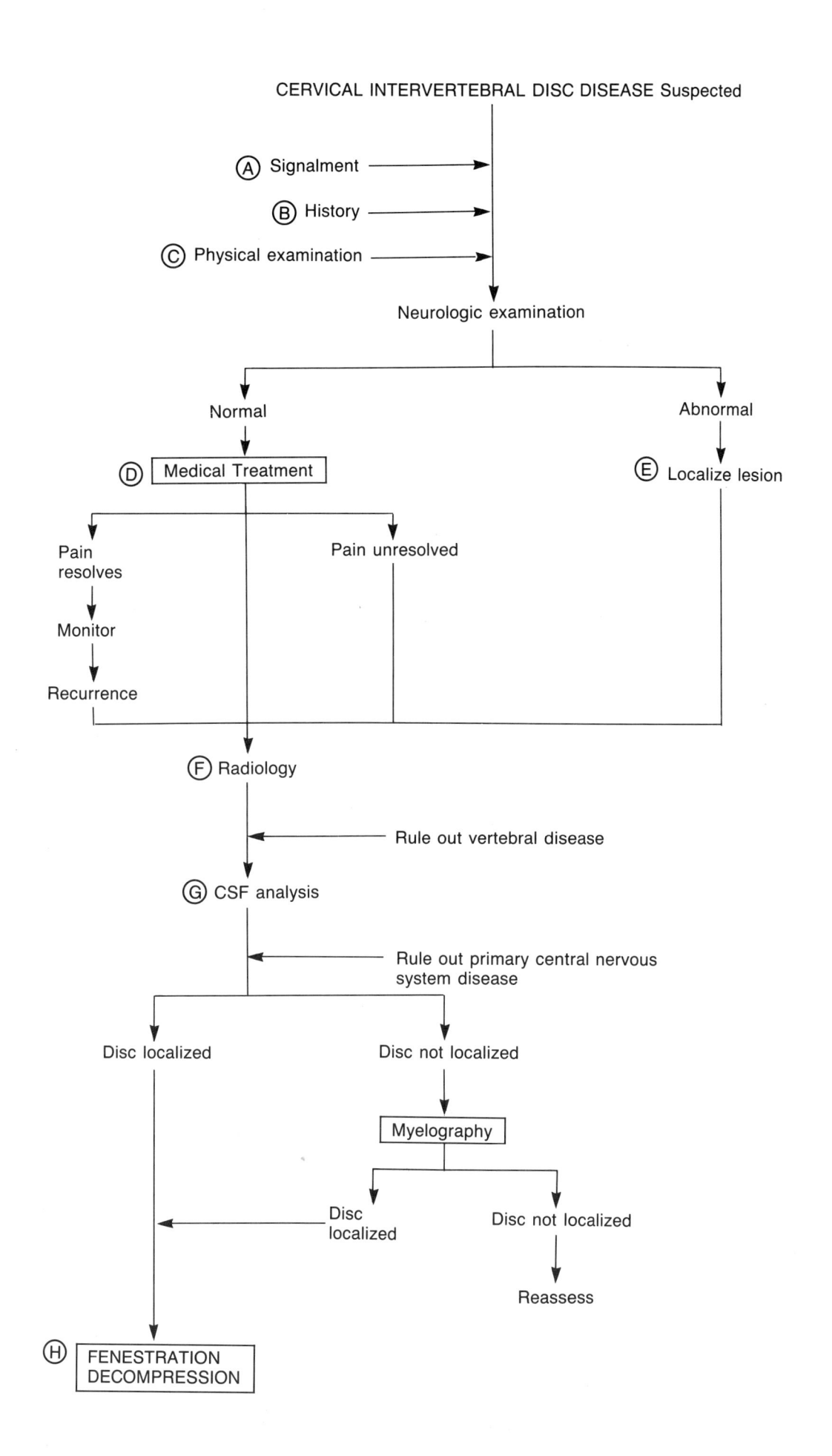

CERVICAL INTERVERTEBRAL DISC DISEASE Suspected

- (A) Signalment
- (B) History
- (C) Physical examination

→ Neurologic examination

- Normal → (D) **Medical Treatment**
  - Pain resolves → Monitor → Recurrence
  - Pain unresolved
- Abnormal → (E) Localize lesion

→ (F) Radiology ← Rule out vertebral disease

→ (G) CSF analysis ← Rule out primary central nervous system disease

- Disc localized
- Disc not localized → **Myelography**
  - Disc localized
  - Disc not localized → Reassess

→ (H) **FENESTRATION DECOMPRESSION**

THORACOLUMBAR INTERVERTEBRAL DISC DISEASE

Joane Parent
Laura L. Smith-Maxie

A. The breed most commonly affected by type I thoracolumbar disc degeneration is the Dachshund, in which the clinical disease generally appears at 3 to 6 years of age. Other frequently affected breeds are the small Poodle breeds, Beagles, Cocker Spaniels, Shih Tzus, Lhasa Apsos, and Basset Hounds. Type II disc disease is seen more commonly in the German Shepherd and the Labrador Retriever. It is a senile degeneration seen in dogs over 5 years of age.

B. Type I disc disease is usually acute in nature, whereas type II is generally chronic and causes a progressive focal myelopathy.

C. A thorough physical examination is essential. Focal hyperesthesia along the vertebral column and lameness (caused by compression of spinal root or nerve) are signs suggestive of intervertebral disc disease (IVDD). Fever may be present as a result of focal subarachnoid hemorrhage or of ascending-descending myelomalacia.

D. An animal with normal neurologic status can have severe spinal cord compression. With a slowly progressive lesion, tremendous compensation can occur in the central nervous system. Both type I and type II disc disease can present in this manner.

E. The patient that is presented with loss of pain sensation of more than 24 hours duration has a remote chance of recovery. Even if pain sensation is preserved, the animal with lower motor neuron deficits has a guarded prognosis.

F. In our opinion, IVDD is a surgical disease. In many cases, there is a mass effect (disc material within the vertebral canal), which, if not treated surgically, may cause irreversible spinal cord damage. Medical treatment is palliative and may offer only temporary relief. However, because of cost considerations or lack of facilities, surgery may not be possible. Dexamethasone (0.25 mg per kilogram three times a day), administered in decreasing dosages, can help to reduce local inflammation. Although the prognosis is guarded initially, paraplegic dogs (even without pain sensation), when treated medically, can recover slowly over an 8 to 12 week period.

G. Always perform spinal radiographs under general anesthesia. Lateral and dorsoventral views of the suspected area should be taken, but survey radiographs may not be diagnostic.

H. Perform cerebrospinal fluid (CSF) analysis prior to myelography in order to rule out myelopathies other than disc disease. In extradural disease, the CSF analysis results should be normal. In acute, severe, focal compression, neutrophils and red cells may be present, but cell count and protein concentration are most likely to be within normal limits. In ascending-descending myelomalacia, neutrophils are seen on cytology, along with an increase in CSF cell count and protein concentration.

I. Myelography should be performed each time spinal surgery is contemplated.

J. If the radiographic study substantiates spinal cord compression or swelling, decompressive laminectomy should be performed, followed by prophylactic fenestration. Fenestration may be performed at the same time as the laminectomy or as a separate procedure 6 to 12 weeks later. The prognosis varies, based on the severity and duration of the lesion.

K. If the radiographic study does not demonstrate spinal cord compression, prophylactic fenestration alone is performed.

Reference

Oliver JE, Lorenz MD. Handbook of veterinary neurologic diagnosis. Philadelphia: WB Saunders, 1983:152.

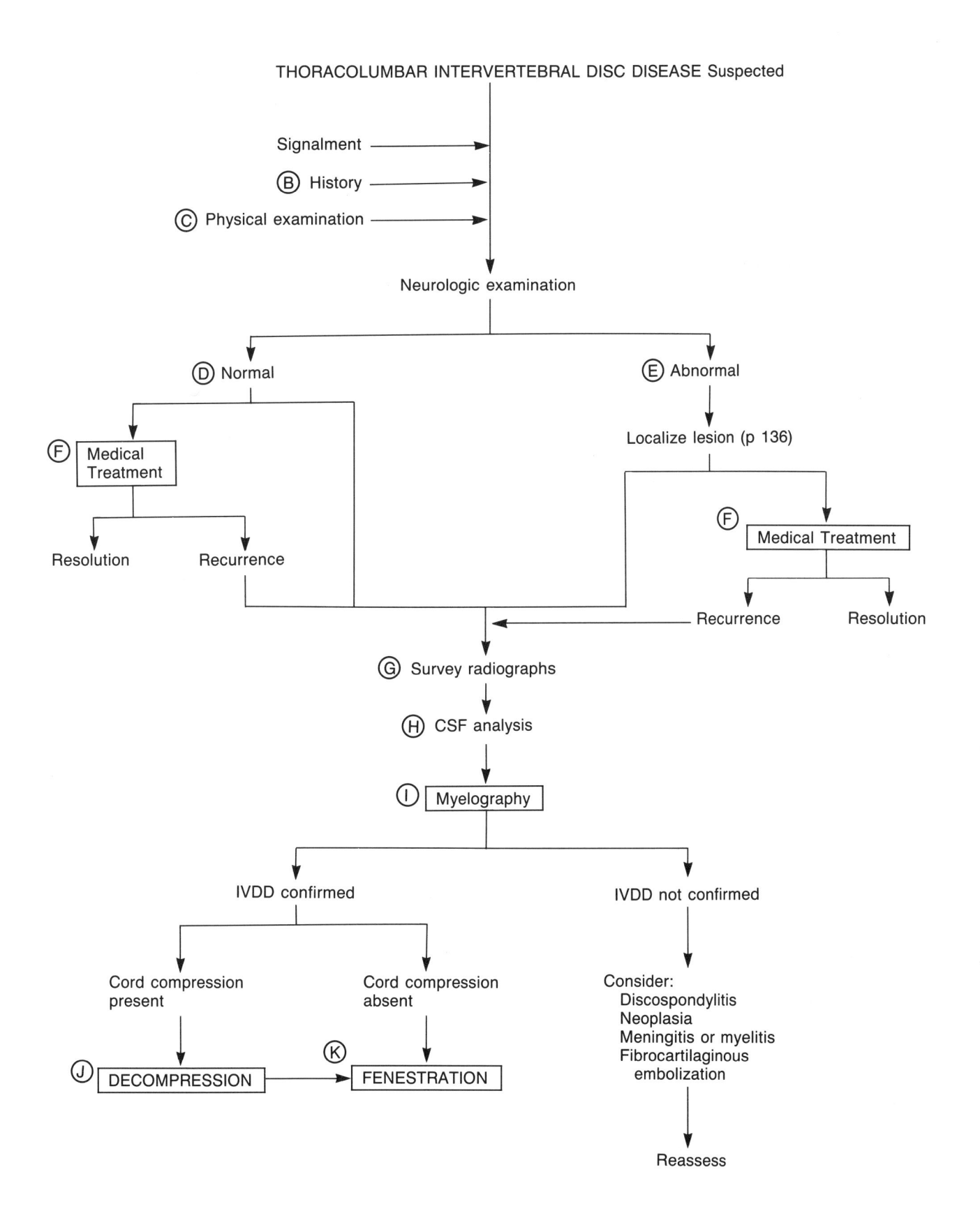

THORACOLUMBAR INTERVERTEBRAL DISC DISEASE Suspected

- Signalment
- Ⓑ History
- Ⓒ Physical examination

↓

Neurologic examination

- Ⓓ Normal
  - Ⓕ Medical Treatment
    - Resolution
    - Recurrence
- Ⓔ Abnormal
  - Localize lesion (p 136)
    - Ⓕ Medical Treatment
      - Recurrence
      - Resolution

↓

Ⓖ Survey radiographs

Ⓗ CSF analysis

Ⓘ Myelography

- IVDD confirmed
  - Cord compression present
    - Ⓙ DECOMPRESSION
  - Cord compression absent
    - Ⓚ FENESTRATION
- IVDD not confirmed
  - Consider:
    - Discospondylitis
    - Neoplasia
    - Meningitis or myelitis
    - Fibrocartilaginous embolization
  - Reassess

143

PERIPHERAL NERVE DISEASE (MONONEUROPATHY)

Joane Parent
Susan M. Cochrane

A. Perform complete neurologic examination in order to determine the limb(s) and nerve(s) affected.

B. Oil-base injectable products are the most likely cause of injury.

C. Causes of surgical nerve injury include perineal hernia repair, pelvic osteotomy, and pelvic and humeral fracture repair.

D. Entrapment may occur from callus and scar formation or following a surgical procedure.

E. The salient feature of the cauda equina syndrome is lumbosacral pain, which may be the only abnormal finding. It can be accompanied by intermittent lameness and abnormal tail and anal sphincter function. The prognosis is guarded if there is urinary incontinence.

F. In any chronic lameness wherein radiographic and joint studies have been normal, a nerve sheath tumor should be considered. Nerve sheath tumors have a tendency to invade the spinal canal. A myelogram should be performed even if there is no sign of spinal cord involvement.

G. In acute cases, explore the nerve involved, and perform debridement and fat grafting. The prognosis is guarded if there is loss of pain sensation.

H. Nonsteroidal anti-inflammatory drugs, glucocorticoids, and rest have all been advocated, but decompressive laminectomy at L7 to S1 is the treatment of choice.

I. Brachial plexus avulsion is by far the most common traumatic peripheral nerve injury in small animals. In most cases, the avulsion is at the spinal cord level. Occasionally, there is secondary spinal cord swelling, which results in contralateral foreleg and hind leg paresis. Horner's syndrome may accompany this injury. It is not infrequent to observe avulsion of the ventral roots with sparing of the dorsal roots. In such a case, there is decreased motor function in the limb, but good pain perception, and the limb may be salvaged by arthrodesis of the carpal joint. When pain perception is absent up to the elbow, the prognosis is very poor.

J. Lumbosacral injury is uncommon. The prognosis is similar to that for brachial plexus avulsion.

K. Sacrococcygeal injury is seen most commonly in cats. The main clinical signs are absence of sensory and motor function of the tail, with partial or complete loss of urethral and anal sphincter function. Occasionally, there is sciatic weakness. The prognosis for recovery is poor if there is loss of urinary control and anal tone. Amputation of the tail is often required.

L. Electromyography (EMG) is helpful in the diagnosis of this syndrome. In addition to the muscles of the tail, muscles innervated by the sciatic and femoral nerves should be evaluated bilaterally.

M. Tomography, intraosseous venography, epidorography, and, occasionally, myelography may be rewarding.

N. Glucocorticoid therapy for 2 to 7 days (0.25 mg per kilogram one to three times daily). If there is urinary incontinence, the bladder must be expressed frequently.

References

Bailey CS. Patterns of cutaneous anesthesia associated with brachial plexus avulsions in the dog. JAVMA 1984; 185:889.

Bradley RL, Withrow SJ, Synder SP. Nerve sheath tumors in the dog. AAHA 1982; 18:915.

Chambers JN, Hardie EM. Localization and management of sciatic nerve injury due to ischial or acetabular fracture. AAHA 1986; 22:539.

Oliver JE, Selcer RR, Simpson S. Cauda equina compression from lumbosacral malarticulation and malformation in the dog. JAVMA 1978; 173:207.

Tarvin G, Prata RG. Lumbosacral stenosis in dogs. JAVMA 1980; 177:154.

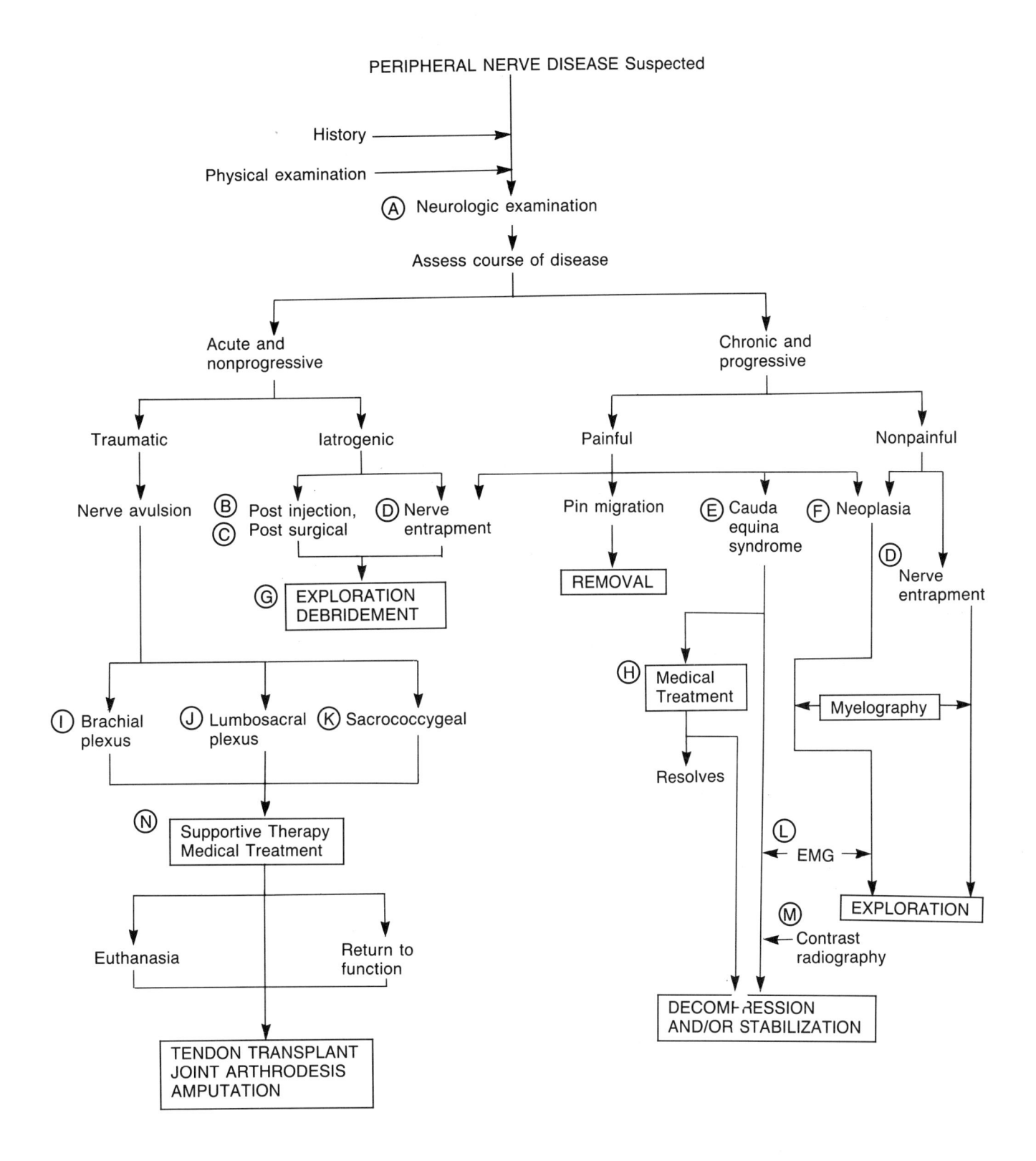

```
                        PERIPHERAL NERVE DISEASE Suspected
                                      │
                    History ──────────→│
                    Physical examination ──→│
                                      │
                              (A) Neurologic examination
                                      │
                                      ▼
                              Assess course of disease
                      ┌───────────────┴───────────────┐
                      ▼                               ▼
              Acute and                         Chronic and
              nonprogressive                    progressive
              ┌───────┴──────┐                ┌───────┴────────┐
              ▼              ▼                ▼                ▼
          Traumatic      Iatrogenic        Painful         Nonpainful
              │         ┌────┴────┐     ┌────┼─────┐          │
              ▼         ▼         ▼     ▼    ▼     ▼          ▼
        Nerve avulsion (B) Post  (D) Nerve  Pin   (E) Cauda  (F) Neoplasia
                        injection, entrapment migration equina         │
                       (C) Post surgical              syndrome       (D) Nerve
                              │                │         │         entrapment
                              ▼                ▼         │
                       (G) EXPLORATION      REMOVAL      │
                           DEBRIDEMENT                   ▼
                                                  (H) Medical
          ┌──────┬──────────┬──────────┐            Treatment ──→ Myelography
          ▼      ▼          ▼          ▼                │
       (I) Brachial (J) Lumbosacral (K) Sacrococcygeal  ▼
          plexus      plexus                         Resolves
              │                                        │
              ▼                                        │   (L) ← EMG →
       (N) Supportive Therapy                          │            │
           Medical Treatment                           │   (M)      ▼
          ┌─────┴─────┐                                │   ← Contrast  EXPLORATION
          ▼           ▼                                │     radiography
       Euthanasia  Return to                           ▼
                   function                    DECOMPRESSION
                      │                        AND/OR STABILIZATION
                      ▼
              TENDON TRANSPLANT
              JOINT ARTHRODESIS
              AMPUTATION
```

145

HEAD TILT

Joane Parent

A. It is important to distinguish acute nonprogressive conditions from progressive ones. The idiopathic feline and canine vestibular syndromes are peracute and self-limiting. Infectious otitis media-interna progressively worsens. Aminoglycosides can produce vestibular nerve degeneration. Otitis media-interna is common in the Cocker Spaniel. The cat also has a high incidence of middle-inner ear infection secondary to mite infestation. The idiopathic vestibular syndrome of the dog usually occurs in elderly canines; whereas the congenital disorder appears around 3 to 4 weeks of age.

B. Particular attention is given to the ear examination. Sedation or general anesthesia should be used if the patient does not allow adequate visualization of the ear canals and tympanic membranes. If infection is present, a sample is taken for culture and sensitivity.

C. Head tilt is the salient feature of central and peripheral vestibular disorders. The most important step is differentiating between the peripheral and central forms.

D. In peripheral vestibular disease, the head tilt may be accompanied by abnormal nystagmus or balance loss (with leaning, rolling, or falling). The nystagmus is horizontal or rotatory and does not change with head position. Horner's syndrome and facial paralysis may also be present.

E. In central vestibular disease, the head tilt may be accompanied by abnormal nystagmus that may be horizontal, rotatory, or vertical and that may change with head position. Concomitant signs of other brain stem abnormalities are usually present; these are depression (indicating reticular formation involvement), incoordination, and cranial nerve deficits. As a rule, central vestibular disease carries a guarded to poor prognosis.

F. Obtain bullae radiographs under heavy sedation or general anesthesia; take open-mouth and left and right oblique views.

G. With intracalvarial extradural tumors, the cerebrospinal fluid (CSF) analysis is normal on cytologic examination. Vascular accidents, although poorly documented in the central nervous system of dogs, can also go undetected on CSF analysis.

H. In otitis media-interna, radiographs of the bullae may be normal. Because infection can ascend through the auditory tube, the external ear canal can be normal. Broad-spectrum antibiotics that cross the blood-brain-barrier (trimethoprim-sulphonamide, chloramphenicol) should be given for at least 6 to 8 weeks.

I. Most of the peripheral vestibular diseases fall in this category. Syndromes such as canine geriatric vestibular disease, feline vestibular neuropathy, and congenital vestibular disorder are self-limiting, and medical treatment is unnecessary. However, tranquilizers are sometimes required in order to prevent self-inflicted trauma which may be caused by falling and rolling. Head tilt is not well compensated for in domestic species. It does improve, but often persists for the animal's life.

J. If medical treatment of otitis media has failed, or if a neoplasm is suspected, surgical exploration is necessary. A ventral approach is preferable. Culture and sensitivity and biopsy of the bulla(e) are taken. In cases of infectious disease, drains are positioned and left in place for 7 to 10 days; antibiotic therapy is continued for 6 to 8 weeks.

References

DeLahunta A. Vestibular system-special proprioception. In: De Lahunta A, ed. Veterinary neuroanatomy and clinical neurology. 2nd ed. Philadelphia: WB Saunders, 1983; 238.

Oliver JE, Lorenz MD. Handbook of veterinary neurologic diagnosis. Philadelphia: WB Saunders, 1983: 227.

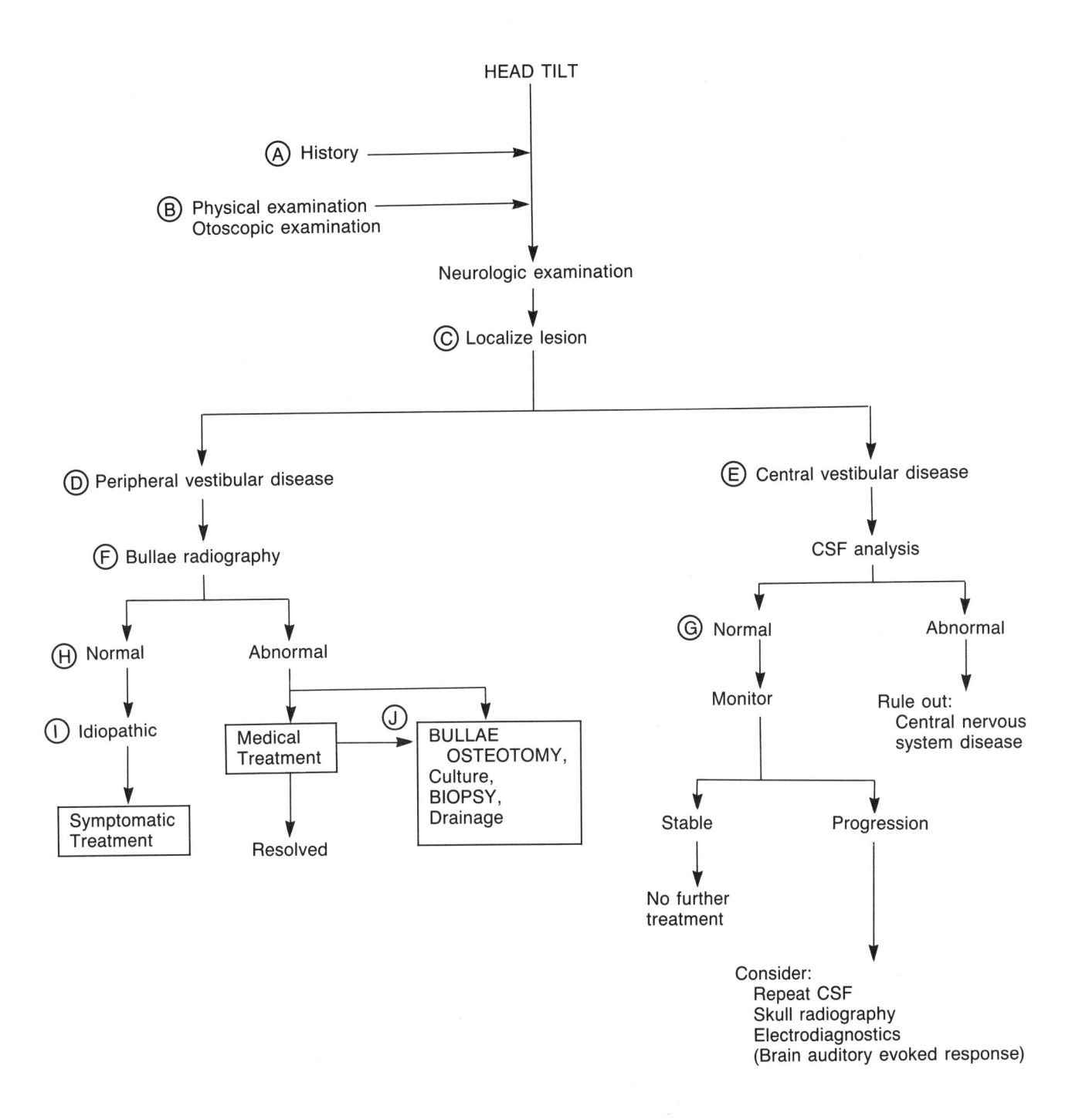

HEAD TILT

- (A) History
- (B) Physical examination / Otoscopic examination
- Neurologic examination
- (C) Localize lesion

(D) Peripheral vestibular disease
- (F) Bullae radiography
  - (H) Normal
    - (I) Idiopathic
      - Symptomatic Treatment
  - Abnormal
    - Medical Treatment → Resolved
    - (J) BULLAE OSTEOTOMY, Culture, BIOPSY, Drainage

(E) Central vestibular disease
- CSF analysis
  - (G) Normal
    - Monitor
      - Stable → No further treatment
      - Progression → Consider: Repeat CSF, Skull radiography, Electrodiagnostics (Brain auditory evoked response)
  - Abnormal
    - Rule out: Central nervous system disease

DEEP RED EYE

Melanie M. Williams
Bernhard M. Spiess

A. An owner may present an animal because redness of the ocular tissues has been noticed. This may be the only abnormality, or there may be ocular pain, discharge, increased lacrimation, blepharospasm, or photophobia. Preliminary examination reveals hyperemia of the ocular tissues, termed "red" eye. Further categorization of the hyperemia is helpful in diagnosing the ocular disease.

B. Conjunctival or superficial hyperemia imparts a diffuse, bright red color to the tissue. Individual conjunctival vessels are small, bright red, tortuously branched, and difficult to discern as individual vessels. When the conjunctiva is elevated with blunt forceps, the vascularity (redness) can be seen to move with the elevated conjunctiva. Application of dilute epinephrine (1:100,000) results in blanching of the conjunctival vessels within 15 seconds. Injection of conjunctival vessels in the absence of deep vessel injection is indicative of an extraocular eye disease such as conjunctivitis, keratitis, or keratoconjunctivitis.

C. Deep or episcleral (ciliary) vessels reside in the episclera and supply both this tissue and the anterior uvea. They appear as deep red, discrete, relatively straight vessels that run parallel to one another and perpendicular to the limbus. These vessels disappear from view approximately 1 mm posterior to the limbus. When the conjunctiva is elevated with blunt forceps, the episcleral vessels do not elevate, but remain fixed in position. Topical application of dilute epinephrine (1:100,000) does not result in blanching of episcleral vessels within 15 seconds. Deep vessel injection is indicative of scleral, deep corneal, or intraocular eye disease such as uveitis or glaucoma (Fig. 1).

D. Intraocular pressure (IOP) is most frequently evaluated by means of Schiotz's indentation tonometry. This procedure involves application of Schiotz's tonometer to the animal's cornea following topical corneal anesthesia. The animal's nose is positioned skyward, and the footplate of the tonometer is positioned entirely on the cornea with no bulbar conjuctival contact. The edge of the footplate should be flush with the corneal surface, and the tonometer must sit perpendicular to the corneal surface. An average of three measurements is calculated. The three measurements should approximate each other. If a 5.5 g-weight is used, a reading on the tonometer scale of 3 to 4 is normal in the canine and feline. If converted to mm of Hg, this is equivalent to 20 to 24 mm Hg on the human chart (chart accompanying the tonometer) or 33 to 38 mm Hg on the canine chart. IOP should be recorded as follows: first give the weight of the tonometer, then the reading on the scale on the tonometer, and finally the conversion to mm Hg (conversion chart utilized), e.g., 5.5 g:3:20 mm Hg (human chart).

E. Episcleritis refers to inflammation of the episclera, which may be present in a focal, nodular, or diffuse form. The conjunctiva and episcleral vessels appear to be injected locally or diffusely. Thickening of the episcleral tissues and invasion of the limbic cornea occur. Hypotony presumably results from a decreased resistance to aqueous humor outflow in the dilated scleral vascular outflow channels. An immune-mediated etiology is suspected. Therapy consists of anti-inflammatory medications such as corticosteroids, which are administered topically, subconjunctivally, and/or parenterally. The disease frequently becomes chronic or recurrent. The majority of cases remain limited to the anterior episclera.

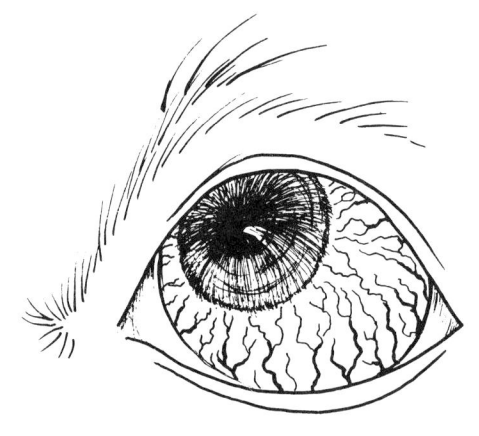

Figure 1 Deep vascular hyperemia due to injection of episcleral/ciliary vessels.

References

Dice PF. The canine cornea. In: Gelatt KN, ed. Textbook of veterinary ophthalmology. Philadelphia: Lea & Febiger, 1981: 343.

Helper LC. The canine nictitating membrane and conjunctiva. In: Gelatt KN, ed. Textbook of veterinary ophthalmology. Philadelphia: Lea & Febiger, 1981:330.

Keller WF. The canine anterior urea. In: Gelatt KN, ed. Textbook of veterinary ophthalmology. Philadelphia: Lea & Febiger, 1981:375.

Slatter DH. Cornea and sclera. In: Slatter DH, ed. Fundamentals of veterinary ophthalmology. Philadelphia: WB Saunders, 1981:347.

Slatter DH. Glaucoma. In: Slatter DH, ed. Fundamentals of veterinary ophthalmology. Philadelphia: WB Saunders, 1981:455.

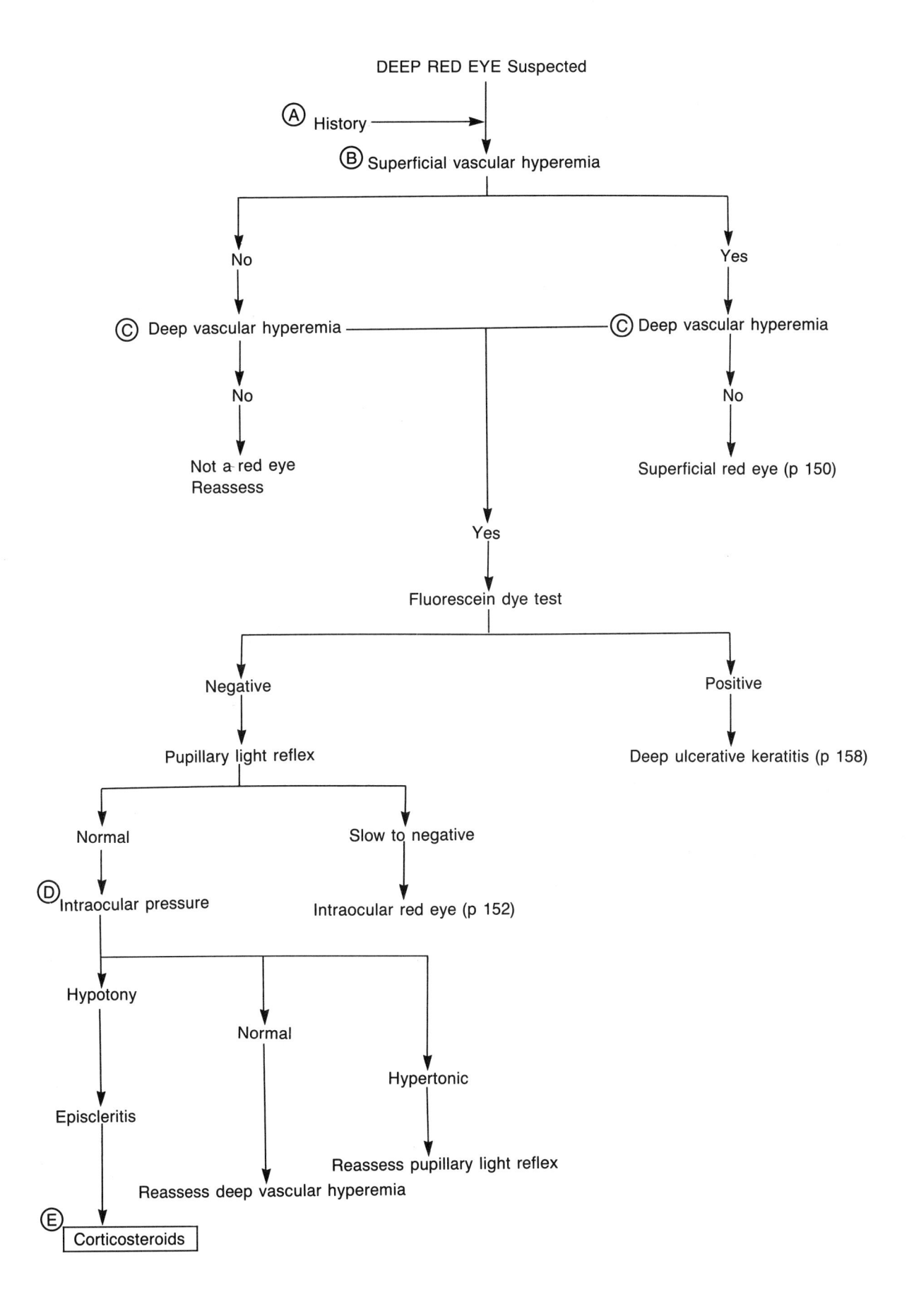

```
                    DEEP RED EYE Suspected
                              │
              Ⓐ History ──────▶│
                              ▼
                  Ⓑ Superficial vascular hyperemia
                    │                    │
                   No                   Yes
                    │                    │
                    ▼                    ▼
        Ⓒ Deep vascular hyperemia ──┐   Ⓒ Deep vascular hyperemia
                    │               │         │
                   No               │        No
                    │               │         │
                    ▼               │         ▼
            Not a red eye           │   Superficial red eye (p 150)
              Reassess              │
                                    ▼
                                   Yes
                                    │
                                    ▼
                          Fluorescein dye test
                              │            │
                          Negative      Positive
                              │            │
                              ▼            ▼
                    Pupillary light    Deep ulcerative keratitis (p 158)
                        reflex
                    │           │
                 Normal    Slow to negative
                    │           │
                    ▼           ▼
        Ⓓ Intraocular    Intraocular red eye (p 152)
            pressure
         │      │      │
      Hypotony Normal Hypertonic
         │      │      │
         ▼      ▼      ▼
    Episcleritis  Reassess    Reassess pupillary
         │       deep vascular    light reflex
         │       hyperemia
         ▼
    Ⓔ [Corticosteroids]
```

149

SUPERFICIAL (EXTRAOCULAR) RED EYE

Melanie M. Williams
Bernhard M. Spiess

A. An owner may present an animal because redness of the ocular tissues has been noted. This may be the only abnormality noted, or there may be mention of ocular pain, discharge, increased lacrimation, blepharospasm, or photophobia.

   Preliminary examination reveals a red eye. The features of the vasculature that impart the redness to the ocular tissues are indicative of superficial or conjunctival hyperemia, without deep or episcleral hyperemia. Superficial vascular hyperemia alone is indicative of extraocular disease, i.e., disease of the conjunctiva, cornea, or both. Conjunctival or superficial hyperemia imparts a diffuse, bright red color to the tissue. Individual conjunctival vessels are small, bright red, tortuously branched, and difficult to discern as individual vessels. When the conjunctiva is elevated with blunt forceps, the vascularity (redness) can be seen to move with the elevated conjunctiva. Application of dilute epinephrine (1:100,000) results in blanching of the conjunctival vessels within 15 seconds. Injection of conjunctival vessels in the absence of deep vessel injection is indicative of an extraocular eye disease such as conjunctivitis, keratitis, or keratoconjunctivitis.

   Deep or episcleral (ciliary) vessels reside in the episclera and supply both this tissue and the anterior uvea. They appear as deep red, discrete, relatively straight vessels that run parallel to one another and perpendicular to the limbus. These vessels disappear from view approximately 1 mm posterior to the limbus. When the conjuctiva is elevated with blunt forceps, the episcleral vessels do not elevate, but remain fixed in position. Topical application of dilute epinephrine (1:100,00) does not result in blanching of episcleral vessels within 15 seconds. Deep vessel injection is indicative of scleral, deep corneal, or intraocular eye disease such as uveitis or glaucoma.

B. The Schirmer I tear test measures the flow of tears, in millimeters, for a 60 second period. The tear production measured in the Schirmer I tear test is basal flow plus reflex flow. The reflex portion is stimulated by the irritative presence of the strip that contacts the conjunctiva and/or cornea. The average Schirmer I result in the canine and feline is 15 mm or greater. A measurement of 10 mm or greater is not likely to result in clinical eye disease unless the Schirmer tear test II value is low.

C. The Schirmer II tear test is performed under topical anesthesia of the cornea and conjunctiva. Anesthesia eliminates the reflex tear production and results in an evaluation of the basal tear production. Two minutes after instillation of topical anesthesia, the inferior conjunctival sac is gently swabbed with a sterile cotton applicator. A Schirmer tear test strip is inserted and tear production is measured after 60 seconds. A measurement of 8 mm or greater is considered normal in the canine and feline. A measurement of 5 to 8 mm may not result in clinical eye disease. At less than 5 mm, clinical eye disease (conjunctivitis or keratoconjunctivitis) is common.

References

Dice PF. The canine cornea. In: Gelatt KN, ed. Textbook of veterinary ophthalmology. Philadelphia: Lea & Febiger, 1981:343.

Gelatt KN, Gwin RM. Canine lacrimal and nasolacrimal systems. In: Gelatt KN, ed. Textbook of veterinary ophthalmology. Philadelphia: Lea & Febiger, 1981:309.

Helper LC. The canine nictitating membrane and conjunctiva. In: Gelatt KN, ed. Textbook of veterinary ophthalmology. Philadelphia: Lea & Febiger, 1981:330.

Slatter DH. Conjunctiva. In: Slatter DH, ed. Fundamentals of veterinary ophthalmology. Philadelphia: WB Saunders, 1981:275.

Slatter DH. Lacrimal system. In: Slatter DH, ed. Fundamentals of veterinary ophthalmology. Philadelphia: WB Saunders, 1981:323.

SUPERFICIAL RED EYE Suspected
↓
(A) Superficial vascular hyperemia

- Absent → Reassess
- Present → (A) Deep vascular hyperemia
  - Present → Reassess (p 148)
  - Absent → (B) Schirmer I tear test
    - < 10 mm per minute → Keratoconjunctivitis sicca (p 162)
    - > 10 mm per minute → (C) Schirmer II tear test
      - < 8 mm per minute → Keratoconjunctivitis sicca (p 162)
      - > 8 mm per minute → Fluorescein dye test
        - Negative → Conjunctivitis (p 156)
        - Positive → Superficial ulcerative keratitis (p 158)

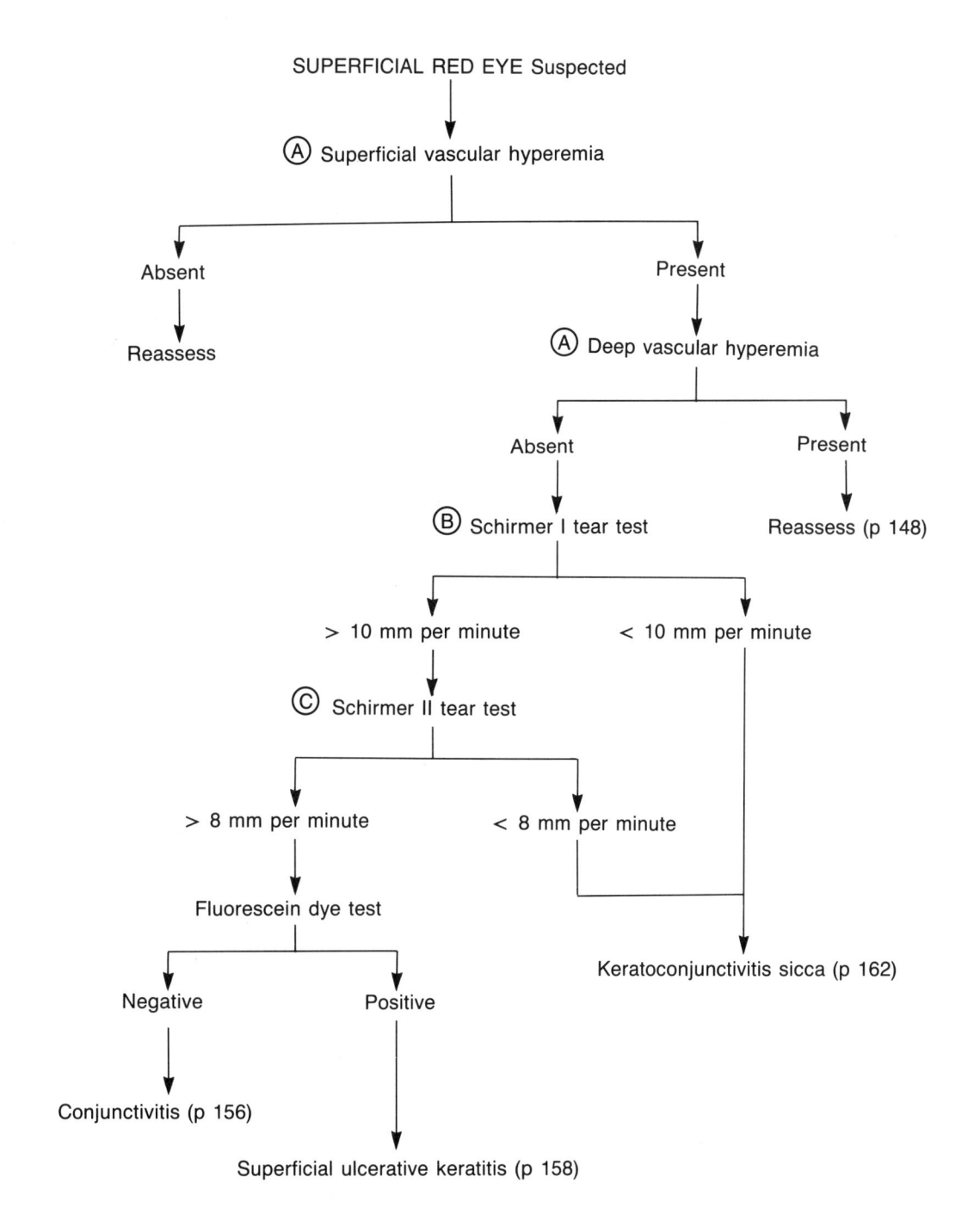

INTRAOCULAR RED EYE

Melanie M. Williams
Bernhard M. Spiess

A. Deep vessel injection is indicative of scleral, deep corneal, or intraocular eye disease such as uveitis or glaucoma.

B. Uveitis produces a hypotonic eye on account of decreased aqueous humor production by the inflamed ciliary body and decreased scleral vascular resistance to aqueous humor outflow. Glaucoma produces a hypertonic eye caused by impaired outflow of aqueous humor at the level of the filtration angle or at the pupil. Chronic uncontrolled glaucoma can eventually cause pressure destruction of the ciliary body epithelium, which results in decreased aqueous humor production, commonly termed "burnt-out" glaucoma. The intraocular pressure is low or normal.

C. Inflammatory cells and fibrin from uveitis may block aqueous humor flow through the pupil (posterior synechia) or may obstruct the filtration angle, which can result in secondary glaucoma.

D. Common primary uveal intraocular tumors include melanoma, and ciliary body adenoma and adenocarcinoma. Common metastatic neoplastic diseases of the uveal tissue are lymphosarcoma and feline leukemia-associated neoplasia.

E. Observation of Purkinje-Sanson's images (P-S images) assists in the localization of lens position. Lens dislocation may cause glaucoma by interfering with aqueous humor drainage. Alternatively, glaucoma can lead to megaloglobus, zonular rupture, and lens dislocation. A dislocated lens can move about within the ocular cavities. Movement may be minimal or extensive and may result in further vitreal displacement or periodic pupil blockage and filtration angle impairment. This labile situation can produce fluctuations in IOP.

F. The following drug therapy is recommended for immune-mediated uveitis: a steroidal anti-inflammatory drug given topically; a systemic nonsteroidal anti-inflammatory drug (ASA 25 mg per kilogram twice a day); a parasympatholytic mydriatic—cycloplegic given topically (atropine 1 percent every 1 to 4 hours); a sympathomimetic mydriatic topically (dipivefrin HCl-epinephrine 0.1 percent every 12 hours); and systemic antibiotic prophylaxis or specific treatment if there is an infective component.

G. Drug therapy for embolic infectious uveitis, or intraocular infection is as follows: specific therapy for the systemic septicemia, i.e., antibiotics given systemically and topically; and a nonsteroidal anti-inflammatory agent PO, a parasympatholytic mydriatic—cycloplegic given topically (atropine), and a sympathomimetic mydriatic given topically (dipivefrin HCl-epinephrine 0.1 percent) as outlined in F.

H. In the case of glaucoma secondary to uveitis, the following drug therapy is recommended: an osmotic diuretic provided that the uveitis is quiescent, (mannitol IV 1 to 2 g per kilogram); a steroidal anti-inflammatory drug given topically (every 4 to 8 hours); a systemic nonsteroidal anti-inflammatory drug PO,(ASA 25 mg per kilogram given twice a day); a sympathomimetic mydriatic topically (dipivefrin-epinephrine given every 12 hours); a carbonic anhydrase inhibitor PO, (acetazolamide 10 to 25 mg daily divided into two or three times a day doses, methazolamide 2 to 10 mg daily divided into two doses, dichlorphenamide 10 to 15 mg daily divided in two daily doses); and cyclocryotherapy once the uveitis is quiescent.

I. Primary intraocular neoplasia may produce a glaucoma. Melanoma, adenoma, and adenocarcinoma are the most common tumors. Glaucoma therapy is only a temporary measure, and enucleation is eventually required for the animal's comfort.

J. "Burnt-out" or "end-stage" glaucoma usually appears as a megaloglobus eye that is normotensive or hypotonic; therefore, glaucoma therapy is not required. If there is exposure keratitis from the megaloglobus, lubricating medications, tarsorrhaphy, or enucleation may be required.

K. In the case of glaucoma with labile intraocular pressure on account of lens mobility, drug therapy is as follows: give an osmotic diuretic (mannitol IV) and a carbonic anhydrase inhibitor as outlined in H; and give a sympathomimetic mydriatic (dipivefrin HCl-epinephrine 0.1 percent - see F) and/or a cholinergic miotic (pilocapine) topically (1 to 2 percent twice to three times daily). Avoid cholinergic miotics with anterior lens luxation (see L). With posterior lens luxation a cholinergic miotic may help retain the lens in the posterior segment of the globe. Perform cyclocryotherapy in a visual eye; consider cyclocryotherapy, pharmacologic ablation of the ciliary body, intrascleral prosthesis, or enucleation in the case of an irreversibly blind eye.

L. Glaucoma secondary to anterior lens luxation or subluxation should be treated as follows: give an osmotic diuretic (mannitol) and a carbonic anhydrase inhibitor as outlined in H and perform surgical lens removal in an anterior chamber lens luxation. Give a cholinergic miotic if the lens is in the posterior chamber and not obstructing the pupil; give a sympathomimetic mydriatic (dipivefrin-epinephrine) if the pupil is blocked by lens dislocation (see F); and perform cyclocryotherapy. Consider pharmacologic ablation of the ciliary body, intrascleral prosthesis, or enucleation in the case of an irreversibly blind eye.

M. The following therapy is recommended for primary glaucoma: an osmotic diuretic (mannitol IV-see H); a carbonic anhydrase inhibitor PO (see H); a cholinergic miotic topically (pilocarpine-see K); a sympathomimetic mydriatic topically (dipivefrin HCl-epinephrine 0.1 percent-see H).

References

Brightman AH, Vestre WA, Helper LC, Tomes JE. Cryosurgery for the treatment of canine glaucoma. JAAHA 1982; 18:319.

```
INTRAOCULAR RED EYE Suspected
                │
              (A) Deep vascular hyperemia
              ┌───┴───┐
          Positive  Negative
              │       │
       Fluorescein   Reassess (p 148)
        dye test
       ┌────┴────┐
   Positive    Negative
       │          │
   Reassess   Pupillary light reflex
   (p 158)    ┌────┴────┐
         Slow or negative  Normal
              │              │
          Pupil Size    Reassess (p 148)
       ┌──────┴──────┐
  Mild constriction  Miotic
       │               │
  (B) Intraocular   (B) Intraocular
      pressure          pressure
      (p 148)           (p 148)
   ┌───┴───┐        ┌────┴────┐
 Hypertony Hypotony Hypotony Hypertony
     │        │       │          │
 Glaucoma          Uveitis   (C) Glaucoma
 likely                          secondary
 secondary                       to uveitis
 to anterior                        │
 lens luxation               (H) Therapy
 or subluxation
              Systemic
              evaluation for:
           ┌──────┴──────┐
        Neoplasia    Septicemia
```

(D) Uveitis secondary to neoplasia of iris or ciliary body

Present ─── Absent ─── Present
              │
         Immune-mediated
         uveitis likely
              │
         (F) Therapy

Embolic infectious uveitis
         (G) Therapy

(L)
Osmotic Diuretic (Mannitol IV)
LENS REMOVAL
and/or Carbonic Anhydrase
Inhibitor
Sympathomimetic topically
(Epinephrine)

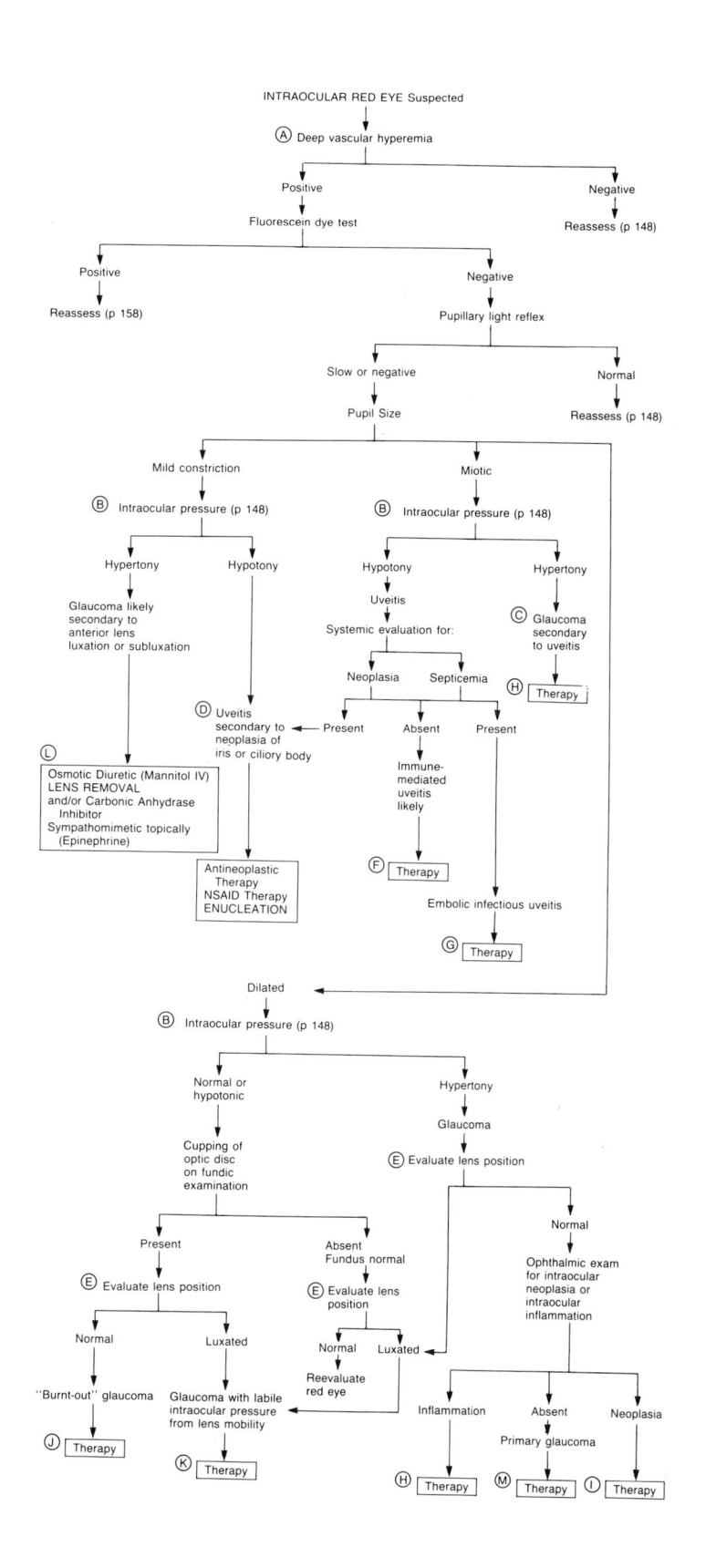

Antineoplastic Therapy
NSAID Therapy
ENUCLEATION

Dilated
│
(B) Intraocular pressure (p 148)
┌────┴────┐
Normal or hypotonic   Hypertony
│   │
Cupping of optic disc Glaucoma
on fundic examination │
┌────┴────┐   (E) Evaluate lens position
Present Absent   ┌────┴────┐
│   Fundus normal Luxated Normal
(E) Evaluate   │   │
lens position   │   Ophthalmic exam
┌───┴───┐   │   for intraocular
Normal Luxated   │   neoplasia or
│   │   │   intraocular
"Burnt-out" Glaucoma with   inflammation
glaucoma   labile intraocular ┌───┬───┐
(J) Therapy pressure from   Inflammation Absent Neoplasia
            lens mobility   Primary
            (K) Therapy   glaucoma
(E) Evaluate lens position
┌───┴───┐
Normal Luxated
│
Reevaluate red eye

(H) Therapy   (M) Therapy   (I) Therapy

Gelatt KN, Keller WF. The canine anterior uvea. In: Gelatt KN, ed. Textbook of veterinary ophthalmology. Philadelphia: Lea & Febiger, 1981:375.

Moyer I, Cook CS, Peiffer RL, Nasisse MP, Harling DE. Indications for and complications of pharmacological ablation of the ciliary body for the treatment of chronic glaucoma in the dog. JAAHA 1986; 22:319.

Slatter DH, ed. Uvea. In: Fundamentals of veterinary ophthalmology. Philadelphia: WB Saunders, 1981:409.

Vestre WA. Use of cyclocryotherapy in management of glaucoma in dogs. Mod Pract Feb 1984: 93.

CLOUDY EYE

Melanie M. Williams
Bernhard M. Spiess

Localization of an ocular opacity can be simplified by ascertaining its proximity to the Purkinje-Sanson images. When a focal light beam is directed into the eye, the light reflects off three surfaces. The first reflection (P-S #1) is upright, bright, and located on the convex corneal surface. The second reflection (P-S #2) is smaller, greyish, upright, and located on the anterior lens capsule. The third reflection (P-S #3) is tiny, grey, inverted, and located on the posterior lens capsule. If the light source is moved from side to side, the P-S #1 and #2 move with the light source; whereas the third P-S image moves in the opposite direction to the light source. An ocular opacity may be localized at the level of a particular P-S image or between two P-S images.

A. Corneal cloudiness produces an opacity at the level of P-S #1.

B. The anterior chamber and its contents correspond to the space between P-S #1 and P-S #2.

C. In uveitis, elevated aqueous humor protein and inflammatory cells produce cloudiness. Excessive amounts of protein and cells may settle ventrally and produce a white mass (pus) in the anterior chamber (hypopyon). Occasionally, lipids produce a cloudy aqueous humor. For this to occur, there must be a breakdown of the blood-aqueous barrier (uveitis).

D. The edematous area is localized to the ulcer and the immediate surrounding corneal stroma.

E. The lens is assessed as P-S #2 and #3 and the space between the two.

F. Elevated intraocular pressure causes corneal haze due to edema. The sodium-potassium pump, located in the corneal endothelial cells, functions subnormally under the influence of elevated intraocular pressure. Thus aqueous humor that normally enters the cornea is not pumped back into the anterior chamber. This effect, combined with a pressure-driven increase in aqueous humor entrance into the cornea, produces a diffuse corneal edema.

G. Uveitis produces a corneal haze on account of failure of the corneal endothelial sodium-potassium pump to remove aqueous humor that enters the cornea. Keratic precipitates, which adhere to the corneal endothelium in uveitis, also contribute to corneal haze.

H. A cataract is any opacity of the lens or its capsule. An anterior capsular cataract is an opacity at the level of P-S image #2. A posterior capsular cataract is an opacity at the level of P-S image #3. A nuclear or cortical cataract occurs behind P-S image #2 and may, if extensive, obliterate P-S image #3. Therapy for a cataract is lens extraction, provided that the cataract is primary (i.e., not caused by other ocular disease), blinding, and in an eye with normal retinal function.

I. Vitreal opacity appears posterior to P-S image #3.

J. Inflammatory exudate in the anterior vitreous can be identified without the aid of an ophthalmoscope as white flocculent material. Posterior vitreal exudate may produce a whitish or cloudy reflex through the pupil, but may require an ophthalmoscope for clear examination.

K. Cataract of the anterior lens capsule is most commonly associated with a posterior synechia from uveitis or occasionally from a persistent pupillary membrane (PPM).

L. Persistent pupillary membranes that cause corneal cloudiness are identified as white or brown strands; these strands originate from the iris face and cross the anterior chamber to the posterior surface of the cornea (corneal endothelium), or occasionally to the anterior surface of the lens. Therapy is not usually indicated.

M. The normal retina cannot be examined without the use of an ophthalmoscope. Retinal elevation or detachment displaces the retina anteriorly, which can then be identified without an ophthalmoscope as a grey veil of tissue that contains red blood vessels. Therapy depends upon the etiology of the retinal detachment. The most common etiologies include posterior uveitis, neoplasia, hypertension with renal or thyroid disease, trauma, and heredity.

N. Corneal epidermalization appears as vascularity, fibrosis, and eventually pigmentation as the corneal tissue becomes epidermis-like. Lipid deposition appears as white crystalline deposits in the cornea and may be secondary (associated with antecedent corneal vascularity) or primary (without antecedent corneal vascularization). If there is a vascular component, decrease scarring by the use of a topical steroid. Lipid deposition is not affected by this therapy, but if superficial within the cornea, can be removed by superficial keratectomy if vision is being impaired. In primary lipid dystrophy, redeposition occurs in the cornea.

O. Primary corneal endothelial dystrophy occurs more commonly in female middle-aged Boston Terriers; however, it has been noted in Chihuahuas and aged dogs of various other breeds. Hyperosmolar NaCl ophthalmic drops or ointment (2 to 5 percent) are required several times daily in order to minimize bulla formation and subsequent ulceration.

References

Dice PF. The canine cornea. In: Gelatt KN, ed. Textbook of veterinary ophthalmology. Philadelphia: Lea & Febiger, 1981:343.

Gelatt KN. The canine glaucomas. In: Gelatt KN, ed. Textbook of veterinary ophthalmology. Philadelphia: Lea & Febiger, 1981:390.

Keller WF. The canine anterior uvea. In: Gelatt KN, ed. Textbook of veterinary ophthamology. Philadelphia: Lea & Febiger, 1981:375.

Slatter DH. Cornea and sclera. In: Slatter DH. Fundamentals of

```
                                    CLOUDY EYE
                                         │
                                         ▼
                                    Assess cornea
                          ┌──────────────┴──────────────┐
                          ▼                             ▼
                      (A) Cloudy                     Clear
                          │                             │
                          ▼                             ▼
                  Fluorescein eye test          (B) Assess anterior chamber
                   ┌──────┴──────┐                 ┌────┴────┐
                   ▼             ▼                 ▼         ▼
                Positive      Tonometry        (C) Cloudy   Clear
                   │                               │           │
                   ▼                               ▼           ▼
               (D) Ulcerative                  Tonometry   (E) Assess lens
                   keratitis
```

Tonometry branches:
- Elevated intraocular pressure → (F) Glaucoma (p 152)
- Normal → (L) Examine for persistent pupillary membrane (PPM)
- Hypotonic → (G) Uveitis → Medical Therapy (p 152)
- Normotensive or hypertensive → Uveitis with secondary glaucoma → Medical Therapy (p 152)

Assess lens:
- Cloudy → (H) Cataract → Assess pupil
  - Normal → Cataract → LENS EXTRACTION
  - (K) Synechia → Cataract with associated uveitis (p 152)
  - (L) PPM with focal cataract
- Clear → (I) Assess vitreal cavity
  - Clear → Reassess commencing at cornea
  - (J) Inflammatory exudate → Posterior uveitis
  - (M) Grey veil of tissue with vessels → Retinal detachment

(L) Examine for persistent pupillary membrane (PPM):
- Present → Corneal scar with associated endothelial attachment of PPM
- Absent → Examine for corneal vascularity
  - Present → (N) Corneal scarring with epidermalization and/or secondary lipid deposition → Steroid Therapy / SUPERFICIAL KERATECTOMY
  - Absent:
    - Crystalline deposit centrally or paracentrally in the cornea → (N) Primary corneal lipid deposition (lipid corneal dystrophy)
      - No treatment
      - Impaired vision → SUPERFICIAL KERATECTOMY
    - Diffuse haze often with cobblestoned pattern → (O) Primary endothelial dystrophy with corneal edema
      - NaCl Ophthalmic Drops or Ointment
      - Secondary corneal ulcer → Ulcerative Keratitis Therapy (p 158)

veterinary ophthalmology. Philadelphia: WB Saunders, 1981:347.

Slatter DH. Uvea. In: Slatter DH, ed. Fundamentals of veterinary ophthalmology. Philadelphia: WB Saunders, 1981:409.

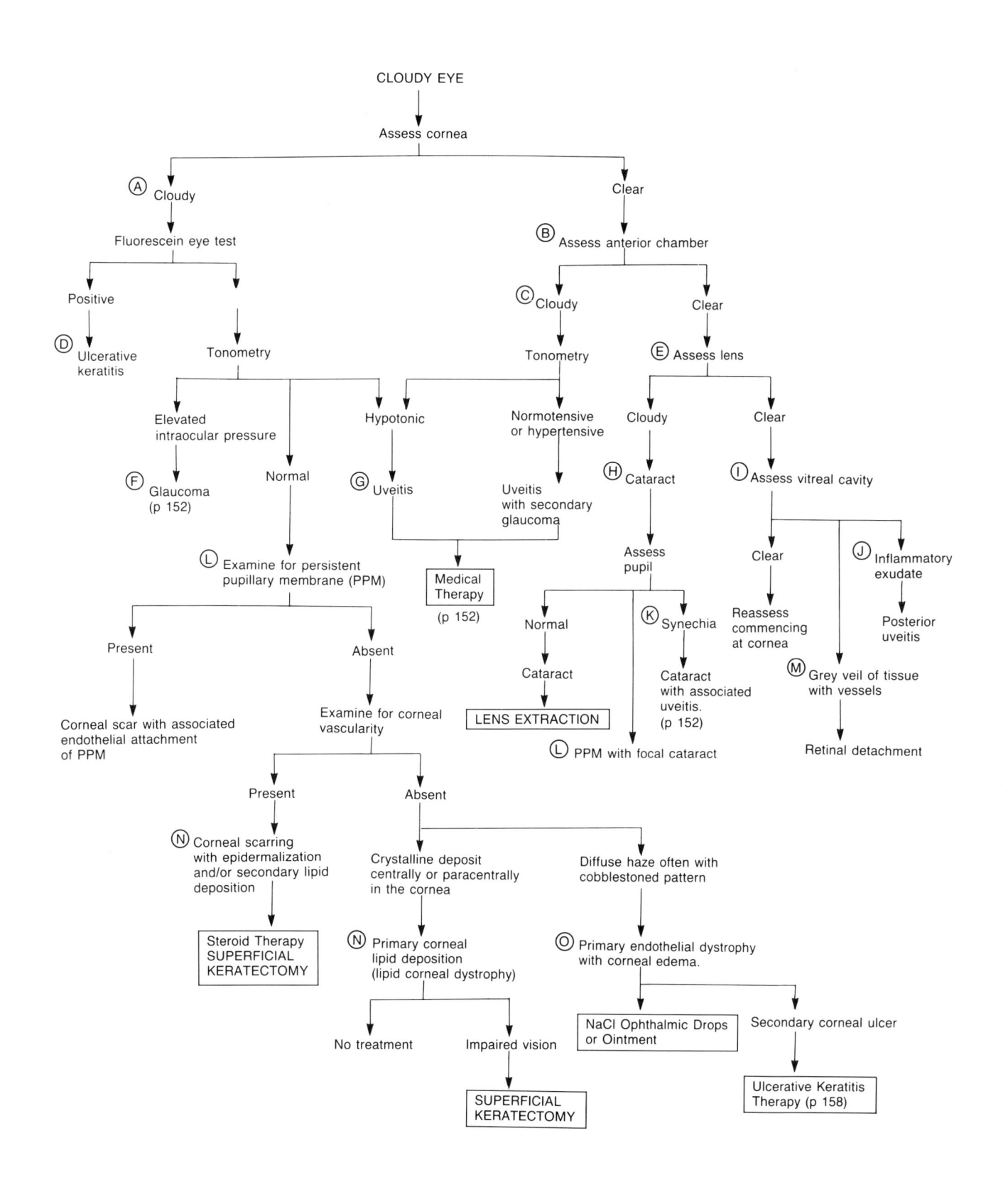

CONJUNCTIVITIS

Melanie M. Williams
Bernhard M. Spiess

A. Injection of conjunctival vessels in the absence of deep vessel injection (episcleral and/or ciliary) is indicative of extraocular eye disease. Conjunctival hyperemia imparts a diffuse, bright red color to the conjunctiva. Individual conjunctival (superficial) vessels are small, bright red, tortuously branched, and difficult to discern. When the conjunctiva is elevated with blunt forceps, the vascularity (redness) can be seen to move with the elevated conjunctiva. Application of dilute epinephrine (1:100,000) results in blanching of the conjunctival vessels within 15 seconds of application.

B. Deep vessel injection is indicative of scleral, deep corneal, or intraocular eye disease. Episcleral and ciliary vessels reside in the episclera. When injected, they appear as deep red, discrete, relatively straight vessels that run parallel to one another and perpendicular to the limbus. These vessels disappear from view approximately 1 to 2 mm posterior to the limbus. When the conjunctiva is elevated with blunt forceps, the episcleral vessels do not elevate, but remain fixed in position. Topical application of dilute epinephrine (1:100,000) does not result in blanching of episcleral vessels within 15 seconds.

C. Conjunctival scrapings and specific culture for chlamydia, herpes virus, or mycoplasma support the diagnosis.

D. The nasolacrimal excretary system is evaluated for patency by passage of fluorescein dye and by cannulation and saline flushing.

E. Meibomian gland openings should be identified on the eyelid margin. Gently squeeze the eyelid (general anesthesia may be required) in order to express glandular and ductule contents which are normally a milky fluid. Abnormal contents or enlarged white ducts suggest glandular infection or impaction. Examine abnormal glandular content cytologically and by culture and sensitivity in order to assist therapeutic drug choice.

F. Extraocular diseases such as sinusitis, dermatitis, otitis externa, dental abscessation, and systemic diseases can cause secondary conjunctivitis.

G. Transient conjunctivitis is common in the canine, especially in working dogs following field or water work. Irritants such as wind, dust, vegetation, and particulate matter are often the inciting agents.

H. Conjunctival neoplasms include squamous cells carcinoma and plasmoma. Plasmoma is a controversial term that implies plasma cell infiltration of the conjunctiva. This produces a chronic, persistent conjunctivitis that is seen most commonly in German Shepherd dogs. Other neoplasms include hemangioma, hemangiosarcoma, and melanoma.

References

Gelatt KN. The canine nictitating membrane and conjunctiva. In: Gelatt KN, ed. Textbook of veterinary ophthalmology. Philadelphia: Lea & Febiger, 1981:330.

Slatter DH. Conjunctiva. In: Slatter DH, ed. Fundamentals of veterinary ophthalmology. Philadelphia: WB Saunders, 1981:275.

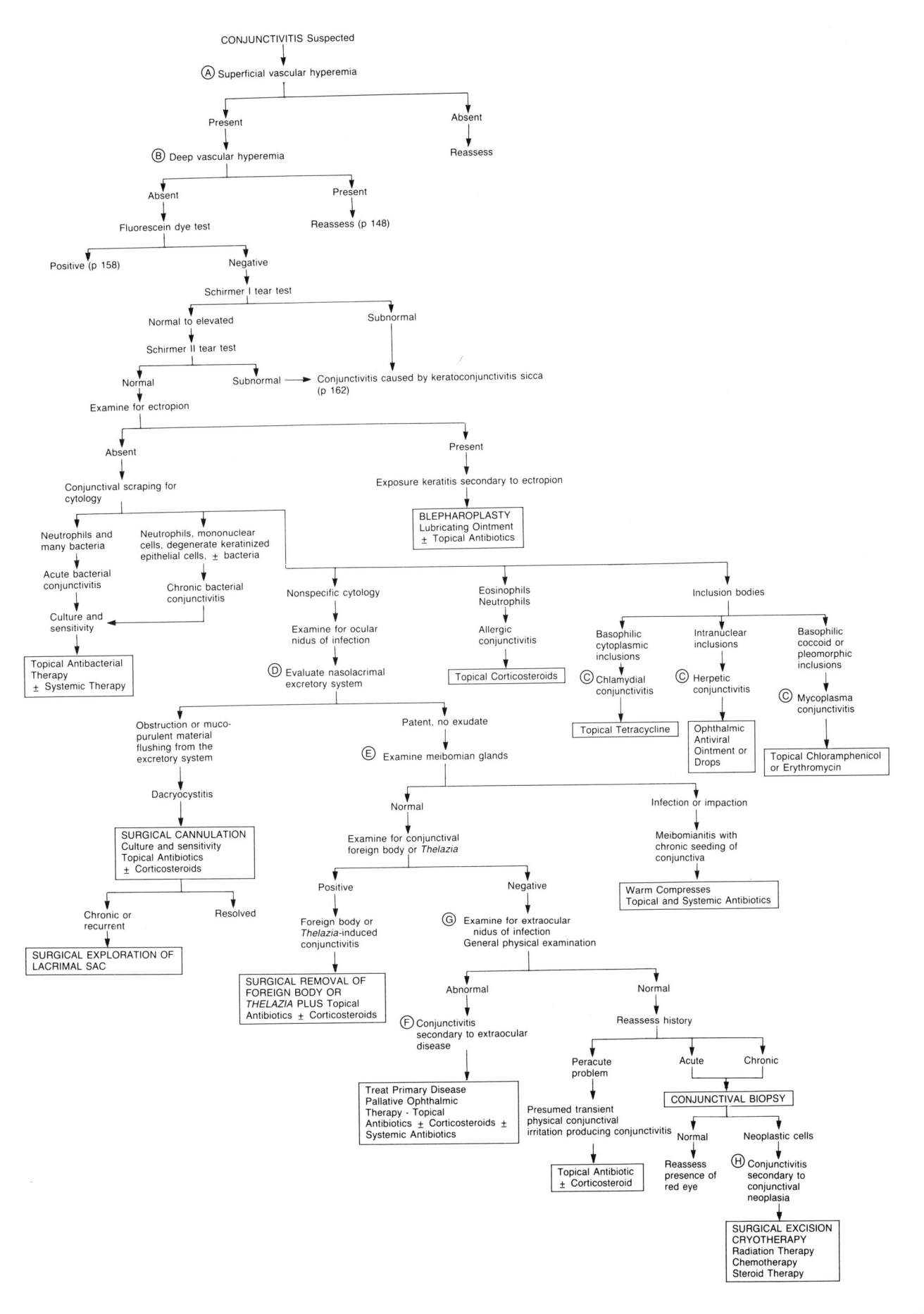

```
CONJUNCTIVITIS Suspected
            │
            ▼
   Ⓐ Superficial vascular hyperemia
       │                │
    Present          Absent
       │                │
       ▼             Reassess
   Ⓑ Deep vascular hyperemia
       │                │
    Absent           Present
       │                │
       ▼           Reassess (p 148)
   Fluorescein dye test
       │                │
   Positive (p 158)  Negative
                        │
                        ▼
                  Schirmer I tear test
                   │              │
          Normal to elevated   Subnormal
                   │              │
                   ▼              ▼
           Schirmer II tear test   Conjunctivitis caused by keratoconjunctivitis sicca (p 162)
            │            │
         Normal      Subnormal ──► (above)
            │
            ▼
      Examine for ectropion
       │                │
    Absent           Present
       │                │
       ▼          Exposure keratitis secondary to ectropion
  Conjunctival scraping for cytology
                              │
                              ▼
                        BLEPHAROPLASTY
                        Lubricating Ointment
                        ± Topical Antibiotics
```

- Neutrophils and many bacteria → Acute bacterial conjunctivitis → Culture and sensitivity → **Topical Antibacterial Therapy ± Systemic Therapy**
- Neutrophils, mononuclear cells, degenerate keratinized epithelial cells, ± bacteria → Chronic bacterial conjunctivitis
- Nonspecific cytology → Examine for ocular nidus of infection → Ⓓ Evaluate nasolacrimal excretory system
- Eosinophils Neutrophils → Allergic conjunctivitis → **Topical Corticosteroids**
- Inclusion bodies:
  - Basophilic cytoplasmic inclusions → Ⓒ Chlamydial conjunctivitis → **Topical Tetracycline**
  - Intranuclear inclusions → Ⓒ Herpetic conjunctivitis → **Ophthalmic Antiviral Ointment or Drops**
  - Basophilic coccoid or pleomorphic inclusions → Ⓒ Mycoplasma conjunctivitis → **Topical Chloramphenicol or Erythromycin**

Ⓓ Evaluate nasolacrimal excretory system:
- Obstruction or mucopurulent material flushing from the excretory system → Dacryocystitis → **SURGICAL CANNULATION** Culture and sensitivity, Topical Antibiotics ± Corticosteroids
  - Chronic or recurrent → **SURGICAL EXPLORATION OF LACRIMAL SAC**
  - Resolved
- Patent, no exudate → Ⓔ Examine meibomian glands
  - Normal → Examine for conjunctival foreign body or *Thelazia*
    - Positive → Foreign body or *Thelazia*-induced conjunctivitis → **SURGICAL REMOVAL OF FOREIGN BODY OR THELAZIA PLUS Topical Antibiotics ± Corticosteroids**
    - Negative → Ⓖ Examine for extraocular nidus of infection; General physical examination
      - Abnormal → Ⓕ Conjunctivitis secondary to extraocular disease → **Treat Primary Disease; Palliative Ophthalmic Therapy - Topical Antibiotics ± Corticosteroids ± Systemic Antibiotics**
      - Normal → Reassess history
        - Peracute problem → Presumed transient physical conjunctival irritation producing conjunctivitis → **Topical Antibiotic ± Corticosteroid**
        - Acute / Chronic → **CONJUNCTIVAL BIOPSY**
          - Normal → Reassess presence of red eye
          - Neoplastic cells → Ⓗ Conjunctivitis secondary to conjunctival neoplasia → **SURGICAL EXCISION CRYOTHERAPY Radiation Therapy, Chemotherapy, Steroid Therapy**
  - Infection or impaction → Meibomianitis with chronic seeding of conjunctiva → **Warm Compresses; Topical and Systemic Antibiotics**

ULCERATIVE KERATITIS

Melanie M. Williams
Bernhard M. Spiess

A. The trigeminal nerve forms the afferent arm of the palpebral reflex. The zygomatic (maxillary) branch provides sensory innervation to the lateral canthus, while the ophthalmic branch provides sensory innervation to the medial canthus. The efferent motor arm of the reflex is the facial nerve.

B. Lagophthalmos (incomplete or ineffective eyelid closure) may be caused by an anatomic imbalance between the eyelids, globe, and orbit or by neurologic dysfunction. Poor tear film distribution and excessive evaporation ensues, which results in exposure keratoconjunctivitis.

C. The sensory afferent arm of the corneal reflex is the ophthalmic branch of the trigeminal nerve; the facial nerve provides the motor efferent arm. Lid closure should result.

D. Distichiasis is common in the canine and may be nonoffensive and unrelated to the ulcerative keratitis. In such a case, the distichia require no therapy. If the distichia are the cause of the ulcerative keratitis, they are located on the portion of the lid margin that contacts the ulcerative area during lid movements (Fig. 1).

E. Lagophthalmos caused by an enlarged palpebral fissure occurs in some breeds of dogs, including the American Cocker Spaniel and brachycephalic breeds. A prominent exposed globe which is the result of a shallow bony orbit, occurs in brachycephalics. Exophthalmos that is caused by an orbital space-occupying lesion may occur in any breed. All result in excessive corneal and conjunctival exposure, which is accompanied by lagophthalmos.

F. The afferent arm of the menace reflex is formed by the retina, optic nerve, optic chiasm, optic tract, optic radiation, and visual cortex. The facial nerve provides the motor efferent arm. In a sighted animal, with the aforementioned neurologic structures functional, lid closure results.

G. Facial nerve dysfunction is the cause of lagophthalmos in a sighted animal. Utilize obstacle course and cotton ball testing if a visual abnormality is suspected.

H. Ulcer solution should consist of basic components that include an artificial tear base, plus an antimicrobial agent, plus acetylcysteine for anticollagenase activity. Atropine sulfate may be added if there is a secondary iridocyclitis, as indicated by miosis in the affected eye. Acetylcysteine acts by direct bathing of the ulcer and, therefore, is most effective when applied to the wound rather than over a flap.

I. Corneal erosion syndrome (indolent or recurrent corneal erosions) occurs most frequently in the Boxer breed, but also in middle-aged to older dogs and cats of any breed. The epithelium attempts to slide and mitose in order to cover the defect; however, inadequate basement membrane prevents proper adherence of the epithelium to the underlying stroma. Corneal neovascularizaton is markedly delayed.

J. The use of a conjunctival or membrana nictitans flap is warranted when an ulcer has not healed after 2 weeks of appropriate treatment or if there is a danger of rupture.

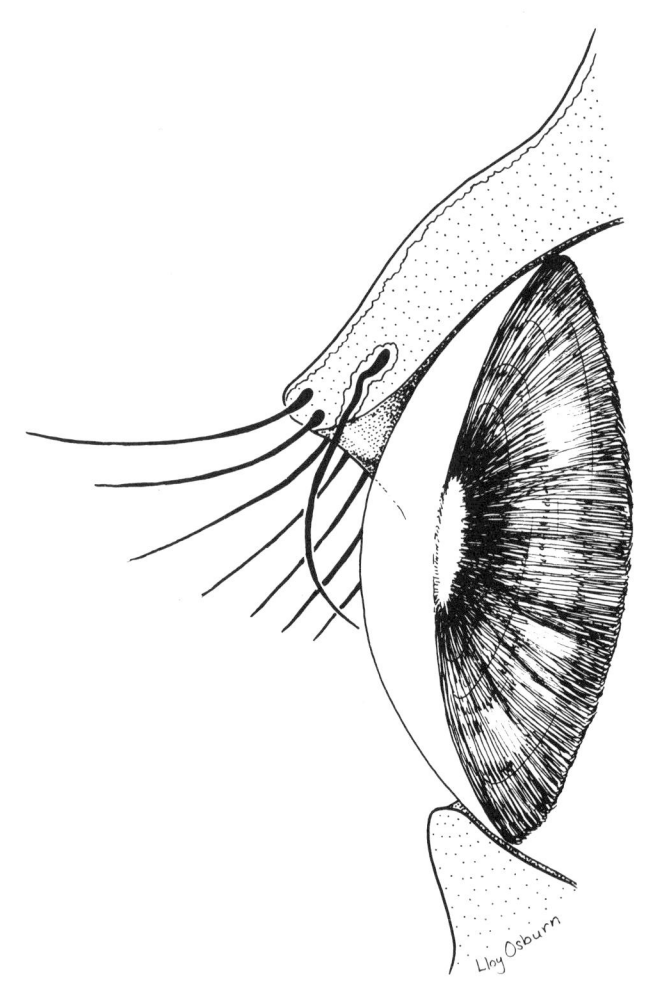

Figure 1 Distichiasis. Aberrant hair emanating from meibomian gland opening resulting in corneal irritation.

References

Dice PF. The canine cornea. In: Gelatt KN, ed. Textbook of veterinary ophthalmology. Philadelphia: Lea & Febiger, 1981:343.

Slatter DH. Cornea and sclera. In: Slatter DH, ed. Fundamentals of veterinary ophthalmology. Philadelphia: WB Saunders, 1981:347.

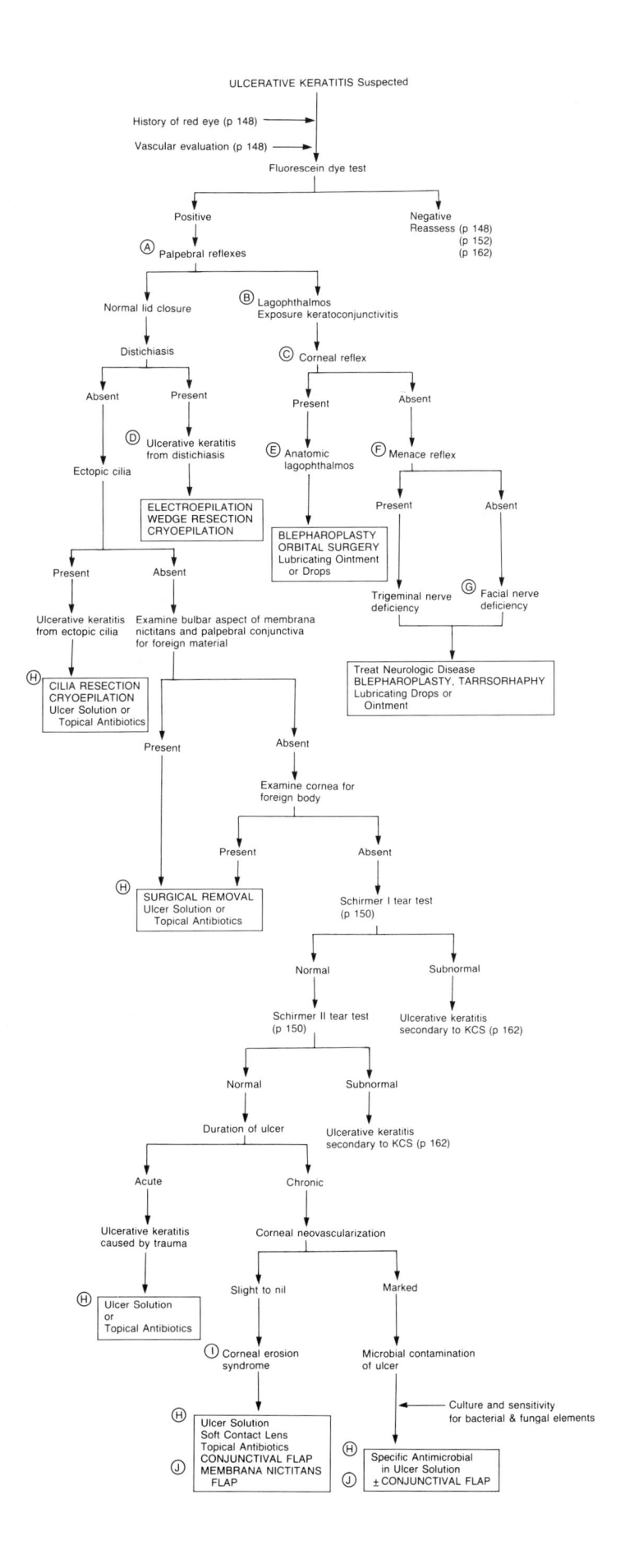

```
ULCERATIVE KERATITIS Suspected
        │
History of red eye (p 148) ──────┐
Vascular evaluation (p 148) ─────┤
                                 ▼
                         Fluorescein dye test
                          │              │
                       Positive       Negative
                          │           Reassess (p 148)
                          ▼                   (p 152)
                    Ⓐ Palpebral reflexes      (p 162)
                    │                    │
            Normal lid closure    Ⓑ Lagophthalmos
                    │              Exposure keratoconjunctivitis
               Distichiasis              │
              │          │         Ⓒ Corneal reflex
           Absent     Present       │            │
              │          │       Present      Absent
         Ectopic     Ⓓ Ulcerative    │            │
          cilia      keratitis   Ⓔ Anatomic   Ⓕ Menace reflex
                    from distichiasis lagophthalmos   │        │
                          │              │         Present   Absent
                    ┌─────────────┐  ┌──────────────┐    │        │
                    │ELECTROEPILATION│ │BLEPHAROPLASTY│ Trigeminal  Ⓖ Facial
                    │WEDGE RESECTION│ │ORBITAL SURGERY│   nerve      nerve
                    │ CRYOEPILATION │ │Lubricating    │ deficiency  deficiency
                    └─────────────┘  │Ointment       │      │        │
        │          │                 │or Drops       │      └────┬───┘
     Present    Absent               └──────────────┘           ▼
        │          │                                    ┌──────────────┐
   Ulcerative  Examine bulbar aspect of membrana        │Treat Neurologic Disease│
   keratitis   nictitans and palpebral conjunctiva      │BLEPHAROPLASTY, TARRSORHAPHY│
   from ectopic for foreign material                    │Lubricating Drops or │
   cilia                │                               │Ointment             │
        │          ┌────┴────┐                          └──────────────┘
        │       Present    Absent
        ▼          │          │
 ┌──────────────┐  │     Examine cornea for
 │Ⓗ CILIA RESECTION│ │     foreign body
 │ CRYOEPILATION│  │      │         │
 │ Ulcer Solution│ │   Present    Absent
 │ or Topical   │  │      │         │
 │ Antibiotics  │  │      ▼      Schirmer I tear test
 └──────────────┘  │ ┌──────────┐   (p 150)
                   │ │Ⓗ SURGICAL │   │         │
                   │ │ REMOVAL  │ Normal   Subnormal
                   │ │ Ulcer Solution│ │       │
                   │ │ or Topical│  Schirmer II  Ulcerative keratitis
                   │ │ Antibiotics│ tear test   secondary to KCS (p 162)
                   │ └──────────┘  (p 150)
                                    │       │
                                 Normal  Subnormal
                                    │       │
                              Duration of  Ulcerative keratitis
                                  ulcer    secondary to KCS (p 162)
                                │      │
                              Acute  Chronic
                                │      │
                       Ulcerative    Corneal neovascularization
                       keratitis       │           │
                       caused by    Slight to nil  Marked
                       trauma          │            │
                          ▼       Ⓘ Corneal    Microbial
                 ┌──────────┐    erosion      contamination
                 │Ⓗ Ulcer   │    syndrome     of ulcer
                 │ Solution │       │            │
                 │ or Topical│      ▼      ◀── Culture and sensitivity
                 │ Antibiotics│ ┌─────────┐    for bacterial & fungal
                 └──────────┘ │Ⓗ Ulcer Solution│  elements
                              │Soft Contact Lens│    │
                              │Topical Antibiotics│  ▼
                              │ⒿCONJUNCTIVAL FLAP│ ┌──────────────┐
                              │ MEMBRANA NICTITANS│ │Ⓗ Specific Antimicrobial│
                              │ FLAP           │  │ in Ulcer Solution │
                              └─────────────┘    │Ⓙ± CONJUNCTIVAL FLAP│
                                                  └──────────────┘
```

WET EYE

Bernhard M. Spiess
Melanie M. Williams

The "wet" eye is a common presenting sign. Often, it is congenital and some of the disorders may have a genetic basis. Treatment in most cases consists of surgical correction of the problem.

A. Inadequate drainage of the tear fluid is called *epiphora* in contrast to *lacrimation*, which is a result of hypersecretion.

B. Entropion and ectropion are frequently diagnosed in several breeds. In most cases surgical correction is easily performed, and the results are usually good.

C. Distichia can be treated by electroepilation and various lid-splitting techniques. The results are not always satisfactory. Recently, cryosurgery has been shown to provide good results. Ectopic cilia, which emerge from the palpebral conjunctiva, can be removed by core biopsy with a small (2 mm) trephine.

D. Lid tumors are frequently found in older dogs. Surgical excision is recommended for small tumors. If large areas of the eyelid are involved, cryosurgery is preferred.

E. The upper and lower puncta can be involved; however, absence or narrowing of the upper punctum rarely causes clinical signs. Flushing of the canaliculi through the open punctum reveals a bleb at the site of the imperforate punctum. The bleb is incised, and patency is maintained with an indwelling polyethylene tube for 2 to 3 weeks (Fig. 1). The lacrimal puncta and canaliculi may be too narrow to allow adequate drainage of tears and may require surgical enlargement.

F. The nasolacrimal duct can be blocked by mucous debris or foreign bodies. Establish patency by repeated flushing and cannulating. Atresia may or may not prove amenable to surgical correction.

G. Blepharospasm and serous discharge are often the only signs in cases of superficial corneal ulceration. In uncomplicated cases the lesion reepithelializes in a few days. In older dogs, and especially in Boxers, epithelial erosions may become a recurrent problem. Application of soft contact lenses for 8 to 14 days provides excellent results in such cases. Alternatively, a topical solution of 5 percent sodium chloride enhances adhesion of the epithelium to the underlying basement membrane and often prevents recurrences.

H. Trichiasis is a condition in which hair that arises from a normal location is misdirected towards the globe. Clipping is sufficient in most cases. Surgical removal of a nasal or facial fold may be indicated in brachycephalic dogs.

I. Eversion of the membrana nictitans is another condition that lends itself to surgical correction. Under general anesthesia, the abnormally curved part of the cartilage is removed. The condition is often complicated by prolapse of the gland of the third eyelid. Removal of the gland may predispose to keratoconjunctivitis sicca and is therefore not recommended. Techniques for suturing the gland back into a normal position have been described and provide excellent results.

References

Blogg JR. Surgical replacement of a prolapsed gland of the third eyelid ("cherry eye")—a new technique. Austr Vet Pract 1979; 9:75.

Gelatt KN, Gwin RM. Canine lacrimal and nasolacrimal systems. In: Gelatt KN, ed. Textbook of veterinary ophthalmology. Philadelphia: Lea & Febiger, 1981:309.

Kaswan RL, Martin CL. Surgical correction of third eyelid prolapse in dogs. JAVMA 1985; 186:83.

Peiffer RL, Gelatt KN, Karpinski LG. The canine eyelids. In: Gelatt KN, ed. Textbook of veterinary ophthalmology. Philadelphia: Lea & Febiger, 1981:277.

Slatter DH. Eyelids. In: Slatter DH, ed. Fundamentals of veterinary ophthalmology, Philadelphia: WB Saunders, 1981:200.

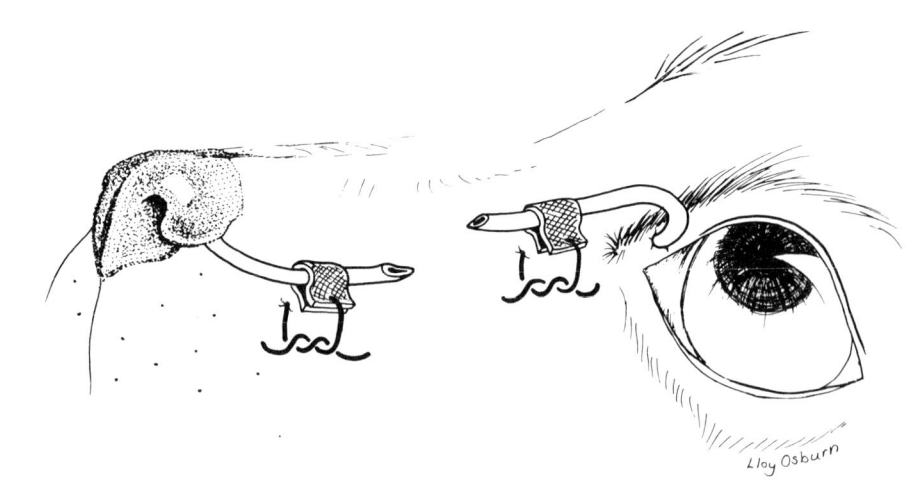

Figure 1 Indwelling nasolacrimal duct catheter to maintain patency.

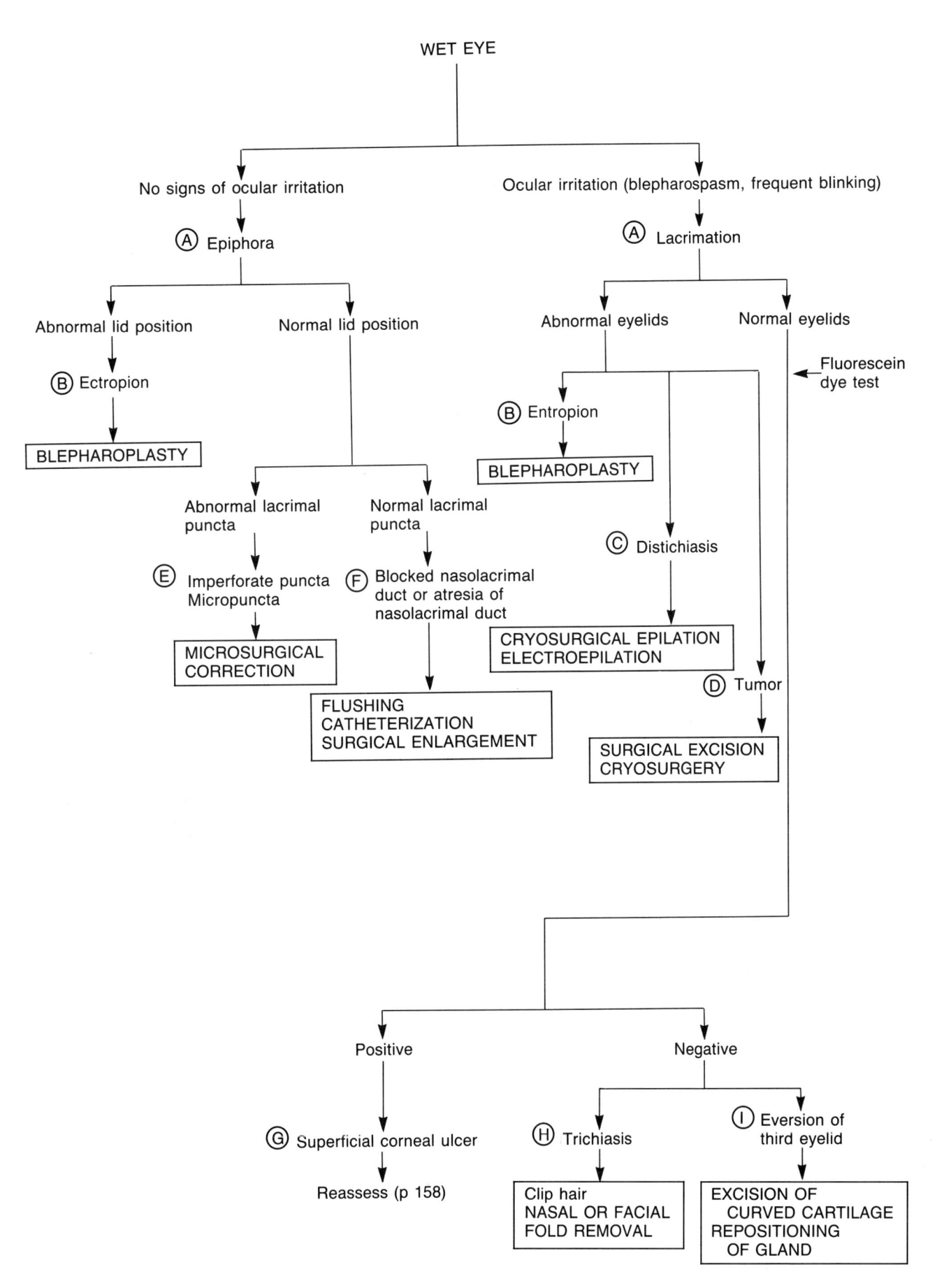

WET EYE

```
                                    WET EYE
                                       │
                ┌──────────────────────┴──────────────────────┐
        No signs of ocular irritation           Ocular irritation (blepharospasm, frequent blinking)
                │                                              │
            Ⓐ Epiphora                                     Ⓐ Lacrimation
                │                                              │
        ┌───────┴───────┐                              ┌───────┴───────┐
  Abnormal lid      Normal lid                    Abnormal         Normal
   position          position                      eyelids         eyelids
        │               │                              │              │
   Ⓑ Ectropion                                    Ⓑ Entropion    ← Fluorescein
        │                                              │              dye test
  ┌───────────┐                                 ┌───────────┐
  │BLEPHARO-  │                                 │BLEPHARO-  │
  │PLASTY     │                                 │PLASTY     │
  └───────────┘                                 └───────────┘
                ┌───────┴────────┐                     │
         Abnormal lacrimal   Normal lacrimal      Ⓒ Distichiasis
              puncta            puncta                 │
                │                 │              ┌──────────────┐
         Ⓔ Imperforate    Ⓕ Blocked naso-     │CRYOSURGICAL   │
           puncta           lacrimal duct        │EPILATION      │
           Micropuncta      or atresia of        │ELECTROEPILATION│
                │           nasolacrimal duct    └──────────────┘
         ┌──────────┐             │                     
         │MICRO-    │       ┌──────────────┐       Ⓓ Tumor
         │SURGICAL  │       │FLUSHING       │            │
         │CORRECTION│       │CATHETERIZATION│      ┌──────────────┐
         └──────────┘       │SURGICAL       │      │SURGICAL       │
                            │ENLARGEMENT    │      │EXCISION       │
                            └──────────────┘      │CRYOSURGERY    │
                                                  └──────────────┘
```

```
                    ┌───────────────┴───────────────┐
                 Positive                        Negative
                    │                               │
         Ⓖ Superficial corneal ulcer      ┌────────┴────────┐
                    │                  Ⓗ Trichiasis    Ⓘ Eversion of
             Reassess (p 158)               │            third eyelid
                                      ┌──────────┐           │
                                      │Clip hair │    ┌─────────────┐
                                      │NASAL OR  │    │EXCISION OF   │
                                      │FACIAL    │    │CURVED CARTILAGE│
                                      │FOLD      │    │REPOSITIONING │
                                      │REMOVAL   │    │OF GLAND      │
                                      └──────────┘    └─────────────┘
```

161

CHRONIC PURULENT OCULAR DISCHARGE

Bernhard M. Spiess
Melanie M. Williams

Unilateral or bilateral purulent ocular discharge is a common presenting complaint.

A. In any case of chronic purulent ocular discharge, material must be collected for bacterial and fungal culture and sensitivity *prior* to the application of topical anesthetics, mydriatics, or dyes, as these solutions have antibacterial activity. Moisten the cotton swab with culture medium prior to collection, in order to increase the yield of organisms.

B. Tear production *must* be evaluated in cases of chronic ocular discharge. A Schirmer test in the unanesthetized eye (Schirmer I) measures both basal and reflex tear production. After topical anesthesia the latter component is eliminated, and basal tear production is measured (Schirmer II). Note that atropine and topical and general anesthesia decrease tear production. In allergic conditions, and in viral and early bacterial infections excessive lacrimation may occur.

C. A fluorescein dye test should be done in any case of ocular inflammation. Sterile fluorescein strips, which are individually packed, are preferred over fluorescein solutions, which may easily be contaminated. Flush excess dye from the eye before examining the result.

D. Mechanical irritation as a cause of ulcerative keratitis must be ruled out; consider foreign bodies, lid malformations, distichiasis, trichiasis, and ectopic cilia.

E. Keratoconjunctivitis sicca (KCS) is a common disease entity in the canine species. The goal of KCS therapy is prevention of corneal desiccation. This can be accomplished by medical therapy, such as artificial tears supplemented by acetylcysteine (a mucolytic agent) and antibiotics. Pilocarpine may be given topically or orally in an attempt to stimulate tear production.

F. Surgical therapy, parotid duct transposition, is indicated if topical medication proves insufficient. In this operation, the duct and the papilla of the parotid salivary gland are dissected free and transposed to the eye, where the papilla is sutured to the lateral aspect of the lower conjunctival sac. Frequent feeding stimulates salivation and lubrication of the eye.

G. In dacryocystitis, inflammatory reactions and discharge are restricted to the medial canthal area, with most of the remaining ocular adnexa uninvolved. Dacryocystitis is often caused by foreign bodies. Repeated flushing of the nasolacrimal duct, under general anesthesia if necessary, may dislodge a foreign body or a mucus plug. Maintain patency of the duct with an indwelling catheter for 2 to 4 weeks, and give systemic and topical antibiotics. The lacrimal sac may have to be opened surgically in order to remove an imbedded foreign body.

H. Conjunctivitis can be caused by bacterial, viral, or fungal organisms; by allergens; by malformation of the eyelids; or by foreign bodies. Conjunctivitis is often associated with systemic diseases. Careful examination and conjunctival scrapings and/or biopsies establish a diagnosis.

I. A large spectrum of skin diseases may involve the eyelids. The most common bacterial organisms found are staphylococci and streptococci. The meibomian glands may harbor bacteria, which are not reached by systemic or topical antibiotics. Frequent manual expression of the glands under topical anesthesia and hot packs are helpful in the management of such conditions.

References

Dice PF. The canine cornea. In: Gelatt KN, ed. Textbook of veterinary ophthalmology. Philadelphia: Lea & Febiger, 1981:343.

Helper LC. The canine nictitating membrane and conjunctiva. In: Gelatt KN, ed. Textbook of veterinary ophthalmology. Philadelphia: Lea & Febiger, 1981: 330.

Peiffer RL, Gelatt KN, Karpinski LG. The canine eyelids. In: Gelatt KN, ed. Textbook of veterinary ophthalmology. Philadelphia: Lea & Febiger, 1981:277.

Slatter DH. Eyelids. In: Slatter DH, ed. Fundamentals of veterinary ophthalmology. Philadelphia: WB Saunders, 1981.200.

Slatter DH. Conjunctiva. In: Slatter DH, ed. Fundamentals of veterinary ophthalmology. Philadelphia: WB Saunders, 1981:275.

CHRONIC PURULENT OCULAR DISCHARGE

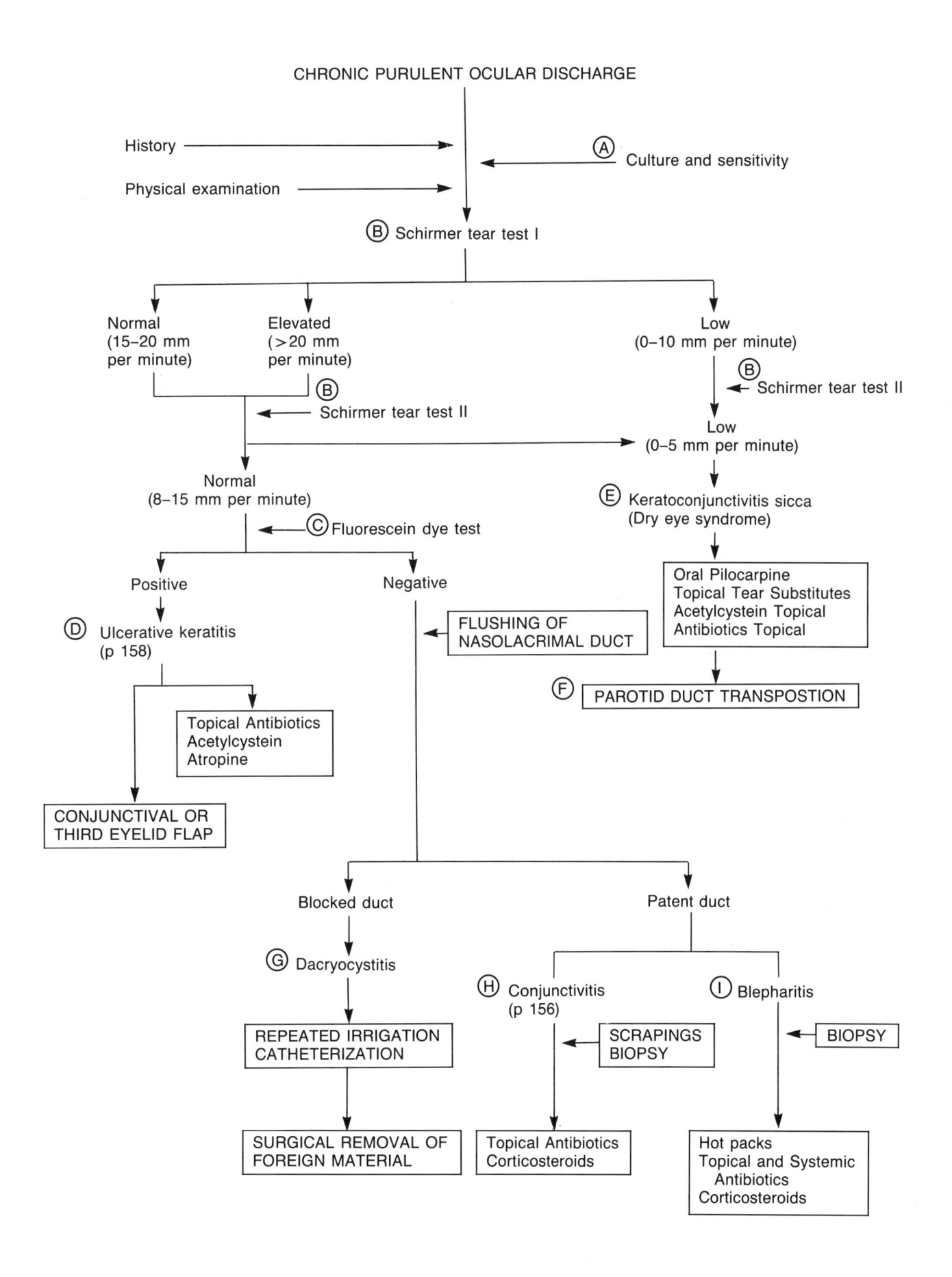

```
History ──────────────────►       ◄────── Ⓐ Culture and sensitivity
Physical examination ─────►
                                  │
                                  ▼
                          Ⓑ Schirmer tear test I
         ┌────────────────────────┼────────────────────────┐
         ▼                        ▼                        ▼
      Normal                  Elevated                    Low
    (15–20 mm               (>20 mm                   (0–10 mm
    per minute)             per minute)              per minute)
         └────────┬───────────────┘                        │
                  ▼  Ⓑ                                     ▼ Ⓑ
                  ◄─── Schirmer tear test II         ◄─── Schirmer tear test II
                  │                                        │
                  ▼                                        ▼
              Normal ────────────────────────────────►   Low
           (8–15 mm per minute)                        (0–5 mm per minute)
                  │                                        │
                  ▼ ◄── Ⓒ Fluorescein dye test            ▼ Ⓔ Keratoconjunctivitis sicca
         ┌────────┴────────┐                               (Dry eye syndrome)
         ▼                 ▼                               │
      Positive          Negative                           ▼
         ▼                 ▲                         ┌─────────────────────┐
     Ⓓ Ulcerative         │                         │ Oral Pilocarpine    │
       keratitis          │  ┌──────────────────┐   │ Topical Tear        │
       (p 158)            │◄─┤ FLUSHING OF      │   │   Substitutes       │
         │                │  │ NASOLACRIMAL DUCT│   │ Acetylcystein       │
         ▼                │  └──────────────────┘   │   Topical           │
   ┌─────────────┐        │                         │ Antibiotics Topical │
   │ Topical     │        │                         └─────────────────────┘
   │ Antibiotics │        │                                 │
   │ Acetylcystein│       │                                 ▼
   │ Atropine    │        │                         Ⓕ ┌─────────────────┐
   └─────────────┘        │                            │ PAROTID DUCT    │
         │                │                            │ TRANSPOSTION    │
         ▼                │                            └─────────────────┘
┌──────────────┐          │
│ CONJUNCTIVAL │          │
│ OR THIRD     │          │
│ EYELID FLAP  │          │
└──────────────┘          │
                ┌─────────┴─────────┐
                ▼                   ▼
           Blocked duct         Patent duct
                ▼             ┌──────┴──────┐
         Ⓖ Dacryocystitis    ▼             ▼
                │          Ⓗ Conjunctivitis  Ⓘ Blepharitis
                │             (p 156)
                │          ◄── SCRAPINGS   ◄── BIOPSY
                │              BIOPSY
                ▼                ▼             ▼
    ┌──────────────────┐   ┌──────────────┐  ┌──────────────────┐
    │ REPEATED         │   │ Topical      │  │ Hot packs        │
    │ IRRIGATION       │   │ Antibiotics  │  │ Topical and      │
    │ CATHETERIZATION  │   │ Corticosteroids │  Systemic        │
    └──────────────────┘   └──────────────┘  │   Antibiotics    │
                │                            │ Corticosteroids  │
                ▼                            └──────────────────┘
    ┌──────────────────┐
    │ SURGICAL REMOVAL │
    │ OF FOREIGN       │
    │ MATERIAL         │
    └──────────────────┘
```

PROTRUDING EYE

Bernhard M. Spiess
Melanie M. Williams

Protrusion of an eye is usually unilateral and is readily recognized by the owner because of the facial asymmetry. It has to be differentiated from bilateral prominence of the eyes in breeds with shallow orbits such as the Pug, Pekinese, and the Shih Tzu.

A. Differentiate by careful examination between true *exophthalmos* (forward displacement of the globe) and *buphthalmos* or megaloglobus (enlargement of a normally located globe).

B. Chronic elevation of intraocular pressure (IOP) leads to irreversible enlargement of the eye, especially in young animals. Chronically elevated IOP often causes secondary corneal lesions if the cornea is no longer protected and lubricated by normal blinking. If the cornea is in good condition, the eye can be eviscerated and an intrascleral silicon prosthesis implanted. This causes the globe to shrink to the size of the chosen implant. Alternatively, the eye may be enucleated.

C. The most common intraocular tumor in dogs is the uveal melanoma. It usually arises from the ciliary body and grows unrecognized until its expansive growth causes secondary glaucoma and megaloglobus. The metastatic potential is very low. If the affected eye becomes painful, treatment consists of enucleation.

D. Exophthalmos and subconjunctival hemorrhage in a dog with a history of trauma suggests retrobulbar hemorrhage, which is usually self-limiting and does not require therapy. However, compression of the optic nerve may affect vision, and a fundic examination may reveal damage to the posterior segment. In rare cases, retrobulbar and subconjunctival hemorrhage may be the presenting sign of warfarin intoxication.

E. Orbital cellulitis and abscessation is common in dogs; the acute onset of exophthalmos differentiates this from other orbital diseases. Other signs of orbital inflammation are pain on opening the mouth, periorbital swelling, chemosis, pyrexia, and anorexia. A fluctuant swelling behind the last upper molar is almost pathognomonic. Drain the orbital abscess through an incision behind the last upper molar. Insert a hemostat into the incision and slowly advance it into the orbit. Systemic antibiotics are used, and a favorable response is usually evident within days.

F. Leakage of saliva from the zygomatic salivary gland or duct, either spontaneously or after trauma, causes inflammation and fibrosis. Mucoceles are usually painless. Drainage from behind the last upper molar reveals a yellow, viscid fluid. Excision of the mucocele and the associated gland is the treatment of choice.

G. A variety of both primary and metastatic neoplasms, e.g., fibrosarcoma, osteosarcoma, meningioma, glioma, and chondrosarcoma, have been reported in dogs. The majority of these tumors are malignant. Exact localization within the orbit can be difficult. Radiography, ultrasonography, and angiography are used to diagnose and localize orbital tumors. Complete removal of all neoplastic tissue by exenteration of the orbit is necessary. Small tumors may be removed with retention of the eye.

H. A pulsating exophthalmos with an orbital "bruit" upon auscultation is diagnostic for an intraorbital arteriovenous (A-V) fistula. Confirm the diagnosis by angiography (p 98). If secondary ocular lesions develop from exposure of the globe, try ligation of the common or the internal carotid artery.

References

Barrie KP, Lavach JD, Gelatt KN. Diseases of the canine posterior segment. In: Gelatt KN, ed. Textbook of veterinary ophthalmology. Lea & Febiger, 1981:474.

Carter JD. Diseases of the canine orbit. In: Gelatt KN, ed. Textbook of veterinary ophthalmology. Lea & Febiger, 1981:265.

Slatter DH. Orbit. In: Slatter DH, ed. Fundamentals of veterinary ophthalmology. Philadelphia: WB Saunders, 1981:662.

PROTRUDING EYE

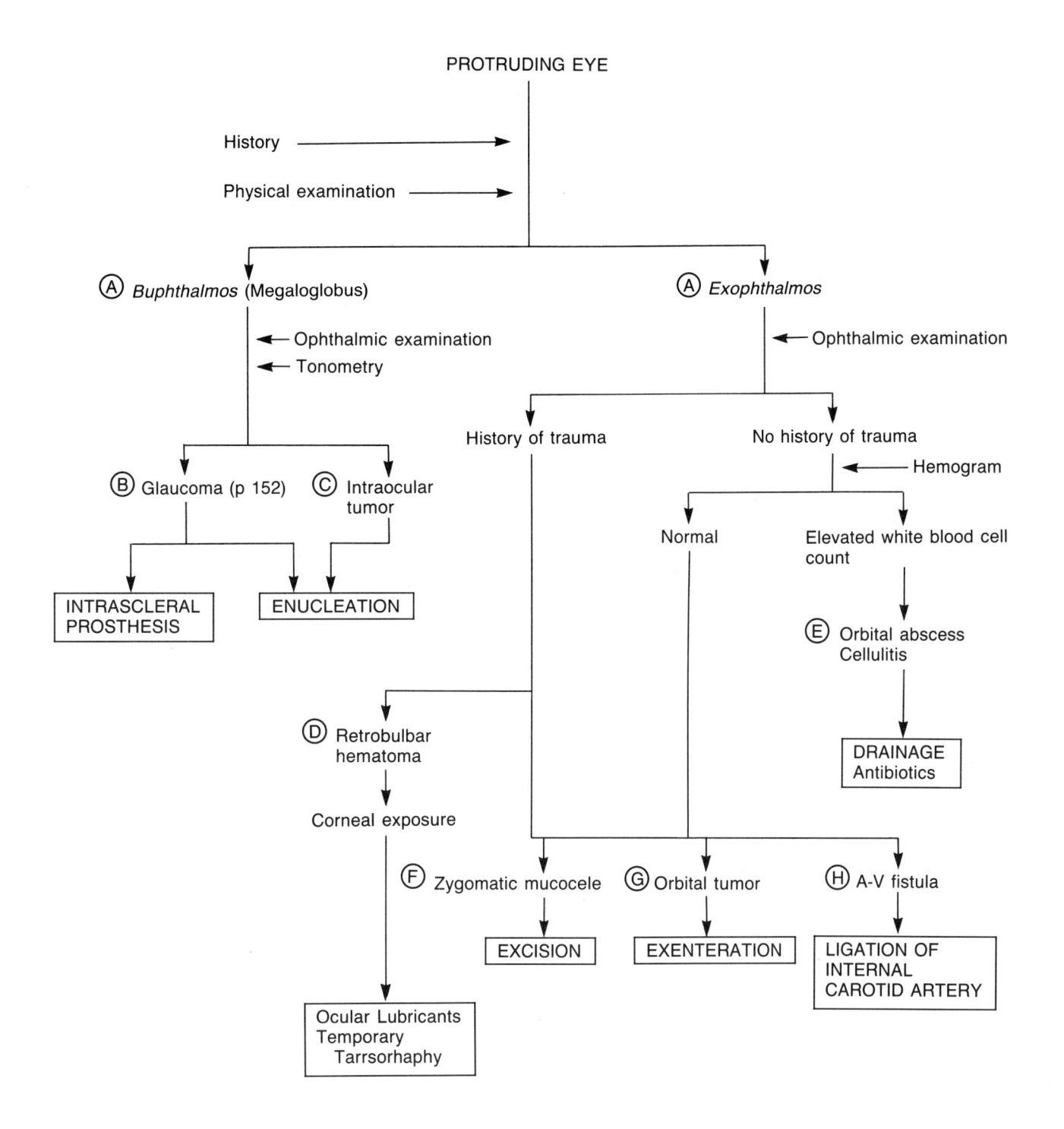

- History
- Physical examination

Ⓐ Buphthalmos (Megaloglobus)
- ← Ophthalmic examination
- ← Tonometry

- Ⓑ Glaucoma (p 152) → **INTRASCLERAL PROSTHESIS** / **ENUCLEATION**
- Ⓒ Intraocular tumor → **ENUCLEATION**

Ⓐ Exophthalmos
- ← Ophthalmic examination

History of trauma
- Ⓓ Retrobulbar hematoma
  - Corneal exposure → **Ocular Lubricants, Temporary Tarrsorhaphy**

No history of trauma
- ← Hemogram

Normal
- Ⓕ Zygomatic mucocele → **EXCISION**
- Ⓖ Orbital tumor → **EXENTERATION**
- Ⓗ A-V fistula → **LIGATION OF INTERNAL CAROTID ARTERY**

Elevated white blood cell count
- Ⓔ Orbital abscess / Cellulitis → **DRAINAGE / Antibiotics**

BLINDNESS

Melanie M. Williams
Bernhard M. Spiess

A complete history is an important part of an ophthalmologic examination, particularly if vision is affected. Remember that unilateral blindness is often not recognized by the owner. Dogs can compensate well for a gradual loss of vision; however, when placed in a strange environment, they appear to suffer a sudden loss of vision. A history of progressive night blindness, behavioral changes, or systemic diseases may be helpful in establishing a diagnosis.

A. Schiotz tonometry is clearly superior to digital tonometry. Normal intraocular pressures (IOP) range from 15 to 28 mm Hg read on a human conversion chart. Determine the IOP in any case of a "red" eye, regardless of pupil size.

B. Inflammation of the uveal tract is often a sign of systemic disease. Uveitis presents with a miotic pupil. Infectious organisms, including *Toxoplasma, Cryptococcus,* and *Blastomyces,* must be eliminated before use of systemic and topical corticosteroids. Early and frequent administration of atropine relieves pain associated with ciliary spasm and prevents formation of posterior synechiae.

C. Glaucoma is the leading cause of blindness in the dog. High IOP for 24 to 48 hours usually results in irreversible retinal damage. Medical therapy is often insufficient and not well tolerated by many dogs. Cyclocryotherapy has consistently led to lowering of IOP by cryonecrosis of the ciliary epithelium. In cases of primary glaucoma, care must be taken to detect early changes of IOP in the other eye.

D. Retinitis can be caused by systemic disease such as distemper, toxoplasmosis, cryptococcosis, blastomycosis, lymphosarcoma, or larva migrans. Infectious agents should be ruled out prior to the use of corticosteroids. Choroiditis and uveitis are usually associated with retinitis.

E. Optic neuritis may or may not involve the optic disc (papillitis). Several systemic diseases can cause optic neuritis including canine distemper, toxoplasmosis, feline infectious peritonitis, reticulosis, orbital cellulitis, and abscessation. If diagnosed early, systemic corticosteroids may restore vision. Some dogs require long-term therapy with low doses of prednisolone in order to prevent a relapse.

F. Neurologic disorders can affect vision. A thorough examination of the cranial nerves often reveals additional neurologic deficits, caused by space-occupying lesions.

G. Retinal vasculature attenuation and tapetal hyper reflectivity are diagnostic for progressive retinal atrophy (PRA). Electroretinography can confirm the diagnosis. These hereditary diseases are untreatable.

H. Corneal disease does not usually result in blindness; however, in neglected cases of chronic superficial keratitis (pannus), corneal pigmentation may eventually involve the entire cornea and affect vision.

References

Barrie KP, Lavach JD, Gelatt KN. Diseases of the canine posterior segment. In: Gelatt KN, ed. Textbook of veterinary ophthalmology. Philadelphia: Lea & Febiger, 1981:474.

Gwin RM, Gelatt KN. The canine lens. In: Gelatt KN, ed. Textbook of veterinary ophthalmology. Philadelphia: Lea & Febiger, 1981:435.

Slatter DH. Lens. In: Slatter DH, ed. Fundamentals of veterinary ophthalmology. Philadelphia: WB Saunders, 1981:489.

Slatter DH. Retina. In: Slatter DH, ed. Fundamentals of veterinary ophthalmology. Philadelphia: WB, Saunders, 1981:538.

Slatter DH. Neuro-ophthalmology. In: Slatter DH, ed. Fundamentals of veterinary ophthalmology. Philadelphia: WB Saunders, 1981:587.

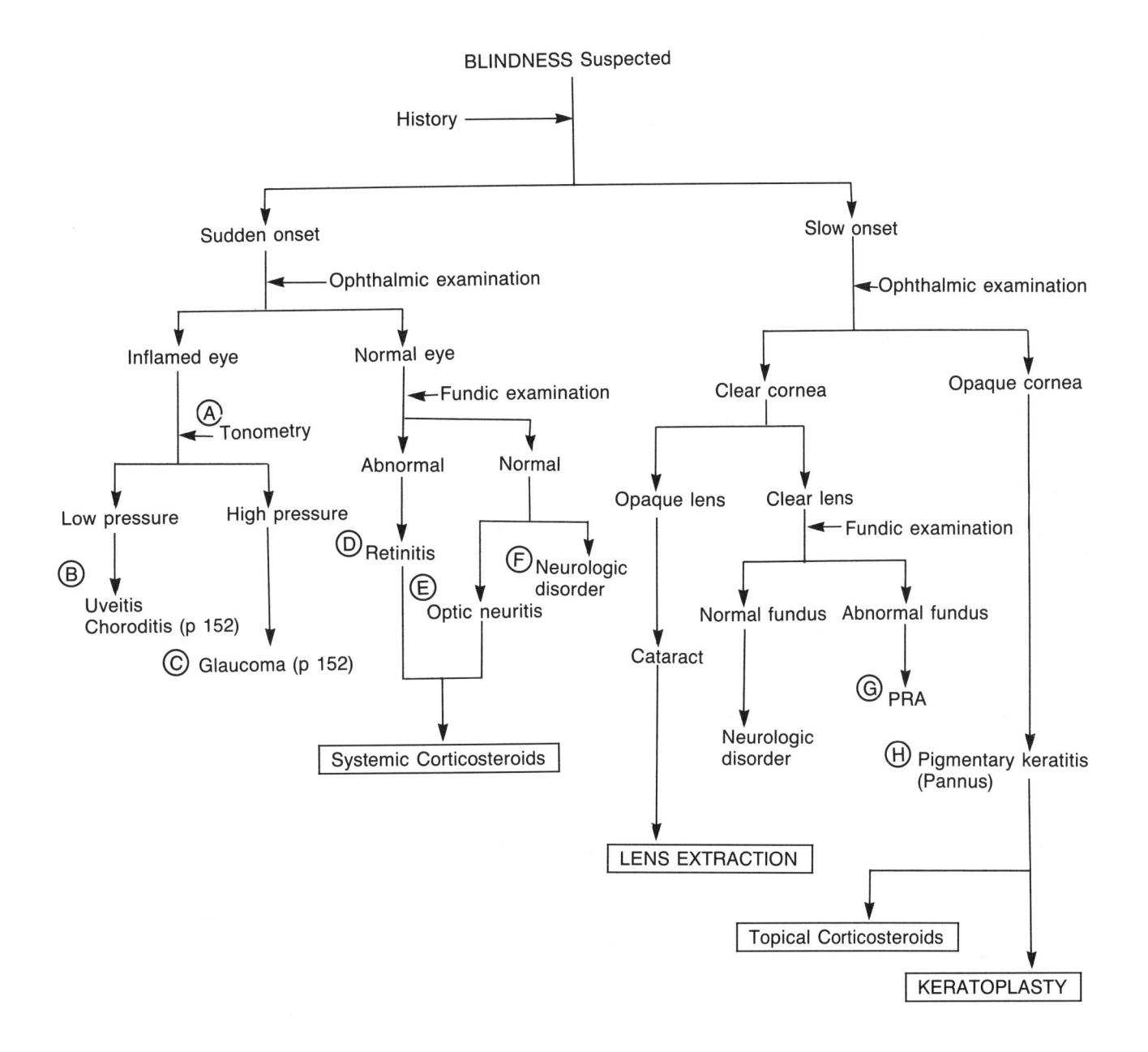

BLINDNESS Suspected

```
                        BLINDNESS Suspected
                               │
                       History ─→
              ┌────────────────┴────────────────┐
         Sudden onset                       Slow onset
         ←─ Ophthalmic examination      ←─ Ophthalmic examination
      ┌──────┴──────┐                      ┌──────────┴──────────┐
  Inflamed eye   Normal eye            Clear cornea         Opaque cornea
      │          ←─ Fundic examination      ┌──────┴──────┐         │
   Ⓐ Tonometry    ┌──────┴──────┐       Opaque lens   Clear lens    │
   ┌──┴──┐     Abnormal      Normal         │       ←─ Fundic exam  │
 Low    High      │              │          │       ┌────┴────┐     │
pressure pressure Ⓓ Retinitis  Ⓕ Neurologic │   Normal    Abnormal  │
   │       │       Ⓔ            disorder    │   fundus    fundus    │
 Ⓑ       Ⓒ       Optic neuritis             │      │         │      │
Uveitis  Glaucoma                         Cataract │       Ⓖ PRA     │
Choroditis (p 152)                           │  Neurologic            │
(p 152)      │                               │  disorder   Ⓗ Pigmentary
             │                               │             keratitis
             ↓                               │             (Pannus)
      ┌─────────────┐                        ↓                │
      │  Systemic   │                ┌───────────────┐        │
      │Corticosteroids│              │LENS EXTRACTION│        │
      └─────────────┘                └───────────────┘        │
                                              ┌──────────────┤
                                              ↓              ↓
                                     ┌────────────────┐ ┌──────────────┐
                                     │    Topical     │ │ KERATOPLASTY │
                                     │Corticosteroids │ │              │
                                     └────────────────┘ └──────────────┘
```

167

ACUTE FULL-THICKNESS WOUND

Craig. W. Miller

A. Ascertain when the animal was injured. The "golden period", during which bacterial multiplication and invasion have not gone beyond the wound margins, is approximately 6 hours after injury. However, time is only one of many factors to be considered; others include the type of contaminating bacteria, the condition of tissues in the area, and the type of foreign debris in the wound.

B. Physical examination should include all body systems. Wounds may be accompanied by serious injury at distant sites or systemic sequelae (e.g., shock caused by hemorrhage), which may be overlooked. As trauma to deep structures may accompany skin wounds, the neurovascular and musculoskeletal structures in the region of the wound should be evaluated.

C. Radiographs of the injured area are indicated if one suspects underlying skeletal damage. Radiographs of distant sites may also be indicated if multisystem trauma is present.

D. First aid should not be overzealous. The priorities are (1) to stop active hemorrhage, (2) to protect the wound from further contamination, (3) to prepare the surrounding skin, and (4) to stabilize underlying skeletal damage. Control hemorrhage by application of a pressure bandage. Occasionally, arterial ligation or repair are necessary to stop blood loss. Tourniquets should not be used to control blood loss from wounded extremities. Initial protection of the wound is necessary in order to reduce additional contamination. A saline-moistened sterile gauze dressing is usually adequate. Clip hair from the surrounding skin, and cleanse the skin using a surgical scrub solution. Discard the wet gauze used to cover the wound, and apply a fresh dressing; delay definitive treatment until the animal is stable. Temporarily immobilize underlying fractures by padded bandages or splints.

E. Note the presence of foreign material, exudate, and devitalized tissue. The type of foreign material present is important (e.g., sand and road dirt produce less wound infection than clay and organic material). A rapid slide technique has been described for early detection of wound contamination and may be useful when deciding between primary and delayed closure.

F. Pressurized lavage, using a 35 ml syringe and 18 gauge needle held 5 cm from the wound, is an effective method of reducing bacterial contamination and removing debris from a wound. Dilute chlorhexidine solution or physiologic saline are useful lavage solutions. Debridement is an important component of wound management. Thorough debridement often requires regional anesthesia, or general anesthesia, when the animal is stable. Damaged muscle, fat, and fascia are often amenable to aggressive debridement with little functional loss. Removal of bone is usually restricted to small detached fragments. Skin is not removed unless it is obviously devitalized. Closure is best accomplished using fine monofilament suture material (p 202). Primary closure is optimum in a wound free from contamination. However, more errors are made by closing contaminated or poorly prepared wounds than by delaying closure of clean wounds.

G. Systemic antibiotics are most effective within the first 3 to 4 hours after injury.

H. Delayed primary closure is best done between 4 and 7 days after the injury. Infection rates of contaminated wounds decrease significantly if closure is done 4 days after injury. Delayed primary closure is by definition done prior to the deposition of granulation tissue, which will be apparent 6 to 7 days after injury.

I. Reconstruction consists of covering skin defects that are not amenable to closure with skin flaps or skin grafts. Several types of skin flaps or grafts exist, and each has inherent advantages and disadvanatages (p 172).

References

Johnston DE. Skin and subcutaneous tissues. In: Bojrab MJ, ed. Pathophysiology in small animal surgery. Philadelphia: Lea & Febiger, 1981:405.

Proceedings for wound management and plastic reconstructive surgery. 14th Annual Surgical Forum, Chicago, 1986:8.

Swaim SF. Surgery of traumatized skin: management and reconstruction in the dog and cat. Philadelphia: WB Saunders, 1980:119.

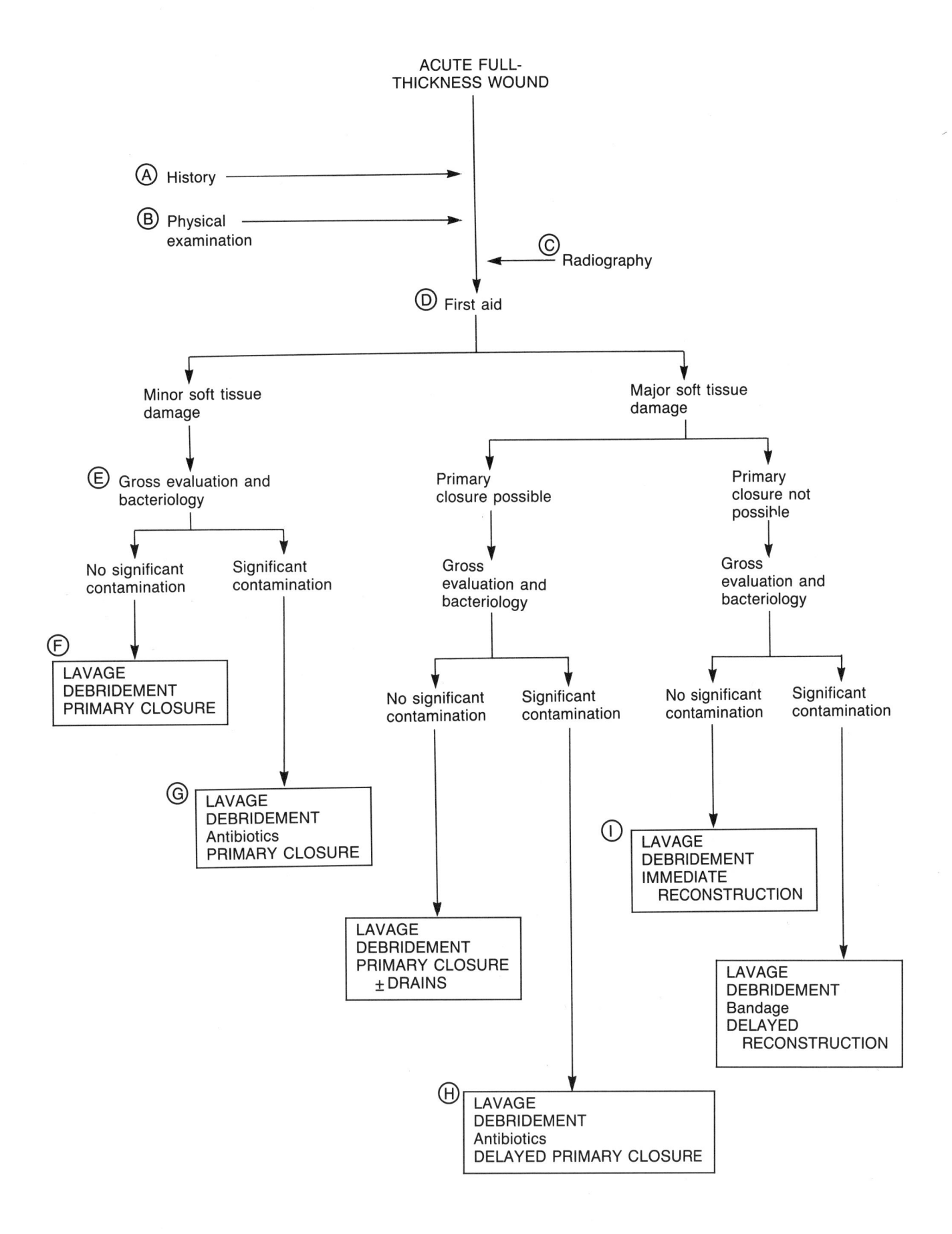

```
                    ACUTE FULL-
                   THICKNESS WOUND
                          │
   (A) History ──────────→│
                          │
   (B) Physical ─────────→│
       examination        │
                          │←──── (C) Radiography
                          ↓
                     (D) First aid
                          │
            ┌─────────────┴─────────────┐
            ↓                           ↓
   Minor soft tissue            Major soft tissue
        damage                       damage
            │                           │
            ↓                 ┌─────────┴─────────┐
   (E) Gross evaluation       ↓                   ↓
       and bacteriology   Primary            Primary
            │             closure            closure not
    ┌───────┴───────┐     possible           possible
    ↓               ↓         │                   │
No significant  Significant   ↓                   ↓
contamination   contamination Gross           Gross
    │               │         evaluation      evaluation
    ↓               │         and bacteriology and bacteriology
(F)                 │              │               │
┌──────────┐        │         ┌────┴────┐     ┌────┴────┐
│ LAVAGE   │        │         ↓         ↓     ↓         ↓
│DEBRIDEMENT│       │      No sig.  Signif.  No sig.  Signif.
│ PRIMARY  │        │      contam.  contam.  contam.  contam.
│ CLOSURE  │        ↓         │         │     │         │
└──────────┘    (G)┌──────────┐         │     │ (I)     │
                   │ LAVAGE   │         │     ↓         │
                   │DEBRIDEMENT│        │  ┌──────────┐ │
                   │Antibiotics│        │  │ LAVAGE   │ │
                   │ PRIMARY  │         │  │DEBRIDEMENT│ │
                   │ CLOSURE  │         │  │IMMEDIATE │ │
                   └──────────┘         │  │RECONSTRUCTION│
                                ┌───────┘  └──────────┘ │
                                ↓                       ↓
                          ┌──────────┐            ┌──────────┐
                          │ LAVAGE   │            │ LAVAGE   │
                          │DEBRIDEMENT│           │DEBRIDEMENT│
                          │ PRIMARY  │            │ Bandage  │
                          │ CLOSURE  │            │ DELAYED  │
                          │ ± DRAINS │            │RECONSTRUCTION│
                          └──────────┘            └──────────┘
                                │
                           (H) ┌──────────┐
                               │ LAVAGE   │
                               │DEBRIDEMENT│
                               │Antibiotics│
                               │DELAYED PRIMARY CLOSURE│
                               └──────────┘
```

169

CHRONIC FULL-THICKNESS WOUND

Craig. W. Miller

A. Take a thorough history in all wound cases. Information regarding the cause, duration, and previous treatment of the wound are important.

B. Physical examination should include the entire body of the patient. Many wounds are accompanied by serious injuries that may not be apparent on cursory examination. Examination of the wound should include evaluation of deeper musculoskeletal and neurovascular structures as a small skin wound may be associated with laceration of arteries, nerves, or tendons. Involvement of these structures alters the prognosis for the wound.

C. Utilize ancillary test when indicated, including radiography both of the wound area (i.e., to evaluate soft tissue or skeletal damage) and of distant sites (e.g., thoracic radiographs in road accident cases). Use contrast radiography in order to delineate chronic draining tracts.

D. The presence of granulation tissue represents the repair or fibroplastic stage of wound healing. Wound closure at this time is termed secondary closure.

E. Note the presence of foreign material, exudate, and necrotic tissue in the wound. The type of foreign material present is important, (e.g., sand and road dirt produce less wound infection than clay and organic material). Bacterial culture and sensitivity is ideal, but decisions to close or to delay closure cannot wait for these results. A rapid slide evaluation for bacterial contamination may be used, particularly during the early decision-making process of wound treatment. Bacterial contamination is important when considering reconstructive techniques, especially free skin grafts.

F. Wound cleansing is the initial step in the treatment process. Pressurized lavage, using a 35 ml syringe and 18 gauge needle with physiologic saline or 0.05 percent chlorhexidine solution, reduces bacterial contamination and removes foreign debris. Damaged muscle, fascia, and fat are often amenable to aggressive debridement with little functional loss. Removal of bone is usually restricted to small detached fragments. Bone curettes or rongeurs can be used to remove imbedded debris from bone. Skin is not removed unless it is obviously devitalized. A staged debridement avoids excision of excess skin when its viability is not certain. A delay of 48 hours often results in a clear demarcation of viable and nonviable skin. Closure is best accomplished using fine monofilament suture material (p 202). Buried suture should be minimized. Dead space should be obliterated either by suture, bandage, or drains.

G. If significant bacterial contamination is present, reduce the number of bacteria prior to closure or reconstruction. This can be accomplished by thorough wound cleansing, lavage, and debridement followed by proper bandaging. Topical antibiotics (gentamycin) or antiseptics reduce bacterial numbers. Systemic antibiotics can be used prior to the formation of granulation tissue, but are not as effective in wounds over 3 to 4 hours old.

H. Reconstruction is the use of skin flaps or skin grafts to cover skin defects not amenable to closure. Several types of skin flaps or grafts can be constructed, and each type has inherent advantages and disadvantages (p 172).

I. Healing by contraction and epithelialization is an effective method of treating contaminated wounds in small animals, especially wounds involving the upper limbs and the torso in which skin mobility is good. As wounds of the lower extremity may be too large to close by wound contraction and the resulting epithelial cover will be thin and easily traumatized, delayed reconstruction may be indicated to cover these wounds.

References

Johnston DE. Skin and subcutaneous tissues. In: Bojrab MJ, ed. Pathophysiology in small animal surgery. Philadelphia: Lea & Febiger, 1981:405.

Proceedings for wound management and plastic reconstructive surgery. 14th Annual Surgical Forum, Chicago, 1986:8.

Swaim SF. Surgery of traumatized skin: management and reconstruction in the dog and cat. Philadelphia: WB Saunders, 1980:119.

CHRONIC FULL-THICKNESS WOUND

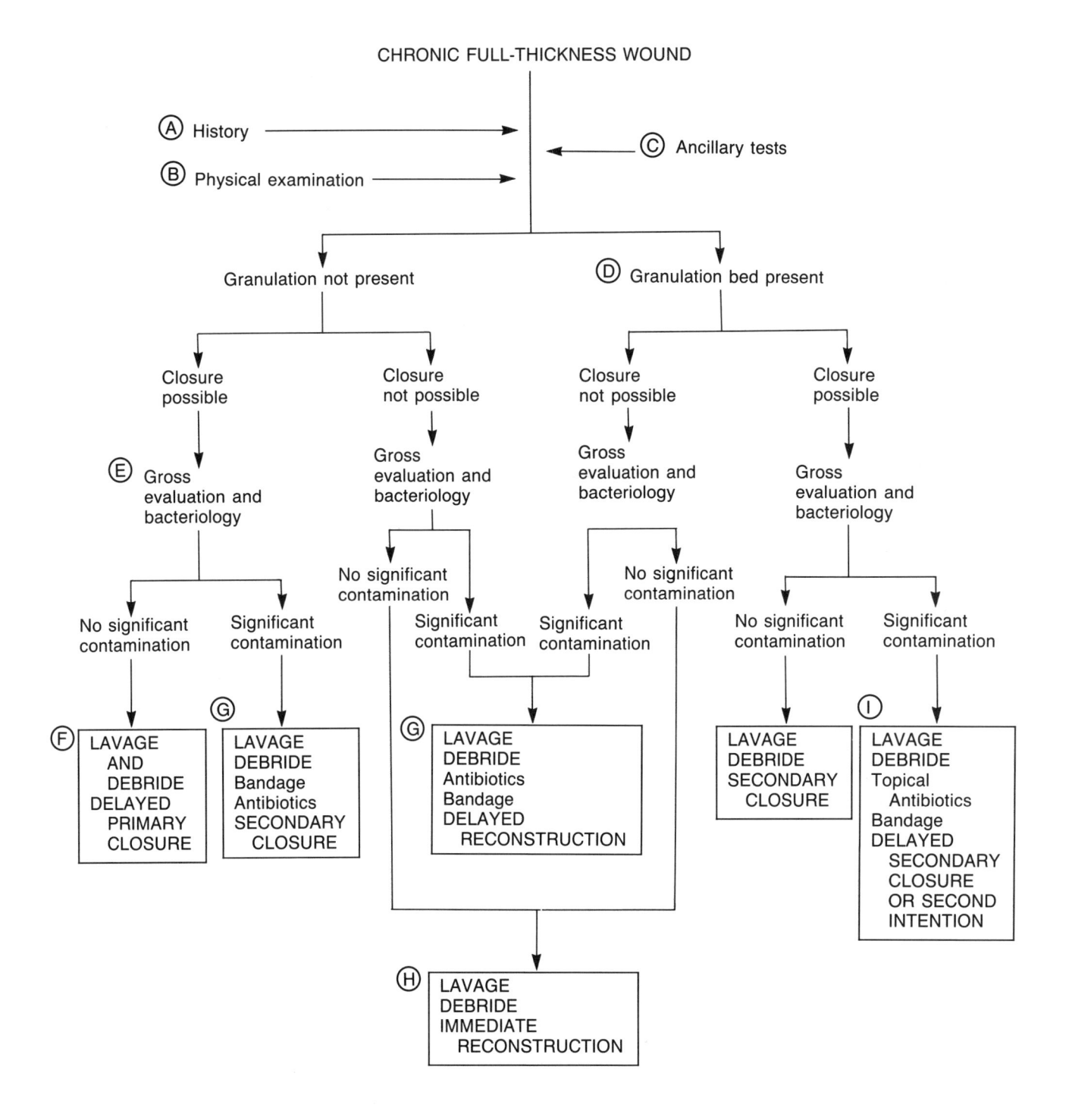

- (A) History
- (B) Physical examination
- (C) Ancillary tests

Granulation not present

Closure possible
(E) Gross evaluation and bacteriology

- **No significant contamination**
  - (F) LAVAGE AND DEBRIDE DELAYED PRIMARY CLOSURE
- **Significant contamination**
  - (G) LAVAGE DEBRIDE Bandage Antibiotics SECONDARY CLOSURE

Closure not possible
Gross evaluation and bacteriology

- **No significant contamination / Significant contamination**
  - (G) LAVAGE DEBRIDE Antibiotics Bandage DELAYED RECONSTRUCTION

(D) Granulation bed present

Closure not possible
Gross evaluation and bacteriology

- **Significant contamination / No significant contamination**
  - (H) LAVAGE DEBRIDE IMMEDIATE RECONSTRUCTION

Closure possible
Gross evaluation and bacteriology

- **No significant contamination**
  - LAVAGE DEBRIDE SECONDARY CLOSURE
- **Significant contamination**
  - (I) LAVAGE DEBRIDE Topical Antibiotics Bandage DELAYED SECONDARY CLOSURE OR SECOND INTENTION

WOUND RECONSTRUCTION

Craig. W. Miller

A. Good local skin mobility exists on the upper extremities and torso of small animals. These areas are conducive to the mobilization of local tissues to cover skin deficits. Poor local skin mobility exists on the face and lower extremities. The skin in these areas is too tight to allow undermining and movement of local skin flaps to cover large defects.

B. The goals of open wound management prior to the construction of a skin flap are to remove foreign or necrotic debris and to decrease bacterial contamination. Lavage and debridement often allows wound cleansing and skin flap reconstruction to be done during the same procedure. Badly contaminated wounds may benefit from staged procedures in which wound cleansing is done first, followed by skin flap reconstruction in 4 to 7 days.

C. A skin flap retains a vascular attachment during its transfer. This endogenous blood supply makes it heartier than a free skin graft. A skin flap can be applied over exposed bone, tendon, nerve, and orthopaedic implants, whereas a free skin graft cannot. Skin flaps are classified by location, configuration, and blood supply. Local flaps are flaps constructed from skin at or near the wound.

D. A free skin graft is completely detached from the body and transferred to a recipient site. Its survival is dependent upon absorption of tissue fluids and neovascularization from the new site. Therefore, a skin graft can neither be placed over a poorly vascularized wound nor over avascular structures such as exposed bone, tendon, nerve, or orthopaedic implants. Full-thickness mesh grafts are most commonly used in small animals.

E. Distant flaps are skin flaps constructed and transferred to distant sites. The most common distant flaps in small animal surgery are bipedicle (pouch) flaps or single pedicle flaps that are constructed on the animal's torso and transferred to an extremity (Fig. 1). Distant flaps can be used over less than optimal wound beds, but they require prolonged bandaging of the extremity to the torso. Some patients will not tolerate the necessary immobilization. Also, joint stiffness can occur if the limb is not immobilized in a physiologic position.

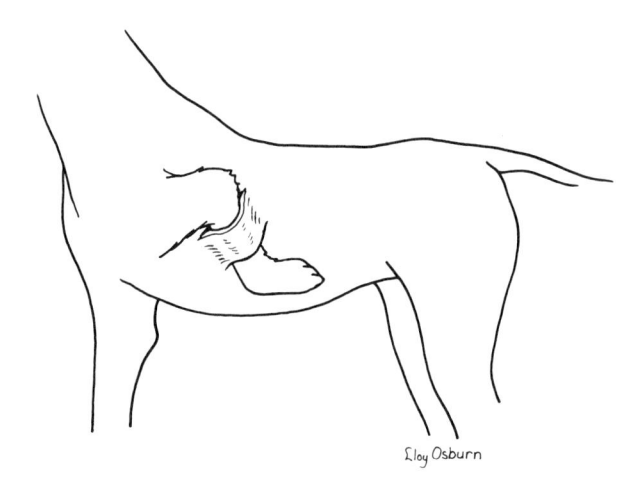

Figure 1 A distant bipedicle thoracic wall skin flap used to cover a forelimb skin defect.

References

Johnston DE. Skin and subcutaneous tissues. In: Bojrab MJ, ed. Pathophysiology in small animal surgery. Philadelphia: Lea & Febiger, 1981:405.

Proceedings for wound management and plastic reconstructive surgery. 14th Annual Surgical Forum, Chicago, 1986:59.

Swaim SF. Surgery of traumatized skin: management and reconstruction in the dog and cat. Philadelphia: WB Saunders, 1980:297.

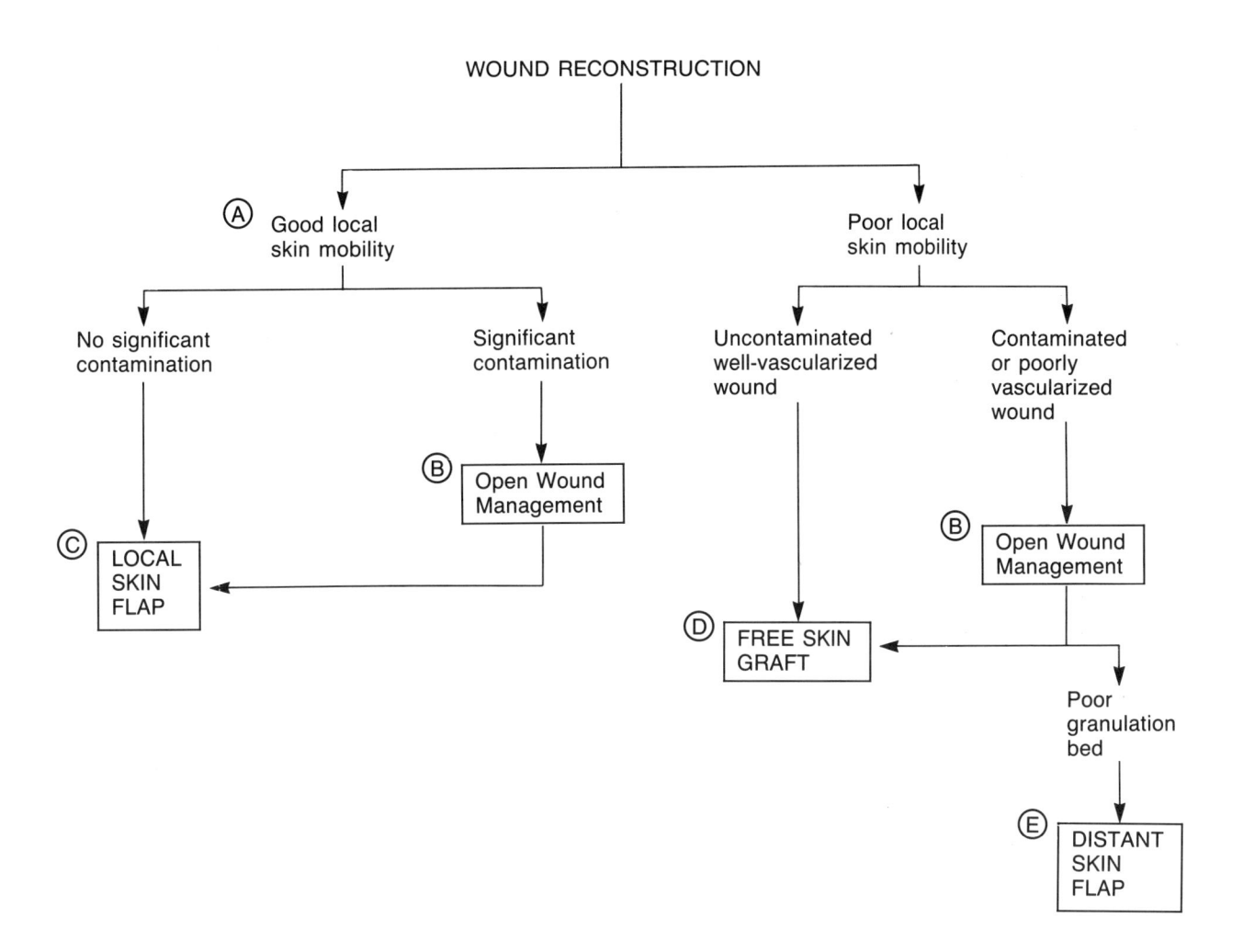

WOUND RECONSTRUCTION

- **A** Good local skin mobility
  - No significant contamination → **C** LOCAL SKIN FLAP
  - Significant contamination → **B** Open Wound Management → LOCAL SKIN FLAP
- Poor local skin mobility
  - Uncontaminated well-vascularized wound → **D** FREE SKIN GRAFT
  - Contaminated or poorly vascularized wound → **B** Open Wound Management → FREE SKIN GRAFT
    - Poor granulation bed → **E** DISTANT SKIN FLAP

THERMAL BURN

Craig W. Miller

A. Burn injuries are classified by depth and extent. The depth of a burn is not always readily apparent in animal patients. Local pain sensitivity, evidence of superficial blood flow, and hair epilation are helpful in the early differentiation of partial versus full-thickness burns (Fig. 1).

B. A burn that involves 15 to 20 percent of the body surface area is considered a major burn and will likely require intensive medical support. A burn involving 40 to 50 percent of the body surface area has a poor prognosis, and euthanasia should be considered.

C. A partial-thickness burn of more than 15 percent of the total body surface area or any significant full-thickness burn requires intensive medical management. Systemic sequelae to thermal burn injuries are diverse and potentially disastrous. Acute complications include hypovolemic shock, electrolyte shifts, protein loss, and hemolysis. These complications cause pathologic changes in multiple organ systems. Correct hypovolemia using intravenous lactated Ringer's solution and 2 percent dextrose. Determine electrolyte and acid-base values and treat accordingly (p 190). Delay blood or plasma administration until the hypovolemia has been corrected and the patient is stable. Corticosteroids may be indicated to counteract adrenal cortical depletion. Systemic antibiotics are indicated in suspected cases of septicemia, but they are not effective in treating infection of the wound itself. Monitor the patient intensively during the post-burn period. A rapid therapeutic response to systemic complications is necessary for patient survival.

D. Closed management of a burn includes wound cleansing, debridement, and application of a dressing. Treating a burn injury by the exposure method (i.e., no dressing) is usually not applicable in veterinary medicine. If a partial-thickness burn involves less than 15 percent of the body surface area, intensive medical support is often not necessary. Initial treatment should include analgesia by intravenous narcotic administration, local cooling if the burn is less than 2 hours old, wound cleansing, debridement, and topical therapy. Many topical agents have been recommended for use in thermal burns. Silver sulfadiazine cream, 0.1 percent gentamicin ointment, and 0.5 percent chlorhexidine solution are among the agents recommended for reduction of local bacterial growth. An 80 percent concentration aloe vera cream has been advocated to prevent thromboxane-mediated vascular occlusion. Whatever topical therapy is chosen, change the dressing daily, lavage the wound, and perform additional debridement if necessary. Closure or reconstruction should be done when the resulting granulation bed appears healthy and free of contamination (p 172).

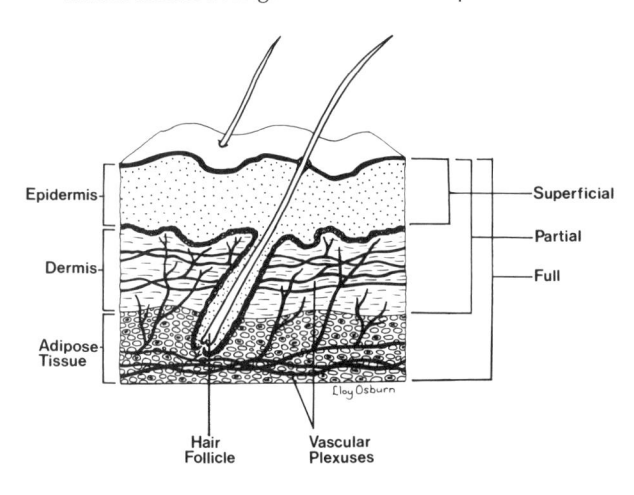

Figure 1 Tissue layers involved in superficial, partial, and full-thickness burns.

References

Davis LE. Initial care of burns and electrical injury. In: Zaslow I, ed. Veterinary trauma and critical care. Philadelphia: Lea & Febiger, 1984:209.

McKeever PJ. Thermal injury. In: Kirk RW, ed. Current veterinary therapy VIII. Philadelphia: WB Saunders, 1983:180.

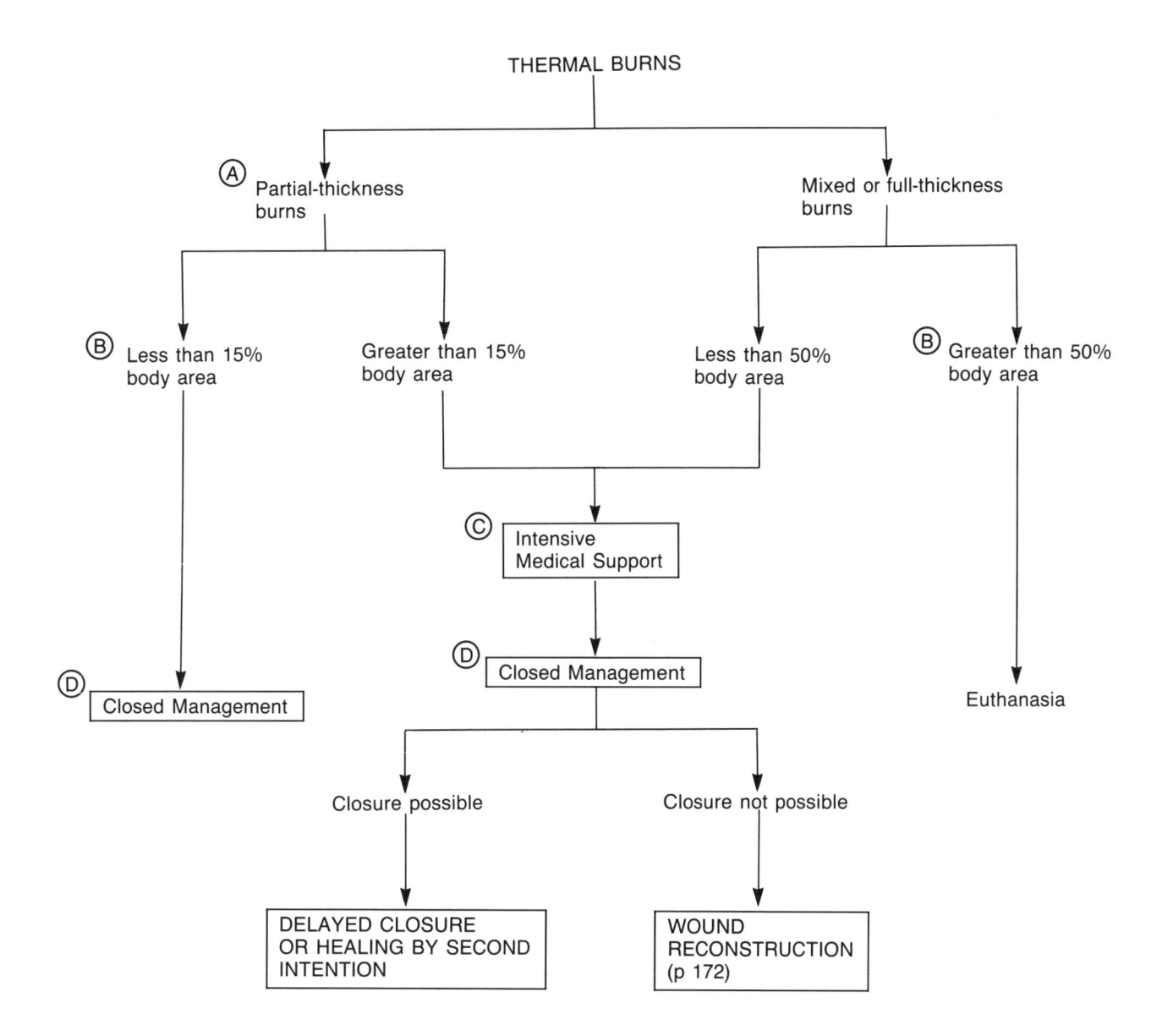

```
                              THERMAL BURNS
                                    |
                    _____|_____
                   |                                 |
              Ⓐ Partial-thickness              Mixed or full-thickness
                 burns                            burns
                   |                                 |
            _____|_____                   _____|_____
           |               |                 |               |
      Ⓑ Less than 15%  Greater than 15%  Less than 50%   Ⓑ Greater than 50%
         body area      body area         body area          body area
           |               |                 |                    |
           |               |_____|                    |
           |                         |                            |
           |                    Ⓒ Intensive                       |
           |                      Medical Support                 |
           |                         |                            |
           |                    Ⓓ Closed Management               |
           |                         |                            |
           |                 _____|_____                    |
           |                |                 |                   |
           ↓            Closure possible   Closure not possible  ↓
      Ⓓ Closed              |                 |              Euthanasia
        Management           ↓                 ↓
                      ┌──────────────┐  ┌──────────────┐
                      │DELAYED CLOSURE│  │   WOUND      │
                      │OR HEALING BY  │  │RECONSTRUCTION│
                      │SECOND         │  │  (p 172)     │
                      │INTENTION      │  │              │
                      └──────────────┘  └──────────────┘
```

SKIN TUMORS

Elizabeth J. Laing

A. Skin tumors commonly present as a "lump" or nonhealing "sore." Tumor duration, rate of growth, associated clinical signs, and response to previous treatment (if any) should be determined. Most skin tumors occur in older animals; however, histiocytomas and multiple fibrosarcomas are common in younger dogs and cats, respectively. Breed predispositions include Poodles (epithelial tumors), Kerry Blue Terriers (pilomatricomas), and Arctic breeds (intracutaneous cornifying epitheliomas).

B. The physical appearance of the lesion is rarely diagnostic. Findings suggestive of certain tumors include pigmentation (melanoma), ulceration (squamous cell carcinoma, mast cell tumor), and cauliflower-like growth (papilloma, squamous cell carcinoma). Rapid growth, ulceration, deep infiltration, and regional lymphadenopathy are often associated with malignancy.

C. Leukocytosis may indicate an inflammatory or infectious process; however, it is also a paraneoplastic sign associated with a variety of tumors. Hypercalcemia, with secondary azotemia, has been reported with adenocarcinomas and squamous cell carcinomas.

D. Radiography is indicated in deep, infiltrating tumors to assess the underlying tissues, and especially bone. Chest films are advised if clinical signs or histology indicate malignancy.

E. Fine-needle cytology is used to differentiate inflammatory, noninflammatory, and neoplastic lesions. If cytology is not diagnostic, pretreatment histology may be necessary. A punch or incisional biopsy is recommended if the results would alter the recommended treatment. Otherwise, an excisional biopsy is preferred.

F. Inflammatory disorders include abscesses, granulomas, eosinophilic plaques, and autoimmune conditions. Cytology reveals a predominance of inflammatory cells.

G. Skin tumors most readily diagnosed by cytology include mast cell tumors, melanomas, and certain epithelial tumors. In other cases, although cytology may differentiate neoplastic from nonneoplastic lesions, further definition of tumor type may not be possible. The extent of the tumor and feasibility of removal are the deciding factors in treatment selection.

H. Noninflammatory, nonneoplastic conditions include epidermal and follicular cysts, sebaceous hyperplasia, dermoids, and fibrous polyps. If necessary, surgical excision is the treatment of choice.

I. Most solitary skin tumors are benign or only locally malignant. Surgical excision is the treatment of choice, provided that at least 1 cm of tumor-free tissue can be removed along all margins. Invasive tumors, such as mast cell tumors and fibrosarcoma, require wider margins. Excised lesions should be submitted for histologic diagnosis. Cryosurgery is used for eyelid and small epithelial tumors. It is contraindicated for large mast cell tumors. Use radiation therapy alone or in combination with surgical excision. Epithelial tumors are generally more radioresponsive than mesenchymal tumors.

J. Benign multiple tumors include papillomas and intracutaneous cornifying epitheliomas. Surgical excision or cryosurgery is indicated for those lesions that cause clinical signs. The most common malignant tumors are mast cell tumors (dogs) and fibrosarcomas (cats). Surgical excision may be palliative for symptomatic lesions, but recurrence is common. Aggressive systemic therapy may improve the clinical response.

K. Systemic tumors with cutaneous manifestations include mast cell tumors (cats) and lymphosarcoma. Tumors that frequently metastasize to the skin include mammary gland carcinoma, hemangiosarcoma, and miscellaneous carcinomas. Unless the primary tumor can be treated, euthanasia is often recommended for humane reasons.

L. Tumors should be histologically diagnosed and staged prior to therapy. Staging may include radiography, CBC, serum chemistry, bone marrow aspirate, and biopsy of regional lymph nodes. Examples of systemic therapy include glucocorticoids and H_2 antihistamines (mast cell tumor), bleomycin (squamous cell carcinoma), and cyclophosphamide-vincristine-prednisone and adriamycin (lymphosarcoma, fibrosarcoma). Other antineoplastic regimes are currently being evaluated.

M. Adjuvant therapy is indicated if surgical excision is incomplete or histology indicates an invasive tumor. Incomplete excision may be treated with wider surgical excision or local radiotherapy. Amputation may be necessary for malignant tumors of the extremities. Castration can decrease the risk of recurrence of perianal gland adenomas. Antineoplastic agents that have been used successfully include glucocorticoids (mast cell tumor), bleomycin (squamous cell carcinoma), and adriamycin (fibrosarcoma). Periodic reevaluation is recommended in tumors with a high incidence of recurrence (fibrosarcoma, hemangiopericytoma, mast cell tumor) and metastasis (squamous cell carcinoma, mucocutaneous melanoma, and perianal adenocarcinoma).

References

Conroy JD. Canine skin tumors. JAAHA 1983; 19:91.
Duncan JR, Prasse KW. Veterinary laboratory medicine - clinical pathology. Ames, IA: The Iowa State University Press, 1977:169.
Perman V, Alsaker RD, Riis RC. Cytology of the dog and cat. South Bend, IN: Am Anim Hosp Assoc Publication, 1979.
Susaneck SJ. Feline skin tumors. Comp Cont Ed 1983; 5:251.
Withrow SJ. Surgical management of skin tumors in dogs and cats. Clinical Veterinary Oncology, Fort Collins, CO: Colorado State University Press, 1983:210.

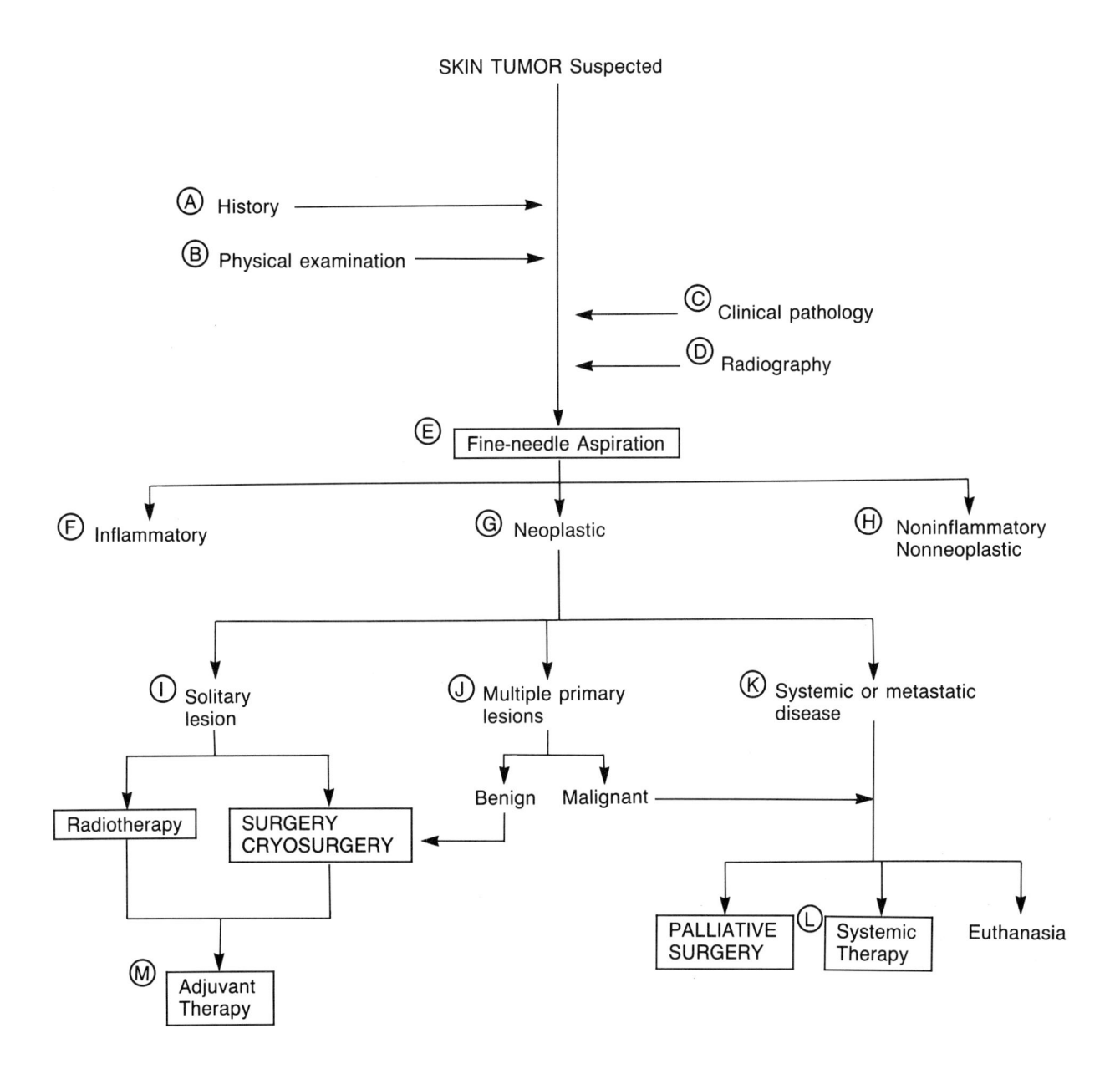

SKIN TUMOR Suspected

- Ⓐ History
- Ⓑ Physical examination
- Ⓒ Clinical pathology
- Ⓓ Radiography
- Ⓔ Fine-needle Aspiration
  - Ⓕ Inflammatory
  - Ⓖ Neoplastic
    - Ⓘ Solitary lesion
      - Radiotherapy
      - SURGERY CRYOSURGERY
        - Ⓜ Adjuvant Therapy
    - Ⓙ Multiple primary lesions
      - Benign
      - Malignant
    - Ⓚ Systemic or metastatic disease
      - PALLIATIVE SURGERY
      - Ⓛ Systemic Therapy
      - Euthanasia
  - Ⓗ Noninflammatory Nonneoplastic

CANINE MAMMARY TUMOR

Elizabeth J. Laing

Mammary tumors are the second most common tumor in dogs. Nearly 60 percent of all mammary tumors are malignant, with adenocarcinoma the most common histologic type. The remaining 40 percent are usually benign mixed tumors. Ovariectomy decreases the risk of tumor development, with surgery prior to the first estrus having maximum benefit. This benefit lessens with age until no protective effect occurs with neutering after 2½ years of age. Therefore, ovariectomy at the time of tumor removal is of questionable value.

A. Mammary tumors usually occur in older female dogs, with a mean age at onset of 10 years. Mammary tumors are rare in males and are often associated with a feminizing testicular tumor. Historic information of prognostic importance includes rate of tumor growth, response to previous therapy, and related systemic signs.

B. The caudal mammary glands are most frequently affected, with multiple tumors occurring in 50 percent of cases. Signs of malignancy include rapid growth, ill-defined borders, ulceration, edema, pruritus, erythema, and fixation to underlying muscle. Regional lymphadenopathy, while often indicative of tumor spread, is of little prognostic significance. Other signs of tumor metastasis may include respiratory distress, lameness, ocular changes, or neurologic deficits. Differentials for mammary swelling include mastitis (lactating bitches), fibrocystic disease, skin tumors, inguinal hernias, and lymphosarcoma.

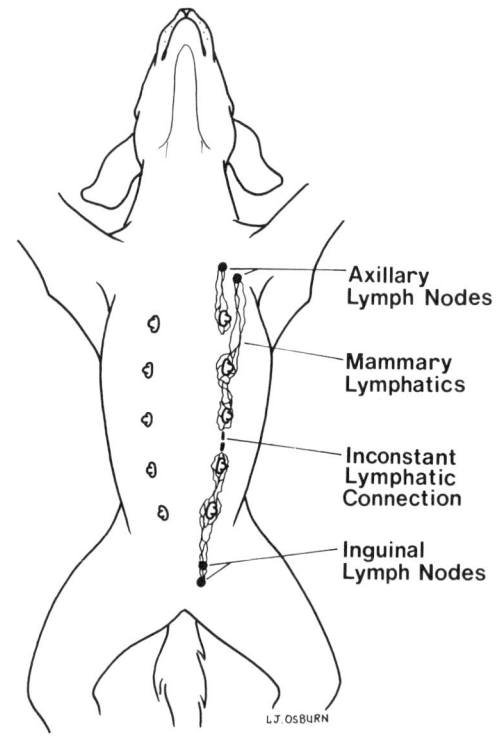

Figure 1 Lymphatic drainage of the five pairs of mammary glands of the dog.

C. A complete blood count (CBC), biochemical profile, and urinalysis are recommended as a preanesthetic screen for older animals. Paraneoplastic syndromes that may be detected include anemia, leukocytosis, disseminated intravascular coagulation, and hypercalcemia. Fine-needle biopsy is not commonly performed. Most tumors contain both benign and malignant cell types. A small cytologic sample may not accurately predict tumor behavior.

D. A ventrodorsal and two opposing lateral chest radiographs are recommended in order to screen for pulmonary metastasis. Lesions may appear as well-defined, soft tissue nodules or as diffuse interstitial densities. Bone metastases usually occur in the humerus, femur, and vertebra. Radiographically, they appear as osteolytic foci with variable periosteal reaction. If nuclear imaging is available, bone scans and lymphoscintigraphy may further define the extent of disease.

E. Mammary tumors are divided into three treatment groups, which are based on tumor size, distribution, and metastatic spread. Local tumors are solitary masses without lymph nodal or distant metastasis. Regional tumors include multiple primary masses or solitary tumors with lymphatic spread. Disseminated tumors include all inflammatory carcinomas and any tumor with distant metastasis.

F. A fine-needle or incisional biopsy is recommended to confirm the diagnosis of inflammatory or metastatic carcinoma. If the tumor is causing local discomfort without systemic signs, attempt palliative excision. Radiotherapy may be tried in localized inflammatory lesions. Antineoplastic chemotherapy and immunotherapy are currently being evaluated in the treatment of metastatic disease. More commonly, euthanasia is recommended because of the poor prognosis and the associated clinical signs.

G. Solitary tumors are most often treated with single gland excision (simple mastectomy) or removal of the gland and draining lymph node (en bloc resection). More radical excision has shown no prognostic advantage over conservative procedures. Postoperative histologic diagnosis is recommended. Local invasion, large tumors (larger than 15 cm), and an infiltrating growth pattern are considered poor prognostic signs. Periodic follow-up is recommended to allow early detection of recurrence.

H. The ideal treatment for regional mammary tumors is not yet known. Surgery should include removal and biopsy of all affected mammary glands. Regional lymph nodes (Fig. 1) (axillary for glands 1, 2, and 3, and superficial inguinal for glands 4 and 5) are generally included in the excision, especially if enlarged. Large tumors (larger than 15 cm), local invasion, and an infiltrating growth pattern are poor prognostic signs. The type of surgery and involvement of regional lymph nodes are not prognostically significant. Periodic follow-up is recommended to allow early detection of recurrence.

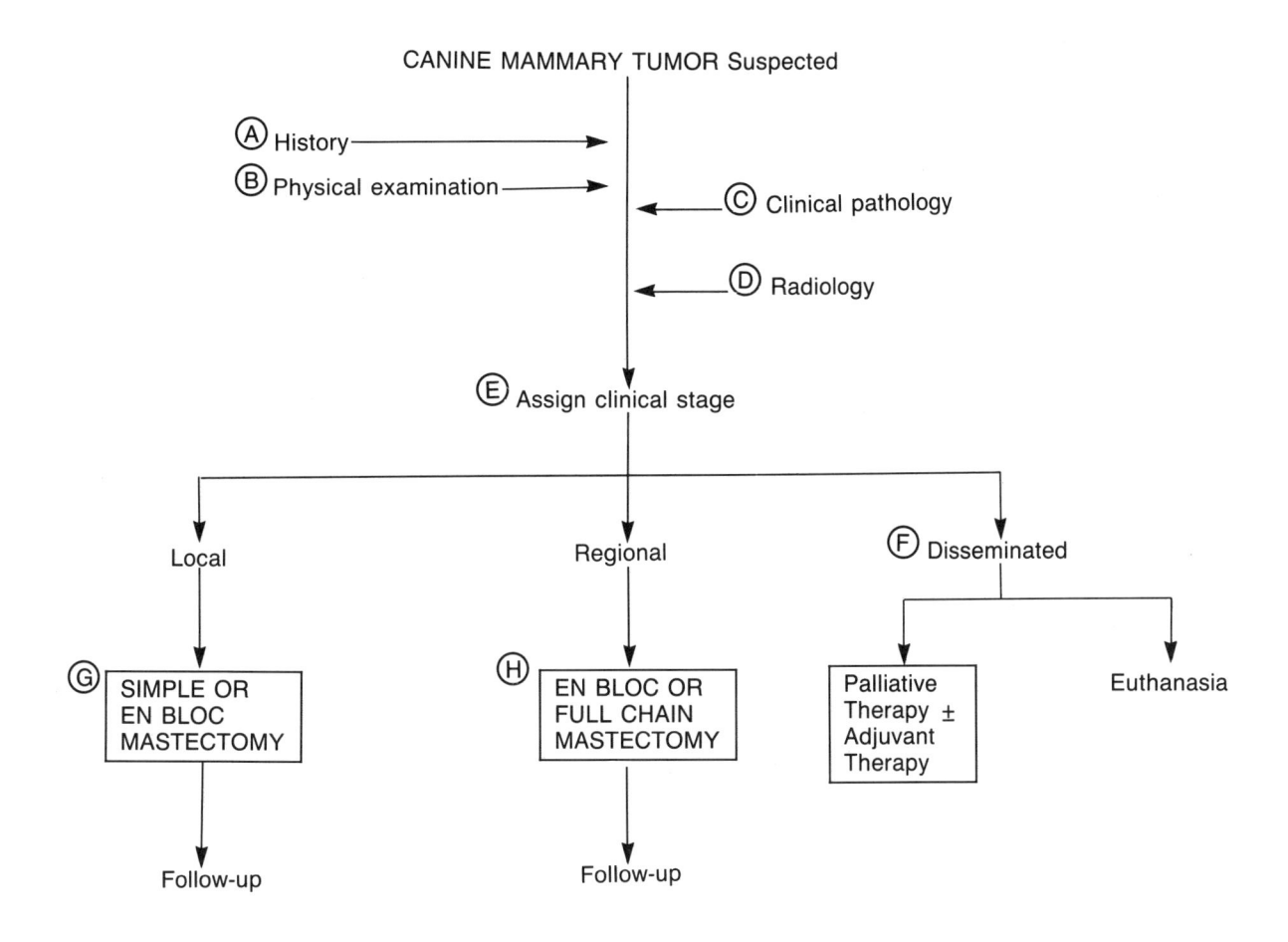

```
                    CANINE MAMMARY TUMOR Suspected
                                │
         Ⓐ History ─────────────▶│
         Ⓑ Physical examination ─▶│◀───── Ⓒ Clinical pathology
                                  │◀───── Ⓓ Radiology
                                  ▼
                         Ⓔ Assign clinical stage
          ┌───────────────────────┼───────────────────────┐
          ▼                       ▼                       ▼
        Local                  Regional              Ⓕ Disseminated
          │                       │                   ┌───┴───┐
          ▼                       ▼                   ▼       ▼
    Ⓖ SIMPLE OR            Ⓗ EN BLOC OR          Palliative  Euthanasia
      EN BLOC                 FULL CHAIN          Therapy ±
      MASTECTOMY              MASTECTOMY          Adjuvant
          │                       │               Therapy
          ▼                       ▼
       Follow-up               Follow-up
```

References

Brodey RS, Goldschmidt MH, Roszel JR. Canine mammary gland neoplasms. JAAHA 1983; 19:61.

Misdorp W, Hart AAM. Prognostic factors in canine mammary cancer. JNCI 1976; 56:779.

Norris AM, Harauz G, Ege GN, Broxup B, Valli VEO, et al. Lymphoscintigraphy in canine mammary neoplasia. Am J Vet Res 1982; 43:195.

Susaneck SJ, Allen TA, Hoopes J, Withrow SJ, Macy DW. Inflammatory mammary carcinoma in the dog. JAAHA 1983; 19:971.

FELINE MAMMARY GLAND TUMOR

Elizabeth J. Laing

The majority of feline mammary tumors are malignant and spread readily to lymph nodes and lungs. Progesterone therapy increases the risk of mammary neoplasia and hyperplasia. Ovariectomy decrease the risk of tumor development, with surgery prior to the first estrous cycle believed to provide maximum benefit. Ovariectomy at the time of tumor removal is of questionable value. Early tumor detection and aggressive therapy are most important in improving survival times.

A. The presenting complaint is usually an asymptomatic mammary mass in a middle-aged to older female cat. Intact females have a seven-fold greater risk compared to neutered females. Mammary tumors are rare in males.

B. All glands are at equal risk of tumor development, with multiple tumors occurring in 60 percent of cases. The cranial two glands drain into the axillary lymph node, whereas the caudal two glands drain into the superficial inguinal node (Fig. 1). Regional lymphadenopathy, large tumors, multiple tumors, and fixation to skin or muscle are associated with advanced disease. Dyspnea or hypertrophic osteopathy may indicate pulmonary metastasis. Other associated problems include uterine disease, ascites, and lymphedema. Differential diagnoses include mastitis in lactating females and fibroepithelial hyperplasia in females 1 to 2 weeks post-estrus.

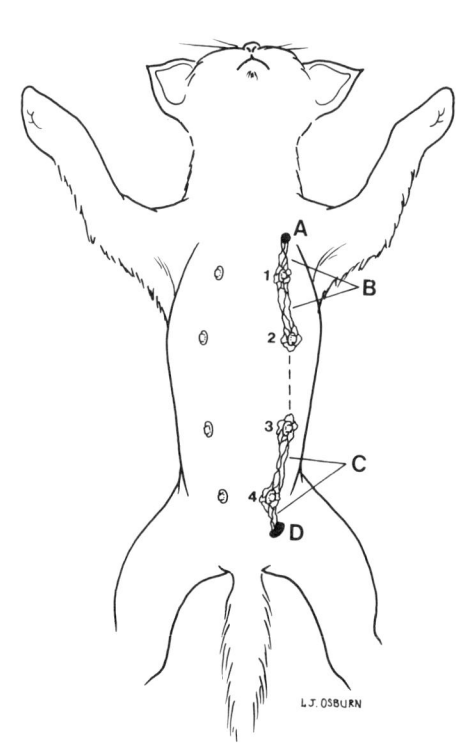

Figure 1 Lymphatic drainage of the four pair of feline mammary glands: *A*, axillary lymph node; *B*, lymphatics connecting the two cranial thoracic mammary glands to the axillary lymph node; *C*, lymphatics connecting caudal two lymph nodes and superficial inguinal lymph node; and *D*, superficial inguinal lymph node.

C. A complete blood count (CBC) and biochemical profile are recommended for all surgical candidates. Anemia and leukocytosis are paraneoplastic syndromes associated with feline mammary tumors. Fine-needle aspirate for cytologic diagnosis is not commonly recommended. Many tumors have extensive areas of necrosis that are difficult to differentiate from inflammatory disorders.

D. Ventrodorsal and left and right lateral chest radiographs are recommended in order to screen for pulmonary metastasis. Abnormal findings may include discrete soft tissue nodules, fluffy interstitial or miliary lesions, pleural effusion, and sternal lymphadenopathy. Early metastatic disease may be indistinguishable from changes of aging or inactive inflammatory lesions.

E. Mammary tumors are divided into four clinical stages, based on tumor size and metastatic spread. Stage multiple tumors individually. Stage 1 tumors are less than 1 cm in diameter and have no detectable lymph node or distant metastases. Benign tumors usually fall in this category. Stage 2 tumors are less than 3 cm in diameter and may have ipsilateral lymph node involvement. Stage 3 includes those tumors larger than 3 cm diameter or any tumor with bilateral lymph node involvement. Stage 4 includes any tumor with distant metastasis.

F. Treatment of stage 4 tumors varies with the clinical signs present. If the tumor is causing local discomfort with no systemic signs of metastasis or other illness, palliative tumor resection may be beneficial. More aggressive therapy includes mastectomy, followed by systemic adjuvant therapy. Although chemotherapy has been beneficial in preliminary trials, the long-term prognosis for these animals is poor.

G. Small solitary tumors may be treated by excision of the affected gland (simple mastectomy) or removal of the gland and draining lymph node (en bloc resection). Since most mammary tumors are malignant, the latter procedure is usually recommended. Histologic diagnosis is essential. If the tumor is benign or of low grade malignancy, periodic follow-up is recommended in order to check for recurrence. If the tumor is highly malignant or lymphatic spread is detected, adjuvant therapy may be beneficial.

H. In cats with malignant tumors, compared to more conservative treatments, radical or full-chain mastectomy has significantly prolonged the disease-free interval. Radical mastectomy removes all four glands on one side plus the ipsilateral axillary and superficial inguinal lymph nodes. In cases of bilateral tumor or lymph node involvement, bilateral surgeries are recommended 3 to 4 weeks apart. Histologic tumor and lymph node diagnosis is essential. If the tumor is highly malignant or metastatic to regional lymph nodes, adjuvant therapy should be considered.

I. Radiotherapy is currently being evaluated in feline mammary tumors. It is of greatest value when used postoperatively for local disease control. Antiestrogen therapy is

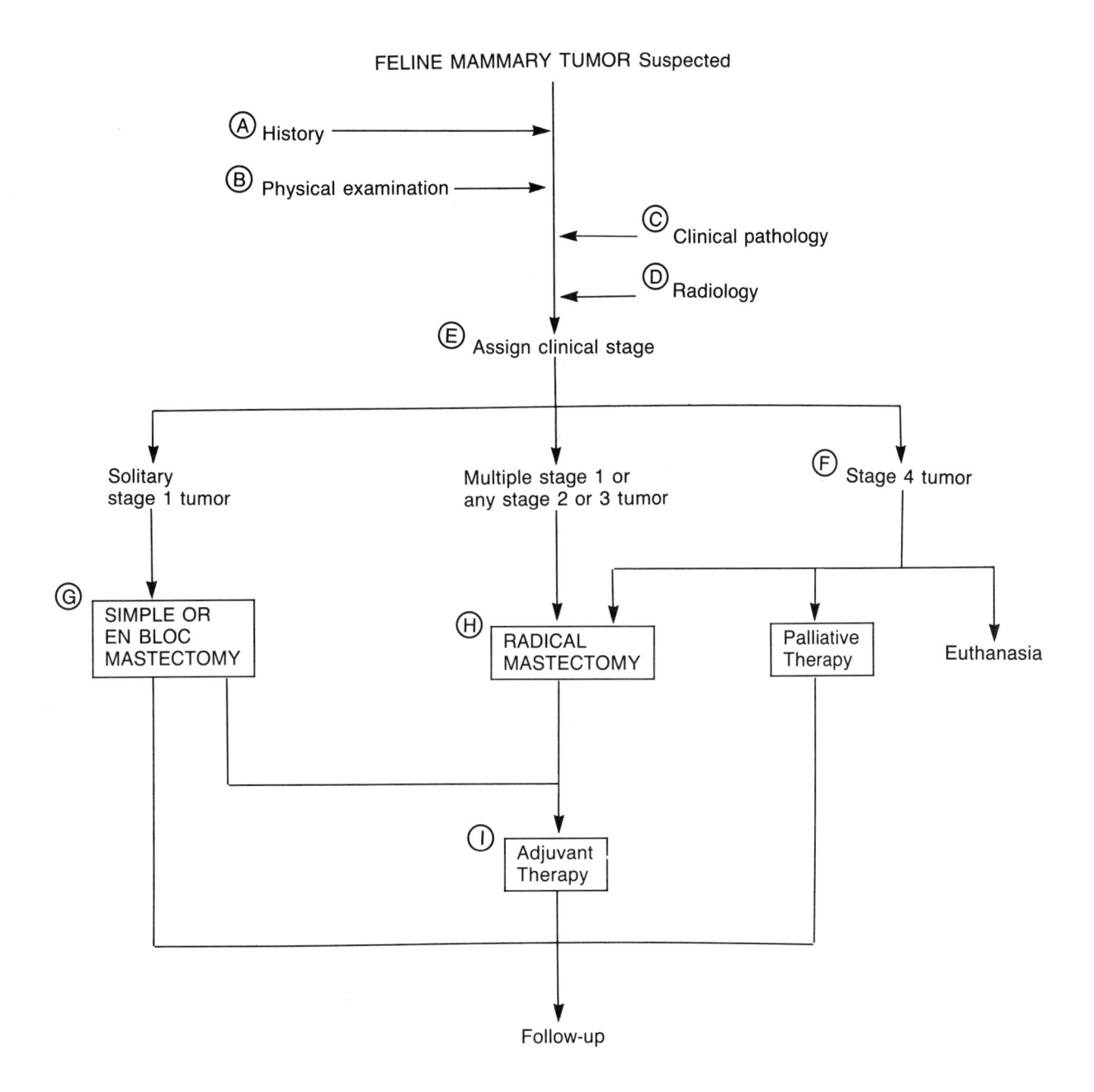

```
                    FELINE MAMMARY TUMOR Suspected
                                    │
        Ⓐ History ──────────────────▶│
                                    │
        Ⓑ Physical examination ─────▶│
                                    │◀────── Ⓒ Clinical pathology
                                    │
                                    │◀────── Ⓓ Radiology
                                    ▼
                          Ⓔ Assign clinical stage
                                    │
          ┌─────────────────────────┼─────────────────────────┐
          ▼                         ▼                         ▼
       Solitary            Multiple stage 1 or         Ⓕ Stage 4 tumor
       stage 1 tumor       any stage 2 or 3 tumor              │
          │                         │                 ┌────────┴────────┐
          ▼                         ▼                 ▼                 ▼
   Ⓖ  ┌─────────┐             Ⓗ ┌─────────┐      ┌──────────┐
      │ SIMPLE OR│                │ RADICAL │      │Palliative│     Euthanasia
      │ EN BLOC  │                │MASTECTOMY│     │ Therapy  │
      │MASTECTOMY│                └─────────┘      └──────────┘
      └─────────┘                      │
          │                            ▼
          │                    Ⓘ ┌──────────┐
          │                       │ Adjuvant │
          │                       │ Therapy  │
          │                       └──────────┘
          │                            │
          └────────────┬───────────────┘
                       ▼
                   Follow-up
```

of questionable value, as most feline mammary tumors are negative for estrogen receptors. Antineoplastic chemotherapy has shown some benefit with minimal toxicity. Frequent follow-up is recommended in order to allow early detection of recurrence.

References

Hayes AA, Mooney S. Feline mammary tumors. Vet Clin North Am (Small Anim Pract) 1985; 15:513.

Jeglum KA, deGuzman E, Young KM. Chemotherapy of advanced mammary adenocarcinoma in 14 cats. JAVMA 1985; 187:157.

MacEwen EG, Hayes AA, Harvey HJ, Patnaik AK, Mooney S, et al. Prognostic factors for feline mammary tumors. JAVMA 1984; 185:201.

Ogilvie GK. Feline mammary neoplasia. Comp Cont Ed 1983: 384.

HYPOTENSION

Doris H. Dyson

A. With hypotension, time is at a premium. Decrease or stop the administration of anesthetic while the history, physical status, and preoperative data are reevaluated. Take a blood sample and process it while further assessment is carried out. If an electrocardiogram (ECG) is not connected, a monitoring strip (lead positioning is of minor importance) should be taken first in order to verify normal rhythm.

B. A blood sample should be taken for determination of baseline data; packed cell volume (PCV), total protein (TP) analysis of blood gases, electrolytes, and glucose. While evaluation of blood oxygen levels can only be made with an arterial sample, venous blood can provide all the other information that is necessary, and it is easier to obtain.

C. Intermittent positive pressure ventilation (IPPV) causes high intrathoracic pressure, which reduces pulmonary blood volume, venous return, and cardiac output. Low blood pressure can result. By reducing tidal volume (TV), and increasing inspiratory flow rate, shorter inspiratory times (1 to 1.5 seconds) allow more time for cardiac filling, although gas distribution may be compromised. As some animals are unable to tolerate the depressive effects of IPPV, allowing them to breath spontaneously at slightly increased CO_2 levels, which stimulate the sympathetic system and increase cardiac output, may be best.

D. Hypotension may be caused by reduced cardiac output or increased capacity for the existing blood volume. Correct loss of blood or a reduction in protein, which maintains fluid in the vascular compartment, with blood or plasma, depending upon the loss involved. Counter minor blood or plasma losses or a reduction in peripheral vascular resistance by rapid fluid therapy, using a balanced electrolyte solution with low potassium levels (4 to 5 mEq per liter). A test dose of 20 ml per kilogram over 15 minutes is usually safe, and the response to therapy can be used to determine the need for more fluids.

E. Hypotension may initially be recognized by a poorly palpable pulse. The lingual artery is a peripheral pulse that may indicate poor blood pressure before it is noted in the femoral. Other techniques may be indicated to monitor these animals when hypotension has been diagnosed. A Doppler technique using a cuff and amplified reflected ultrasound is very useful. An oscillometric technique can also give a reasonable estimate of systolic blood pressure. A systolic pressure of more than 90 mm Hg should be achieved.

F. Septic or endotoxic shock can cause hypotension that may respond to high dose steroids (prednisolone sodium succinate 30 mg per kilogram IV). Plasma or transfusion reactions can result in hypotension. Give transfusions slowly with careful patient monitoring as these reactions can be very acute and may result in cardiac arrest. If a reaction occurs, discontinue the transfusion and maintain the blood pressure with fluids, dextrans, sympathomimetic agents, and calcium.

G. Central venous pressure (CVP) determines the relationship between the blood volume and the cardiovascular system's capacity to hold and move this volume (Fig. 1). A value greater than 10 cm H_2O indicates that the heart is unable to handle the load presented to it. Reduce speed of administration. A value less than 0 cm H_2O indicates inadequate volume with respect to capacity. Restoration of volume with fluids, blood, or plasma is required. Within the normal range, further fluid therapy can safely be continued. Peripheral vasoconstriction may occur in response to a deficiency in blood volume. This can result in adequate venous return (normal CVP), but reduced peripheral perfusion. Tissue perfusion and pulse may be improved by increasing blood volume. The CVP will remain in the normal range as the vasoconstriction is reduced in response to the expanded blood volume.

H. Cardiac stimulants may increase cardiac efficiency. The use of β_1-agonist drugs in low doses results in increased stroke volume. High doses cause tachycardia and vasoconstriction. Dobutamine (5 to 10 μg per kilogram per minute IV) can be given by infusion, adjusting the dose for the desired rise in blood pressure and fall in CVP. Ephedrine (0.02 to 0.04 mg per kilogram IV) results in both α- and β-receptor stimulation and increases norepinephrine release. Calcium gluconate (50 mg per kilogram) is recommended in calcium deficiency or in massive blood transfusions where the anticoagulant reduces calcium availability. Adequate calcium levels are

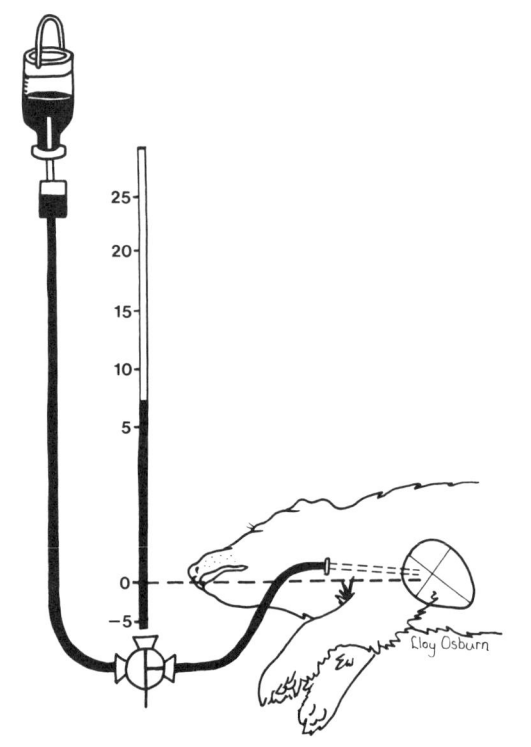

Figure 1 Monometric measurement of central venous pressure in the dog. Note: Dog is in right lateral recumbency.

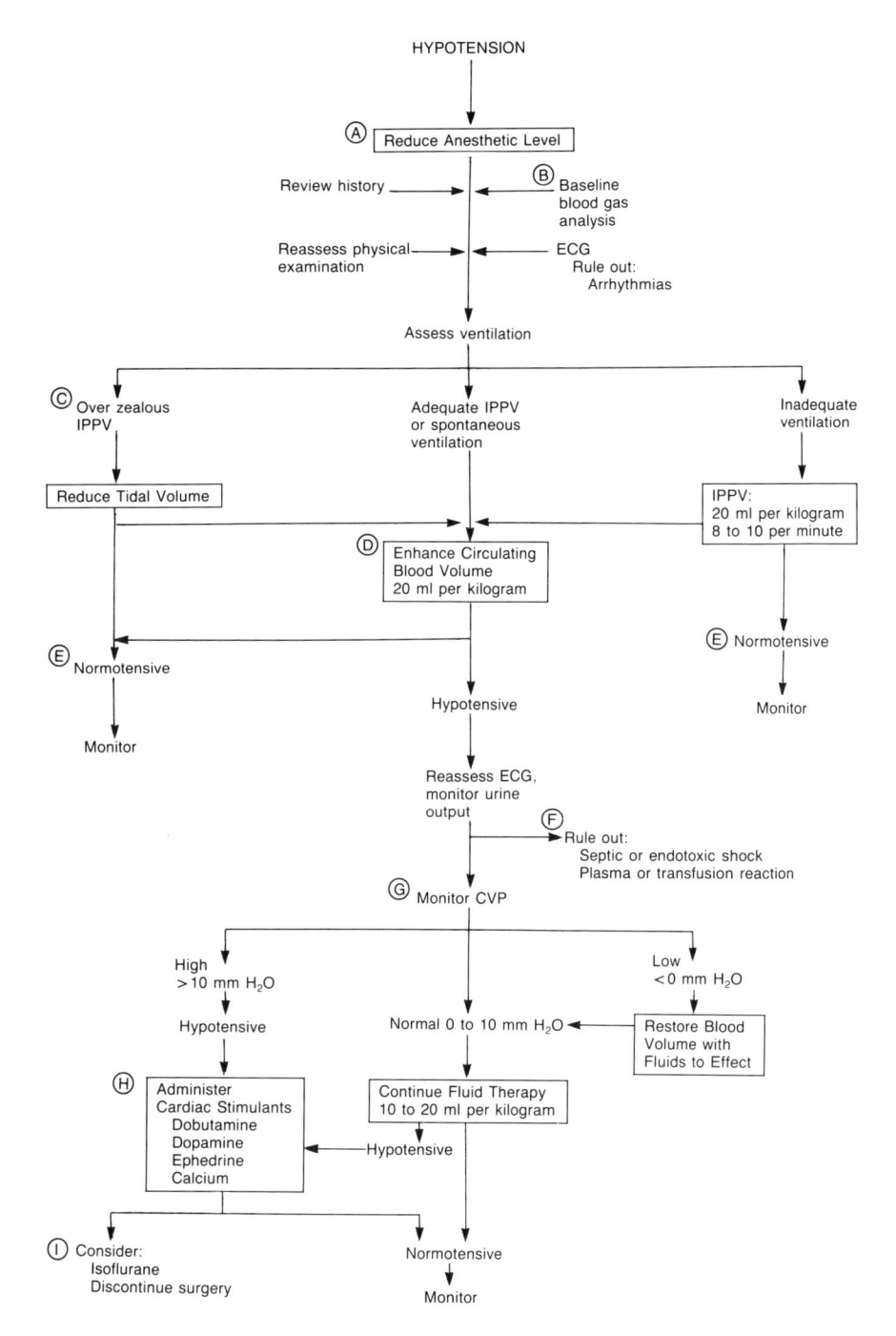

```
                          HYPOTENSION
                              │
                              ▼
                     Ⓐ ┌─────────────────┐
                       │ Reduce Anesthetic Level │
                       └─────────────────┘
         Review history ──→  ←── Ⓑ Baseline blood gas analysis
         Reassess physical ──→  ←── ECG
         examination              Rule out: Arrhythmias
                              │
                              ▼
                        Assess ventilation
        ┌─────────────────────┼─────────────────────┐
        ▼                     ▼                     ▼
   Ⓒ Over zealous      Adequate IPPV           Inadequate
      IPPV             or spontaneous          ventilation
                       ventilation
        │                                            │
        ▼                                            ▼
  ┌──────────────┐                         ┌──────────────┐
  │ Reduce Tidal │                         │ IPPV:        │
  │ Volume       │                         │ 20 ml per kg │
  └──────────────┘                         │ 8 to 10/min  │
        │                                  └──────────────┘
        │         Ⓓ ┌──────────────────┐           │
        │            │ Enhance Circulating │        │
        │            │ Blood Volume        │◀───────┤
        │            │ 20 ml per kilogram  │        │
        │            └──────────────────┘           │
        ▼                     │                     ▼
  Ⓔ Normotensive         Hypotensive           Ⓔ Normotensive
        │                     │                     │
        ▼                     ▼                     ▼
     Monitor           Reassess ECG,            Monitor
                       monitor urine
                       output
                     Ⓕ  → Rule out:
                           Septic or endotoxic shock
                           Plasma or transfusion reaction
                  Ⓖ Monitor CVP
        ┌─────────────┼─────────────┐
        ▼             ▼             ▼
      High         Normal          Low
    >10 mm H₂O   0 to 10 mm H₂O   <0 mm H₂O
        │                          ┌──────────────┐
   Hypotensive                     │ Restore Blood│
        │                          │ Volume with  │
        ▼                          │ Fluids to Effect│
  Ⓗ ┌──────────────┐               └──────────────┘
     │ Administer   │           ┌──────────────────┐
     │ Cardiac      │           │ Continue Fluid   │
     │ Stimulants   │◀──────────│ Therapy 10 to 20 │
     │  Dobutamine  │ Hypotensive│ ml per kilogram │
     │  Dopamine    │           └──────────────────┘
     │  Ephedrine   │
     │  Calcium     │
     └──────────────┘
        │                         Normotensive
        ▼                              │
  Ⓘ Consider:                          ▼
     Isoflurane                    Monitor
     Discontinue surgery
```

required for effective excitation-contraction coupling in the heart.

I. Improve poor cardiac output by reducing the afterload against which the heart must pump. Isoflurane reduces peripheral vascular resistance while maintaining cardiac output and is the inhalant anesthetic of choice in cardiac disease and the severely debilitated animal. Other vasodilators such as phentolamine are contraindicated if the BP remains low. Hypotension may be worsened. If there is persistent difficulty in raising blood pressure, the surgery should be stopped, recovery carried out, and a stable cardiac condition produced before surgery is attempted again. This may require the use of digoxin or reduction of afterload with hydralazine or prazosin in the awake animal.

References

Adams HR. New perspectives in cardiopulmonary therapeutics: receptor-selective adrenergic drugs. JAVMA 1984; 185(9):966.

Harvey RC, Short CE. The use of isoflurane for safe anesthesia in animals with traumatic myocarditis or other myocardial sensitivity. Canine Pract 1983; 10(4):18.

Jennings PB, Anderson RW, Martin AM. Central venous pressure monitoring: guide to blood volume replacement in the dog. JAVMA 1967; 151(10):1283.

Morgan BC, Martin WE, Hornbein TF, Crawford EW, Cruntheroth WG. Hemodynamic effects of intermittent positive pressure respiration. Anesthesiology 1966; 27:584.

APNEA ASSOCIATED WITH ANESTHESIA

Doris H. Dyson

A. Immediately handle acute respiratory arrest at induction by intubation and oxygen (O_2) delivery. A patent airway allows spontaneous breathing to resume without interference (long soft palate obstruction, pharyngeal mucus, or vomitus aspiration). Most animals are induced while breathing room air, which results in an abrupt fall in alveolar O_2 with apnea. Preoxygenation (3 to 5 minutes of high O_2 concentrations by face mask) provides a reserve of O_2, which allows up to 7 minutes of apnea before dangerous hypoxemia occurs. Intermittent positive pressure ventilation (IPPV) on 100 percent O_2 for several breaths immediately following induction apnea enhances the lung O_2, permitting time for reassessment.

B. If the animal is in a stable cardiovascular condition, assess reflexes in order to determine the depth of anesthesia. When apnea accompanies induction, variations may exist depending on the agent used. A light plane of anesthesia permits the patient to breath hold after intubation. Monitor laryngeal sensitivity by observing abdominal movements when the trachea or larynx is externally palpated or the endotracheal tube gently moved. The jaw tone, palpebral and pedal reflexes, or ear flick (in the cat) will also assist in assessing the depth of anesthesia. During maintenance, the response of the dog to the surgical stimulus adds to the anesthetic evaluation. Monitor changes in heart rate and strength of pulse.

C. Once the animal is breathing spontaneously on 100 percent O_2, introduce the maintenance inhalation anesthetic. The transfer from an intravenous induction to the inhalation agent should be carried out over a few minutes to prevent the animal from breath holding in response to a sudden high concentration of pungent gas. Then monitor to ensure that adequate spontaneous ventilation continues.

D. When the animal breath holds during a light anesthetic plane, it is usually easiest to deepen anesthesia with more anesthetic agent. On induction, either use more intravenous agent or control ventilation with increased concentration of the inhalation anesthetic chosen for maintenance. Apnea during maintenance may result from awareness of the endotracheal tube or surgical stimulus. The inhalant agent concentration can be increased or additional analgesia can be achieved with narcotic supplementation. Carry out reassessment of the animal's ability to ventilate spontaneously when reflexes indicate a more suitable level of anesthesia.

E. IPPV is best carried out to provide natural thoracic movement at a rate of 10 times per minute. A tidal volume of 20 ml per kilogram at this rate should provide adequate carbon dioxide removal. Oxygenation of the blood is dependent upon both adequate ventilation with a high O_2 concentration and perfusion of these ventilated areas. It is therefore imperative to maintain cardiac output and blood pressure. Excessively high ventilation volumes or pressures reduce venous return and cardiac output and may cause alveolar rupture. Rapid administration of fluid therapy using a balanced electrolyte solution with low potassium levels can reduce the hypotension that accompanies deeper planes of anesthesia. Give a volume of 20 ml per kilogram over 15 minutes.

F. If spontaneous ventilation occurs after a period of apnea, it is important to evaluate its adequacy. Oxygen levels may be maintained, but carbon dioxide may increase with shallow respirations because of the rebreathing of dead space gases. Occasionally deep, infrequent breaths may allow oxygen and carbon dioxide levels to remain in a physiologically appropriate range. This assessment can be difficult to make in some animals. Blood gas analysis provides accurate judgment if an arterial sample is used. When there is some doubt concerning the ventilation adequacy, IPPV is best carried out for the duration of the surgery.

Reference

Grandy JL, Steffey EP. Anesthesia and the respiratory system. In: Slatter DH, ed. Textbook of small animal surgery. Philadelphia: WB Saunders, 1985:2621.

APNEA

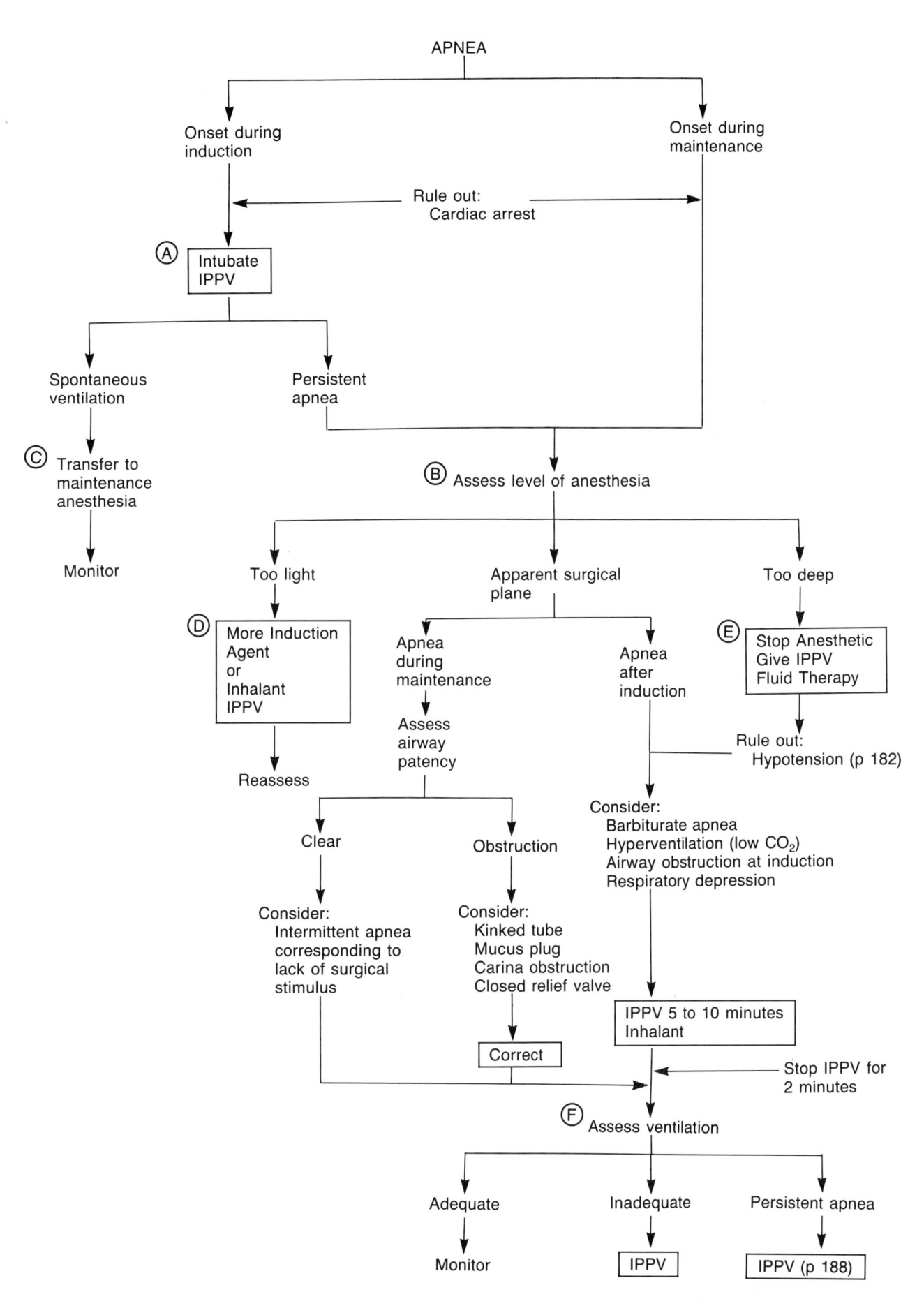

- Onset during induction
- Onset during maintenance

Rule out: Cardiac arrest

(A) Intubate IPPV

- Spontaneous ventilation
  - **(C) Transfer to maintenance anesthesia**
  - Monitor
- Persistent apnea

(B) Assess level of anesthesia

- Too light
  - **(D) More Induction Agent or Inhalant IPPV**
  - Reassess
- Apparent surgical plane
  - Apnea during maintenance
    - Assess airway patency
      - Clear
        - Consider: Intermittent apnea corresponding to lack of surgical stimulus
      - Obstruction
        - Consider: Kinked tube, Mucus plug, Carina obstruction, Closed relief valve
        - Correct
  - Apnea after induction
- Too deep
  - **(E) Stop Anesthetic, Give IPPV, Fluid Therapy**
  - Rule out: Hypotension (p 182)

Consider:
- Barbiturate apnea
- Hyperventilation (low CO_2)
- Airway obstruction at induction
- Respiratory depression

IPPV 5 to 10 minutes Inhalant

Stop IPPV for 2 minutes

(F) Assess ventilation

- Adequate → Monitor
- Inadequate → IPPV
- Persistent apnea → IPPV (p 188)

INTRAOPERATIVE OR POSTOPERATIVE PAIN

Peter J. Pascoe

A. It appears to be beneficial to treat pain before it is sensed. If the animal is allowed to wake up and feel the pain, it is likely to be harder to control. Thus, it is best to give analgesics or nerve blocks before the animal becomes conscious.

B. Nonsteroidal anti-inflammatory drugs (NSAIDs) act by reducing the release of prostaglandins in the injured area; prostaglandins appear to sensitize nociceptive neurons to painful stimuli. Aspirin (25 to 30 mg per kilogram), acetaminophen (25 to 30 mg per kilogram), or phenylbutazone (10 mg per kilogram) can be used in the dog. Cats are more sensitive to these agents, but a single dose of aspirin (20 to 25 mg per kilogram) should not be toxic. Opiates such as meperidine, pentazocine, morphine, oxymorphone, butorphanol, and fentanyl all provide analgesia. Meperidine, pentazocine, and fentanyl have relatively brief activity (1 to 2 hours), whereas the others last for longer than 3 hours. Used preoperatively, they may increase the degree of respiratory depression during anesthesia.

C. Methoxyflurane is a good analgesic and reduces postoperative pain for 6 to 24 hours after surgery.

D. In the head and neck area, it is appropriate to use opiates or NSAIDs because regional nerve blocks are relatively difficult. Topical anesthesia for the cornea or gingiva may be useful, but is brief in duration. In the forelimbs, perform specific nerve blocks for pain relief.

E. Intercostal nerve blocks, using bupivacaine, are relatively easy to perform and give pain relief for 3 hours. Block the two intercostal nerves anterior and the one nerve posterior to the incision by injecting 2 to 3 ml of 0.5 percent bupivacaine along the caudal border of the rib. The total dose of bupivacaine should not exceed 6 mg per kilogram.

F. Epidural analgesia using local anesthetics may provide pain relief for surgery in this area, but also paralyzes motor function in the animal. This can be distressing for animals that expect to be active. Epidural opiates may be used. Morphine at 0.1 mg per kilogram appears to give 16 to 24 hours of pain reduction. The morphine should be diluted to a volume of 1 ml per 5 kilogram.

G. If a cast or bandage causes discomfort, it should be adjusted. Drugs may be useful to control nervous or highly sensitive individuals. Acepromazine (0.03 to 0.05 mg per kilogram IM) may produce good sedation. Diazepam (0.2 to 0.5 mg per kilogram IV) does not sedate the animal but may make it less fearful. Pentobarbital (start with 3 to 5 mg per kilogram) can be given to effect, and the level of sedation can be increased to the point of reanesthetizing the animal if necessary.

References

Bonath KH, Saleh AS. Long term pain treatment in the dog by peridural morphines. Proc 2nd Int Congress Vet Anesth 1985:161.

Lumb WV, Wynn Jones E. Veterinary anesthesia. 2nd ed. Philadelphia: Lea & Febiger, 1984:371.

Taylor PM. Analgesia in the dog and cat. In Pract 1985; 7:5.

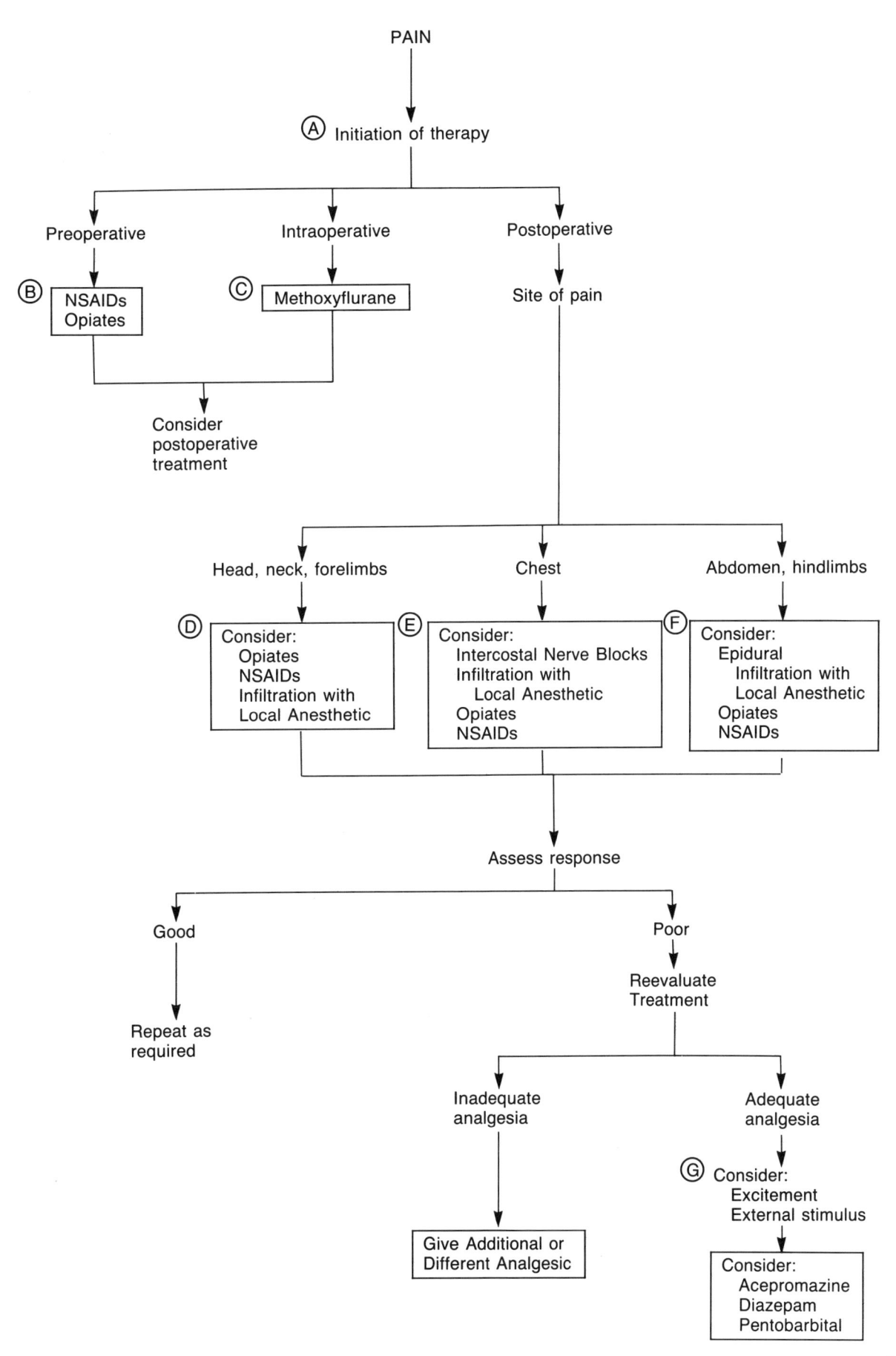

```
                          PAIN
                            │
                            ▼
                    Ⓐ Initiation of therapy
          ┌─────────────────┼─────────────────┐
          ▼                 ▼                 ▼
    Preoperative       Intraoperative     Postoperative
          │                 │                 │
          ▼                 ▼            Site of pain
    Ⓑ ┌─────────┐      Ⓒ ┌──────────────┐
      │ NSAIDs  │        │ Methoxyflurane│
      │ Opiates │        └──────────────┘
      └─────────┘
          │
          ▼
      Consider
      postoperative
      treatment
```

          ┌────────────────────┼────────────────────┐
          ▼   ▼   ▼
   Head, neck, forelimbs   Chest   Abdomen, hindlimbs

Ⓓ Consider: Ⓔ Consider: Ⓕ Consider:
    Opiates   Intercostal Nerve Blocks   Epidural
    NSAIDs   Infiltration with   Infiltration with
    Infiltration with   Local Anesthetic   Local Anesthetic
       Local Anesthetic   Opiates   Opiates
                             NSAIDs   NSAIDs

                         Assess response
                    ┌─────────┴─────────┐
                    ▼   ▼
                  Good   Poor
                    │   │
                    ▼   ▼
               Repeat as   Reevaluate
               required   Treatment
                              ┌────────┴────────┐
                              ▼   ▼
                        Inadequate   Adequate
                        analgesia   analgesia
                              │   │
                              ▼   ▼
                      Give Additional or   Ⓖ Consider:
                      Different Analgesic   Excitement
                                               External stimulus
                                                    │
                                                    ▼
                                               Consider:
                                                 Acepromazine
                                                 Diazepam
                                                 Pentobarbital

POOR RECOVERY

Doris H. Dyson

A. Prevention is the best approach to hypothermia. Very young, old, or small patients are susceptible to significant hypothermia. Prolonged surgery and extensive tissue exposure enhances the danger. Anesthetic requirements lessen, and the animal's ventilatory ability becomes impaired, which results in prolongation of the surgical anesthetic plane during recovery. Rewarming is best carried out over a period of time; this allows the core temperature to equilibrate with that of the surface. Use warm water circulating blankets, warm water bottles, and heat lamps to provide surface warming. With some forms of rewarming caution must be used to prevent burning the animal. Avoid overtreatment (return to 36.5º C). Enriched oxygen breathing during this time compensates for the high metabolic demand of shivering and the reduced tissue O_2 release with hypothermia.

B. With inhalation anesthesia, the best approach to slow recovery is the institution of intermittent positive pressure ventilation (IPPV). Depressed, debilitated, obese, or deeply anesthetized animals have poor ventilatory ability. Administer high flows of 100 percent O_2 in order to wash the anesthetic gases from the circuit, thus preventing rebreathing of expired gases. When the inhalant has been removed from the animal through ventilation, respiration returns quickly, even if the carbon dioxide levels are reduced. IPPV at 8 to 10 per minute and 20 ml per kilogram tidal volume produces adequate ventilation.

C. Barbiturate anesthesia is not ideal for prolonged anesthetic management. Thiobarbiturates redistribute for rapid recovery, but if several doses are given, a saturation point is reached eventually. Metabolism required for recovery is a slow process. Pentobarbital depends completely on metabolism for recovery. Methohexital is the preferred agent when several injections are required since redistribution occurs, but metabolism is very rapid in comparison to the others. Since the active component is prevalent in acidic environments, adequate ventilation and minor alkalinizing of the blood with small doses of bicarbonate (1 to 2 mg per kilogram) result in a lightened anesthetic plane and a more rapid recovery.

D. Xylazine may be reversed partially by the use of yohimbine (0.125 mg per kilogram), which competes specifically with xylazine in the CNS. The use of 4-amino pyridine (0.3 mg per kilogram) results in a degree of CNS excitation that may assist in reversing xylazine. Narcotic premedication may be reversed with naloxone (0.04 mg per kilogram). This dose may be repeated within 3 minutes to achieve the desired effect. Renarcotization is possible because of the short duration of effect. Further reversal may be necessary.

E. Analysis of blood gases may prove helpful in determining other problems (metabolic acidosis, iatrogenic respiratory alkalosis, hypoxia).

F. Innovar-vet or oxymorphone combinations can be reversed using levallorphan (1 mg) or nalorphine (5 mg). These are agonist-antagonists, which reverse the stronger effects of other narcotics, but may allow a small degree of pain relief and respiratory depression to persist. Naloxone (0.04 mg per kilogram) is a true antagonist, possessing no agonistic properties. It reverses not only the respiratory depression and sedation, but also removes analgesia, which may be undesirable. This reversal is warranted in the severely debilitated and when the slightest chance of respiratory depression is intolerable.

G. Competitive neuromuscular blocking agents can be successfully reversed after signs of a partial block appear. This can be determined by using a nerve stimulator or allowing the passage of at least 15 minutes after the correct dose of relaxant is given. Signs of some diaphragmatic movements or weak respiratory efforts help to assess the response to the reversal agent as well as confirm a partial block. Atropine (0.04 mg per kilogram IV) should be given with neostigmine (0.02 to 0.04 mg per kilogram IV) in order to prevent undesirable muscarinic stimulation by neostigmine (salivation, micturition, bradycardia, cardiac arrest).

H. A phase II block can occur with succinyl choline following a high dose or repeated injections in which respiratory function fails to return in the expected time interval (20 minutes in the dog, 5 minutes in the cat). The drug may act as a competitive muscle relaxant and will respond to an anticholinesterase agent. Edrophonium, a test drug, may produce a shorter duration of action although some controversy exists regarding this.

I. The Doxapram test may determine whether persistent central nervous system (CNS) depression or residual neuromuscular block is responsible for the poor recovery. Doxapram (2 mg per kilogram IV) is a central respiratory stimulant that also enhances peripheral chemoreceptor activity. Improved respiration, in the form of increased tital volume, results, if the CNS is depressed by anesthesia and the muscles are able to respond. CNS depression may also be caused by surgical or medical pathology. An unrecognized hypoxic episode during anesthesia can also cause this observation. The animal with poor muscle function caused by a persistent block is unable to improve ventilation after doxapram, but may increase the rate at the expense of tidal volume. This persisteant block may be due to unreversed muscle relaxant, neostigmine overdose, or antibiotic interaction with the muscle relaxant (aminoglycosides).

References

Klein L, Klide AM. Anesthesia and the musculoskeletal system. In: Slatter DH, ed. Textbook of small animal surgery. Philadelphia: WB Saunders, 1985:2675.

Short CE. Practical use of the ultra short-acting barbiturates. New Jersey: Veterinary Learning Systems, 1983:13.

Waterman A. Accidental hypothermia during anesthesia in dogs and cats. Vet Rec 1975; 96:308.

Winnie AP, Collins VJ. The Doxapram test: a new technique for the differential diagnosis of apnea. Anesthesiology 1965; 26:265.

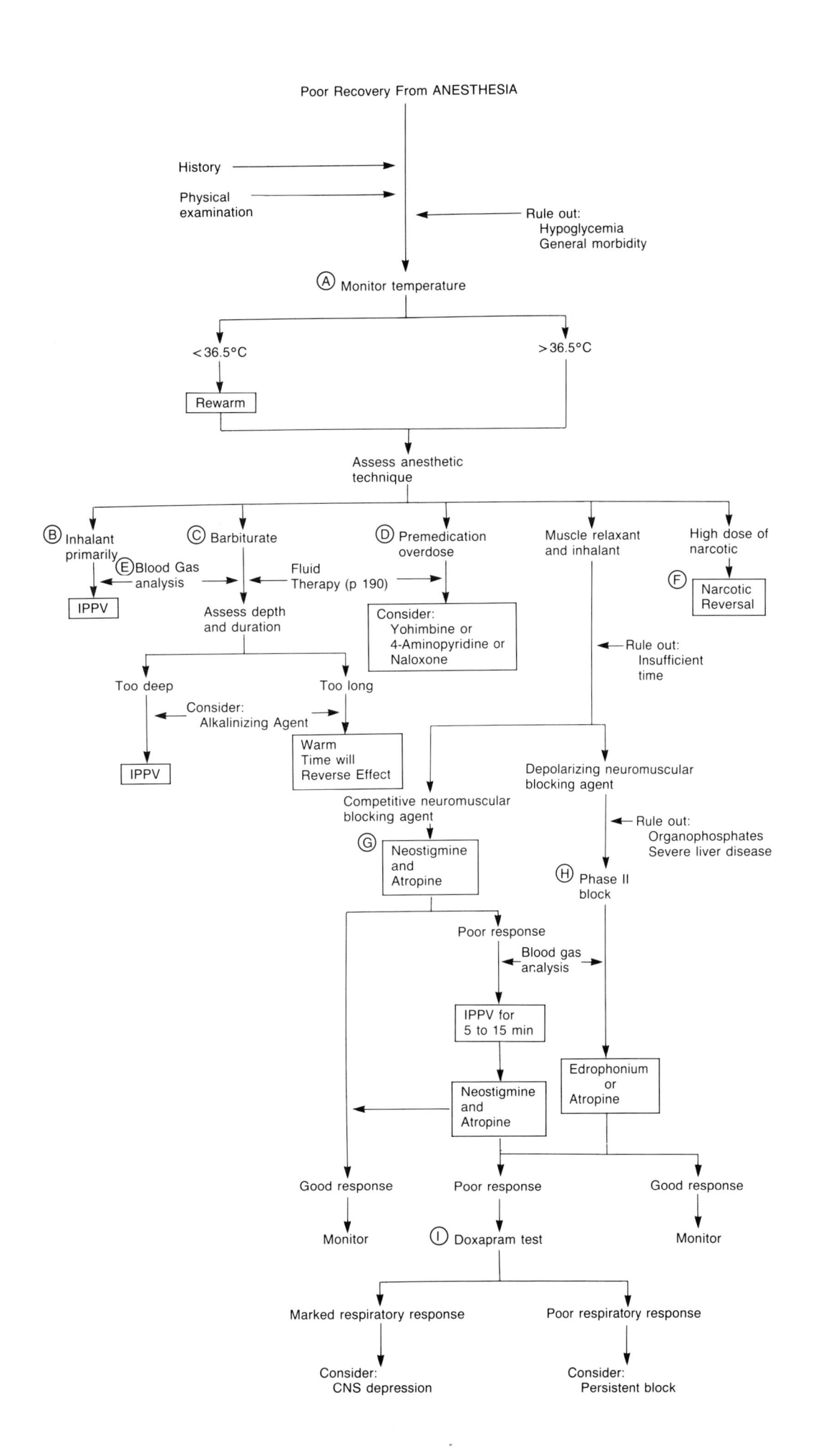

Poor Recovery From ANESTHESIA

History →
Physical examination →

Rule out:
- Hypoglycemia
- General morbidity

(A) Monitor temperature
- < 36.5°C → Rewarm
- > 36.5°C

↓

Assess anesthetic technique

- **(B) Inhalant primarily** → (E) Blood Gas analysis → IPPV
- **(C) Barbiturate** → Fluid Therapy (p 190) → Assess depth and duration
  - Too deep → Consider: Alkalinizing Agent → IPPV
  - Too long → Warm, Time will Reverse Effect
- **(D) Premedication overdose** → Consider: Yohimbine or 4-Aminopyridine or Naloxone
- **Muscle relaxant and inhalant** — Rule out: Insufficient time
  - Competitive neuromuscular blocking agent → **(G) Neostigmine and Atropine**
  - Depolarizing neuromuscular blocking agent — Rule out: Organophosphates, Severe liver disease → **(H) Phase II block**
- **High dose of narcotic** → **(F) Narcotic Reversal**

After Neostigmine and Atropine:
- Poor response → Blood gas analysis → IPPV for 5 to 15 min → Neostigmine and Atropine

Phase II block → Edrophonium or Atropine

Outcomes:
- Good response → Monitor
- Poor response → **(I) Doxapram test**
  - Marked respiratory response → Consider: CNS depression
  - Poor respiratory response → Consider: Persistent block
- Good response → Monitor

FLUID THERAPY

Doris H. Dyson

Simple steps may be taken to develop an individualized fluid therapy schedule that can be applied to both surgical and nonsurgical patients; however this will need frequent reevaluation. Consideration of unexpected ongoing losses within the day may be required, depending upon the stability of the patient's condition.

A. Always perform packed cell volume (PCV), total protein (TP), and urinalysis. Expanded laboratory data allows an improved response to the more accurately calculated fluid therapy. When these tests are not available, choices must be made considering the expected losses with the abnormality presented.

B. Do not allow total protein (TP) to fall below 3.5 to 4.0 g per deciliter. Albumin is the primary protein that maintains oncotic pressure within the vascular compartment. Losses result in a reduction of vascular volume by a fluid shift into interstitial spaces. Pulmonary edema commonly occurs. Correction with fresh or stored plasma should be carried out over 2 hours. The following formula provides a guideline:

$$\frac{\text{desired TP} - \text{recipient TP}}{\text{donor TP}} \times \text{wt (kg)} \times 50 = \text{ml plasma}$$

Give Dextran 70, a commercially available colloid, diluted 1:4 with a balanced electrolyte solution in order to produce a temporary effect beneficial for acute situations, when plasma is not available.

C. Nonbreeding, first transfusion animals can safely be given untyped blood, but a simple crossmatch procedure can be used to reduce the occurrence of an adverse reaction. Heartworm testing is recommended on donor blood. Stored blood is suitable unless the history or coagulation tests indicate that fresh blood is required for platelets or coagulation factors. An animal maintained for the purpose of blood transfusions should be type A negative. Stored blood should be cultured to assure sterility. When blood loss is 10 to 15 percent of the blood volume, replacement fluids alone may be used with careful observation of PCV (>25) and total protein (>3.5 g per deciliter). If blood is given to correct for acute blood losses, administer a balanced, calcium-free electrolyte solution simultaneously in order to decrease viscosity. Fluids must be given in quantities of 3 to 4 times the estimated volume of blood loss in order to compensate for the redistribution that occurs. When PCV or total protein fall below these levels, include blood or plasma in the therapy.

D. When anemia is present, viscosity is not a problem, and blood can be given without concurrent fluids. Dehydration of 5 percent or more is assessed by physical examination (skin turgor, mental status, eye appearance). The degree of dehydration is determined, and fluid replacement is calculated (percent dehydration $\times$ weight (kg) = number of liters required).

E. When potassium levels are normal, 15 to 20 mEq per liter should be included when replacing losses from vomition, diarrhea, or diuresis. Add a similar amount to maintenance fluids. A maximum of 80 mEq per liter can be used with severe deficits, especially if bicarbonate, insulin, or glucose are administered concurrently. Infusion of potassium-containing solutions must not exceed 0.5 mEq per kilogram per hour, and thus, fluids for rapid bolus administration should have only 4 to 5 mEq per liter of potassium. When fluids are slowed to maintenance flows (50 to 90 ml per kilogram per 24 hours), add potassium supplementation as required.

F. Bicarbonate may be required when acidosis is suspected. If the pH is greater than 7.2, then correction of the cause and administration of a balanced electrolyte solution may suffice. If a greater degree of acidemia is present on account of a metabolic (not respiratory) disturbance, then give bicarbonate replacement over a minimum of 30 minutes. [(24 − measured bicarbonate) $\times$ weight (kg) $\times$ 0.3 = mEq of bicarbonate required]. Partial slow replacement with bicarbonate should be carried out if severe metabolic acidosis is present. Animals that have suffered hypoxia or severe hypotension may be treated with bicarbonate (1 to 4 mEq per kilogram) given slowly intravenously. The dose chosen is dependent upon the duration of the hypoxia or hypotension. High fluid therapy is best started in the severely dehydrated patient before bicarbonate replacement in order to prevent overdose caused by the contracted blood volume.

G. Glucose may be considered for very young and very small animals in order to prevent hypoglycemia with concomitant short-term anorexia. Enhanced intracellular transfer of K^+ may be achieved by including 5 percent glucose in the fluids given when hyperkalemia exists or when high potassium-containing fluids are used.

H. Further losses from vomition, diarrhea, diuresis, surgical evaporation, and bleeding must be evaluated and replaced. During surgery, 5 to 10 ml per kilogram per hour fluid therapy can correct evaporative, fecal, urinary, and very minor blood losses.

I. Maintenance fluids should contain the following electrolytes in quantities similar to normal daily losses (40 mEq per liter Na^+, 40 mEq per liter Cl^-, 20 mEq per liter K^+, 20 mEq per liter HCO_3^-. Dextrose (5 g per deciliter) is often included. Dilute balanced electrolyte solutions with 5 percent dextrose solution and a K^+ supplement added to these fluids in order to achieve similar values. Most animals with normal kidney function are forgiving with respect to minor errors in Na^+ concentration. Significant K^+ deficits are commonly produced when balanced elctrolyte solutions with 4 to 5 mEq per liter K^+ are used for long-term therapy.

References

Haskins SC. Blood gases and acid-base balance: clinical interpretation and therapeutic implications. In: Kirk RW, ed. Current veterinary therapy VIII. Philadelphia: WB Saunders, 1983:201.

Killingsworth CP. Use of blood and blood components for the feline and canine patient. Vet Crit Care 1984; 7(1):6.

Waterman A. Practical fluid therapy for small animals. In Pract 1984; 6(5):143.

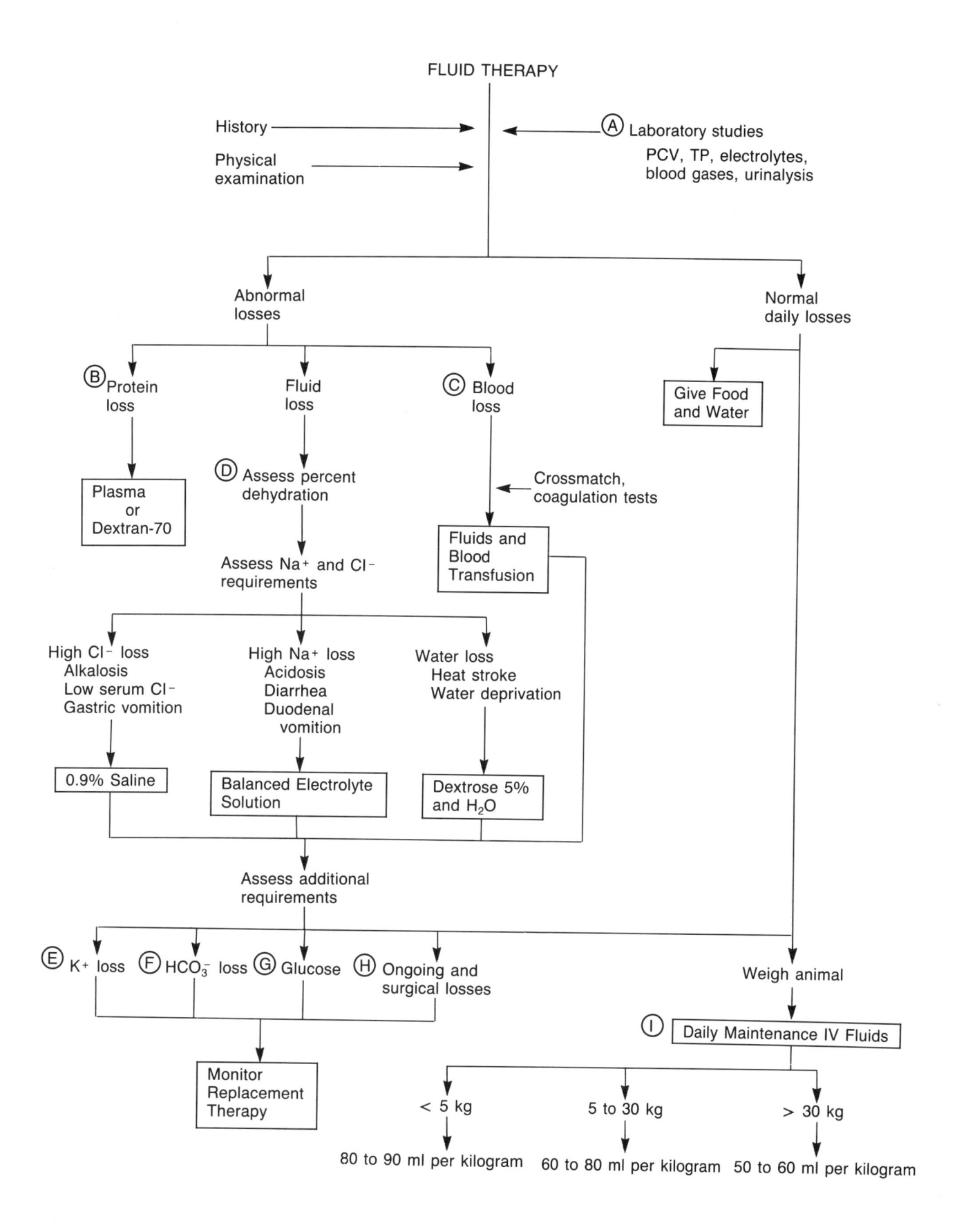

FLUID THERAPY

- History
- Physical examination
- (A) Laboratory studies: PCV, TP, electrolytes, blood gases, urinalysis

Abnormal losses

- (B) Protein loss → Plasma or Dextran-70
- Fluid loss → (D) Assess percent dehydration → Assess Na$^+$ and Cl$^-$ requirements
- (C) Blood loss ← Crossmatch, coagulation tests → Fluids and Blood Transfusion

Assess Na$^+$ and Cl$^-$ requirements

- High Cl$^-$ loss, Alkalosis, Low serum Cl$^-$, Gastric vomition → 0.9% Saline
- High Na$^+$ loss, Acidosis, Diarrhea, Duodenal vomition → Balanced Electrolyte Solution
- Water loss, Heat stroke, Water deprivation → Dextrose 5% and H$_2$O

→ Assess additional requirements:
- (E) K$^+$ loss
- (F) HCO$_3^-$ loss
- (G) Glucose
- (H) Ongoing and surgical losses

→ Monitor Replacement Therapy

Normal daily losses

- Give Food and Water
- Weigh animal → (I) Daily Maintenance IV Fluids
  - < 5 kg: 80 to 90 ml per kilogram
  - 5 to 30 kg: 60 to 80 ml per kilogram
  - > 30 kg: 50 to 60 ml per kilogram

CARDIAC ARREST: DOG OR CAT

Peter J. Pascoe

Cardiac arrest is defined as the state where there is no pulse, no auscultable heart beat, and no breathing. Agonal gasps may occur after the onset of cardiac arrest, but these do not provide adequate ventilation and should not be considered as breathing.

A. Clinical data may affect the therapeutic approach to the arrest. In an acute arrest with no previous suggestion that an arrest was imminent, adequate resuscitation may be achievable without bicarbonate therapy. If the animal has been sick for some time, there may be significant metabolic derangement that requires further therapy.

B. The airway must be clear. If the animal does not have an endotracheal tube in place, insert one. If a tube is not available, a tight-fitting mask can be used, but this may also inflate the stomach. If the animal is already connected to an anesthetic machine, squeezing the rebreathing bag will indicate whether the airway is clear.

C. Early defibrillation works better than late defibrillation. A defibrillator, if available, is used even if the dysrhythmia has not been defined. If defibrillation restores a normal rhythm and an effective pulse, further therapy may be unnecessary. In animals that weigh under 5 kg, spontaneous defibrillation may occur, but this is unlikely in larger animals. Give a single electrical shock at this stage, before beginning massage (Table 1).

D. Carry out external cardiac compression at a rate of 60 to 120 per minute, using the higher frequencies for smaller patients. Ventilate the animal at a rate of 8 to 10 breaths per minute, interposing these breaths between the chest compressions (1 breath per 5 compressions or 2 per 15 if you are on your own).

E. If no IV access is present, give epinephrine by the pulmonary route. This can be achieved by inserting a canine urinary catheter down the endotracheal tube into the bronchi. A dose of 10 to 20 μg per kilogram is recommended. When a venous access is present, give the epinephrine intravenously at 5 to 10 μg per kilogram.

F. Administer fluid therapy (lactated Ringer's or equivalent) at 20 to 90 ml per kilogram in the dog; 10 to 50 ml per kilogram in the cat.

G. Five to 10 minutes of poor circulation may produce more tissue damage than no circulation for this period. In dogs over 15 kg in weight, external massage produces circulation mainly by alterations in intrathoracic pressure rather than by direct cardiac compression. The flow achieved with this method is poor; therefore, internal massage is advocated to improve cerebral and coronary perfusion.

H. With inadequate perfusion, the mucous membranes do not return to a healthy pink colour and no peripheral pulse can be felt. Altering the position of the animal or the point of manual compression may help. A venous access is essential for further therapy. Wrapping the abdomen increases the venous return and fixes the diaphragm, which improves the effect of external cardiac compression. If these measures fail, thoracotomy and internal massage are indicated. Use a thoracotomy also as a diagnostic tool to visually differentiate between fibrillation and no fibrillation, if an ECG is not available.

I. Thoracotomy is performed through the 5th or 6th intercostal space. Ventilation is stopped for the incision through the pleura, and the pericardium is opened to facilitate cardiac massage. To achieve maximum cranial and coronary circulation, slide the index finger of the other hand dorsal to the lungs and compress the aorta against the thoracic vertebrae.

J. Give all drugs intravenously. Epinephrine (5 to 10 μg per kilogram), sodium bicarbonate (0.5 mmol per kilogram), atropine (0.06 mg per kilogram), or dexamethasone phosphate (2 to 4 mg per kilogram) may be helpful.

K. Double the dose of epinephrine used at each repetition.

TABLE 1 Defibrillation

Electrical

  External

< 7 kg	2 watt sec (Joules) per kg
7 to 40 kg	2 to 5 watt sec per kg
>40 kg	5 to 10 watt sec per kg

  Internal:
  0.2 to 0.4 watt sec per kg
  Repeat if fibrillation persists, increasing the dose by up to 50%.

Chemical
  1. 20 to 30 mmol KCl followed by calcium chloride (10 mg per kg) if defibrillation occurs.
  2. 1 mmol per kg KCl plus acetylcholine (6 mg per kg), followed by calcium chloride (10 mg per kg) if defibrillation occurs.
  3. 0.05 mmol per kg KCl plus acetylcholine (0.3 mg per kg) when given intracardiac with the aorta compressed. Follow with calcium chloride (5 mg per kg) if defibrillation occurs.

References

Bircher N, Safar P. A comparison of standard and 'new' closed chest CPR in dogs. Crit Care Med 1981; 9:384.

Ederstrom HE. Ventricular fibrillation susceptibility as related to heart size and maturity. Fed Proc 1976; 35:221.

Ralston SH, Voorhees WD, Babbs CF. Intrapulmonary epinephrine during prolonged cardiopulmonary resuscitation: improved regional blood flow and resuscitation in dogs. Ann Emerg Med 1984; 13:79.

Rudikoff MT, Maughan WL, Effron M, Freund P, Weisfeldt ML. Mechanisms of blood flow during cardiopulmonary resuscitation. Circulation 1980; 61:345.

Yakaitis RW, Ewy GA, Otto CW, Taren DL, Moon TE. Influence of time and therapy on ventricular defibrillation in dogs. Crit Care Med 1980; 8:157.

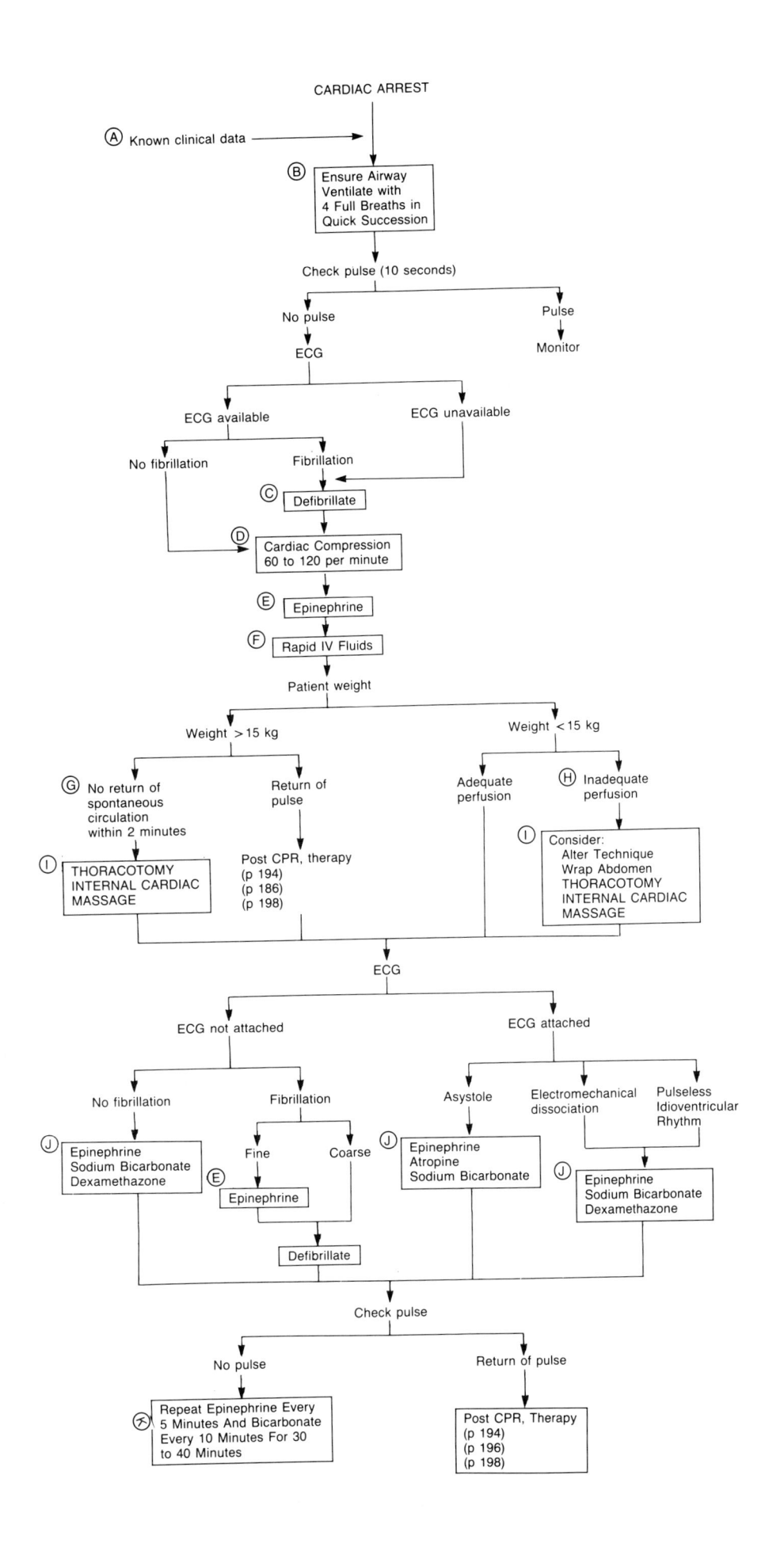

```
                          CARDIAC ARREST
                                │
    Ⓐ Known clinical data ─────▶│
                                ▼
                        Ⓑ ┌──────────────────┐
                          │ Ensure Airway    │
                          │ Ventilate with   │
                          │ 4 Full Breaths in│
                          │ Quick Succession │
                          └──────────────────┘
                                │
                        Check pulse (10 seconds)
                        ┌───────┴────────┐
                     No pulse          Pulse
                        │                │
                       ECG            Monitor
                  ┌─────┴─────┐
           ECG available   ECG unavailable
           ┌──────┴──────┐       │
     No fibrillation  Fibrillation
           │             │
           │          Ⓒ ┌────────────┐
           │            │ Defibrillate│
           │            └────────────┘
           │             │
           ▼             ▼
        Ⓓ ┌──────────────────────────┐
          │ Cardiac Compression       │
          │ 60 to 120 per minute      │
          └──────────────────────────┘
                    │
        Ⓔ ┌────────────┐
          │ Epinephrine│
          └────────────┘
                    │
        Ⓕ ┌────────────────┐
          │ Rapid IV Fluids│
          └────────────────┘
                    │
              Patient weight
       ┌────────────┴────────────┐
   Weight >15 kg            Weight <15 kg
   ┌────┴────┐              ┌────┴────┐
 Ⓖ No return   Return of   Adequate   Ⓗ Inadequate
   of spontaneous  pulse    perfusion   perfusion
   circulation      │                      │
   within 2 minutes │                      ▼
      │         Post CPR, therapy    Ⓘ ┌───────────────┐
      ▼         (p 194)                │ Consider:     │
   Ⓘ ┌──────────┐(p 186)                │ Alter Technique│
     │THORACOTOMY│(p 198)               │ Wrap Abdomen  │
     │INTERNAL   │                      │ THORACOTOMY   │
     │CARDIAC    │                      │ INTERNAL      │
     │MASSAGE    │                      │ CARDIAC       │
     └──────────┘                       │ MASSAGE       │
                                        └───────────────┘
                         │
                        ECG
              ┌──────────┴──────────┐
         ECG not attached       ECG attached
         ┌───────┴────────┐    ┌─────┼─────────┐
     No fibrillation  Fibrillation  Asystole  Electromechanical  Pulseless
         │            ┌───┴────┐     │       dissociation    Idioventricular
         │           Fine    Coarse   │              │         Rhythm
    Ⓙ ┌──────────┐   │        │   ┌─────────┐       │           │
      │Epinephrine│  ▼        │   │Epinephrine│     │     Ⓙ ┌──────────┐
      │Sodium     │ Ⓔ┌────────┐│   │Atropine   │     │       │Epinephrine│
      │Bicarbonate│  │Epinephr││   │Sodium     │     │       │Sodium     │
      │Dexamethaz.│  │ine     ││   │Bicarbonate│     │       │Bicarbonate│
      └──────────┘  └────────┘│   └─────────┘       │       │Dexamethaz.│
                        │     │                             └──────────┘
                        ▼     │
                   ┌────────┐ │
                   │Defibril│ │
                   │late    │ │
                   └────────┘ │
                        │
                    Check pulse
              ┌─────────┴─────────┐
           No pulse           Return of pulse
              │                    │
    ┌────────────────────┐    ┌──────────────┐
  ✈ │Repeat Epinephrine   │   │Post CPR,     │
    │Every 5 Minutes And  │   │Therapy       │
    │Bicarbonate Every 10 │   │(p 194)       │
    │Minutes For 30 to 40 │   │(p 196)       │
    │Minutes              │   │(p 198)       │
    └────────────────────┘    └──────────────┘
```

POST CARDIOPULMONARY RESUSCITATION: CIRCULATORY RESUSCITATION

Peter J. Pascoe

After cardiac arrest it is imperative that circulation be returned to a normal state as rapidly as possible. Establish normal or high normal blood flow and pressure in order to minimize the damage to the brain and myocardium.

A. If hypotension was the original cause of the arrest, adequate fluid loading is necessary. A central venous pressure (CVP) measurement can determine whether the heart is coping with the fluid being returned to it. An absolute value of 15 cm H_2O or less, or a change of less than 5 cm H_2O in 10 minutes, indicates that the heart is coping with the fluid. CVP values of less than 0 cm H_2O indicate inadequate circulatory volume.

B. Dopamine is a $beta_1$ and a dopaminergic stimulator. Dobutamine is a $beta_1$ stimulator. An infusion of either should increase myocardial contractility and raise cardiac output. Give dopamine as a 2 to 10 μg per kilogram per minute infusion in 5 percent dextrose and dobutamine as a 5 to 20 μg per kilogram per minute infusion in 5 percent dextrose.

C. Maintain the blood pH in the range 7.2 to 7.5. If the pH is low and ventilation is adequate (Pco_2 = 20 to 40 mm Hg), use sodium bicarbonate to correct the deficit (base deficit × body weight (kg) × 0.3 = the dose of bicarbonate in mmol). Half of this should be given slowly, and the patient reassessed. If the pH is too high and ventilation is adequate, use an acidifying solution such as sodium chloride (NaCl).

D. Hypokalemia: give potassium chloride (KCl) at a maximum of 0.5 mmol per kilogram per hour to correct this.

Hyperkalemia: calcium chloride ($CaCl_2$) counteracts the effects of the potassium; dextrose and insulin help to drive the potassium into the cell.

Hypocalcemia: this is very rare, and the actual value is probably not as important as the rate of change. Calcium chloride (10 mg per kilogram) can be given slowly as a supplement.

Hypercalcemia: if this occurs, it is probably iatrogenic. Crystalloid diuresis and furosemide may help to reduce the level.

E. If the pulse is still weak, increase the infusion rate of dopamine or dobutamine. The end point for these agents is tachycardia. This produces no further circulatory advantage and increases the stress on the myocardium. Corticosteroids (dexamethasone phosphate 2 to 4 mg per kilogram or prednisolone sodium succinate 30 mg per kilogram) may improve the effect of the above agents. If circulation cannot be maintained with crystalloid solutions, colloidal solutions such as blood, plasma, or dextrans may improve circulation.

References

Adams HR. New perspectives in cardiopulmonary therapeutics: receptor selective adrenergic drugs. JAVMA 1984; 185:966.

Schaer M. Disorders of potassium metabolism. Vet Clin North Am Small Anim 1982; 12:399.

Weil MH, Henning RJ. New concepts in the diagnosis and fluid treatment of circulatory shock. Anesth Analg 1979; 58:124.

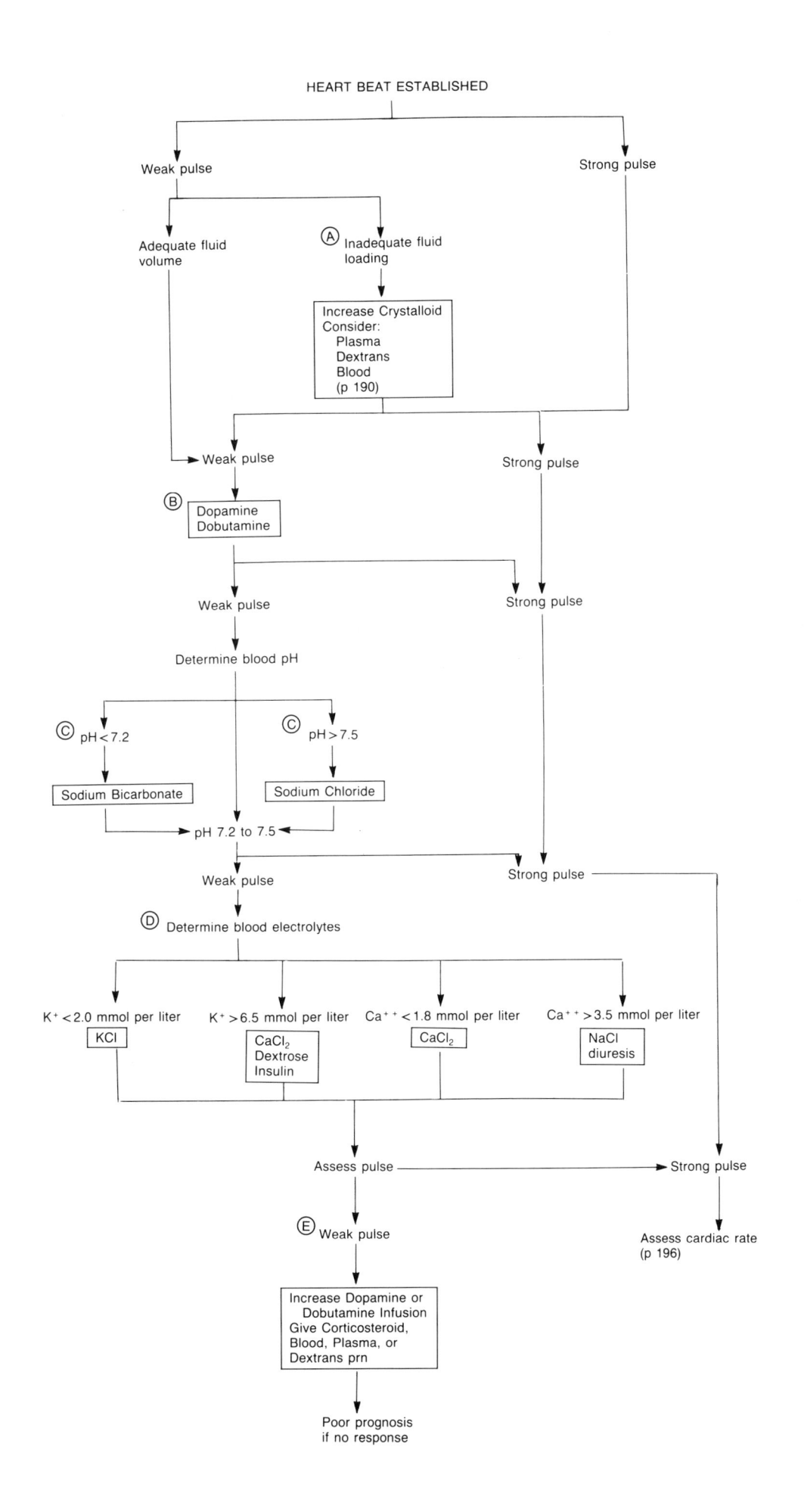

```
                        HEART BEAT ESTABLISHED
                        │
        ┌───────────────┴───────────────┐
    Weak pulse                      Strong pulse
        │
    ┌───┴────────────────┐
Adequate fluid      Ⓐ Inadequate fluid
  volume               loading
                        │
                   ┌────┴────┐
                   │ Increase Crystalloid │
                   │ Consider:            │
                   │   Plasma             │
                   │   Dextrans           │
                   │   Blood              │
                   │   (p 190)            │
                   └──────┬──────┘
        ┌──────────────┬──┴──────────┐
    Weak pulse     Strong pulse
        │
   Ⓑ ┌──────────┐
     │ Dopamine │
     │ Dobutamine│
     └─────┬────┘
      ┌────┴─────────┐
  Weak pulse    Strong pulse
      │
 Determine blood pH
      │
   ┌──┴──┐
Ⓒ pH<7.2   Ⓒ pH>7.5
   │          │
┌──┴──┐   ┌───┴───┐
│Sodium│  │Sodium │
│Bicarb│  │Chloride│
└──┬──┘   └───┬───┘
   └──→ pH 7.2 to 7.5 ←──┘
         │
     Weak pulse ─────────── Strong pulse
         │
   Ⓓ Determine blood electrolytes
         │
  ┌──────┼──────┬──────┐
K⁺<2.0  K⁺>6.5  Ca⁺⁺<1.8  Ca⁺⁺>3.5
 KCl    CaCl₂    CaCl₂    NaCl
        Dextrose          diuresis
        Insulin
         │
     Assess pulse ──────→ Strong pulse
         │                      │
    Ⓔ Weak pulse           Assess cardiac rate
         │                      (p 196)
  Increase Dopamine or
  Dobutamine Infusion
  Give Corticosteroid,
  Blood, Plasma, or
  Dextrans prn
         │
  Poor prognosis
  if no response
```

POST CARDIOPULMONARY RESUSCITATION: RATE AND ARRHYTHMIA CONTROL

Peter J. Pascoe

A. For arrhythmias of ventricular origin, lidocaine and procainamide are the drugs of choice in the dog. Give lidocaine in 1 to 2 mg per kilogram boluses intravenously. If initial control is gained with this, use an infusion of 50 to 70 µg per kilogram per minute lidocaine in sodium chloride or dextrose. Give procainamide (6 to 20 mg per kilogram IM every 4 to 6 hours) as an adjunct to lidocaine therapy if total control cannot be obtained with the latter. Lidocaine does not appear to be any more toxic in normal cats than in any other species, but in cats with cardiomyopathies, cardiac arrest has occurred. Propranolol (0.1 mg per kilogram IV) may be the drug of choice in this instance.

B. Give atropine (0.02 to 0.04 mg per kilogram) or glycopyrrolate (0.01 mg per kilogram) intravenously to counteract vagally induced bradycardia. Use isoproterenol intravenously as a last resort for its positive chronotropic effect (0.5 to 5 µg per minute).

C. Once hypotension and residual catecholamines have been ruled out (the latter have a relatively short half-life), attempt a vagal maneuver (massaging the carotid sinus, external pressure on the eyes). This may convert a sinus tachycardia to normal rhythm and rate. Use propranolol (0.1 to 0.15 mg per kilogram IV) only as a last resort to slow a high heart rate because it is also a negative inotrope and may lead to hypotension.

D. Attain a stable rhythm with a strong beat before further therapy. This is particularly true in cases where open chest massage has been used; the heart should be stable before closure of the thorax is attempted.

References

Chadwick HS. Toxicity and resuscitation in lidocaine or bupivacaine-infused cats. Anesthesiology 1985; 63:385.

Tilley LP. Essentials of canine and feline electrocardiography. 2nd ed. Philadelphia: Lea & Febiger, 1985.

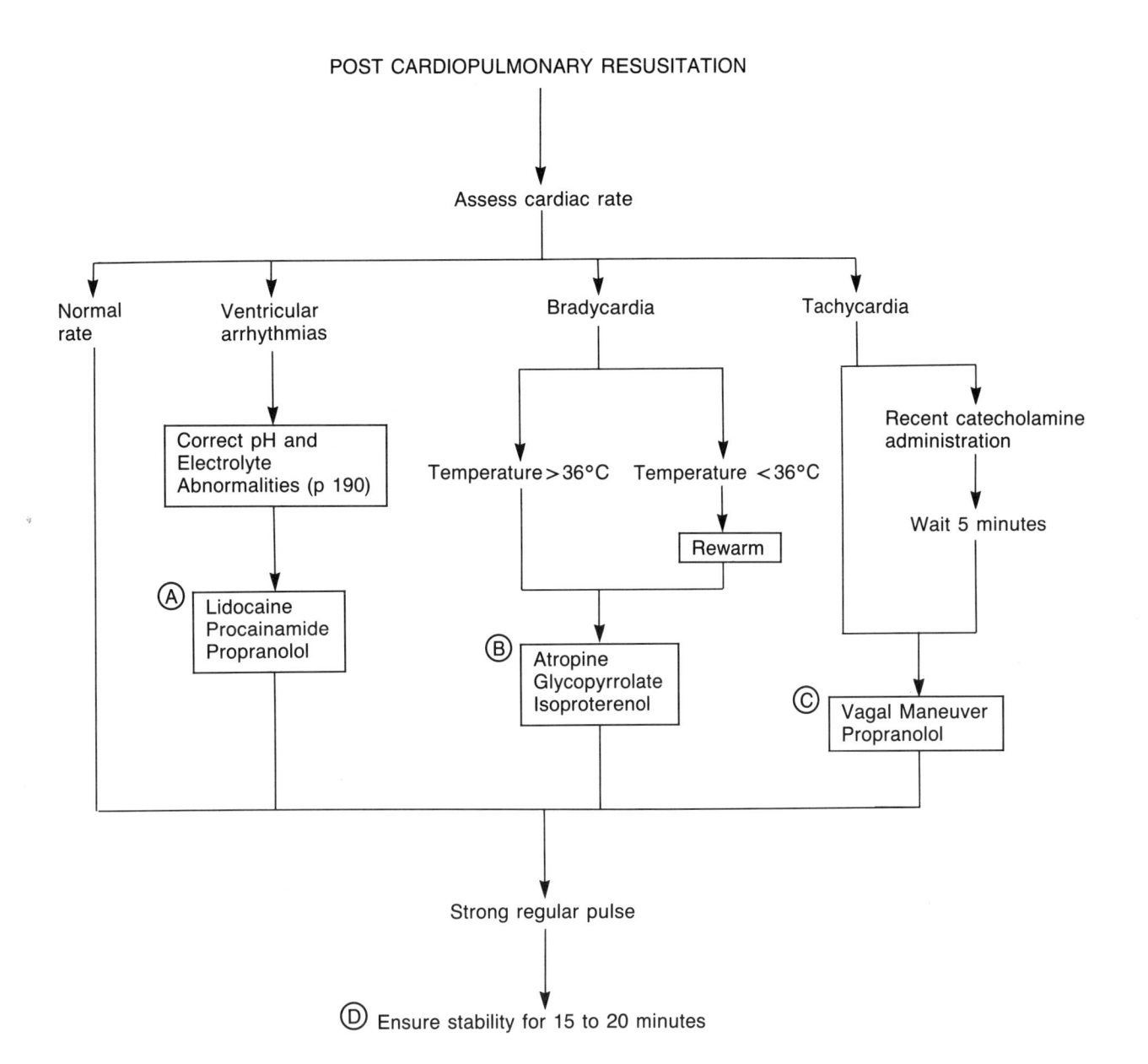

POST CARDIOPULMONARY RESUSITATION

```
                    Assess cardiac rate
         ┌─────────────┬──────────────┬──────────────┐
    Normal      Ventricular       Bradycardia     Tachycardia
     rate       arrhythmias
                     │                                  │
              Correct pH and                    Recent catecholamine
              Electrolyte              ┌────────┴────┐  administration
              Abnormalities (p 190)    │             │         │
                     │           Temperature>36°C  Temperature<36°C
                     │                 │             │    Wait 5 minutes
               Ⓐ Lidocaine             │           Rewarm
                  Procainamide         │             │
                  Propranolol          └──────┬──────┘
                                              │
                                       Ⓑ Atropine
                                          Glycopyrrolate      Ⓒ Vagal Maneuver
                                          Isoproterenol         Propranolol
```

Strong regular pulse

Ⓓ Ensure stability for 15 to 20 minutes

197

POST CARDIOPULMONARY RESUSCITATION: CEREBRAL RESUSCITATION

Peter J. Pascoe

A. Delayed recovery indicates that there was sufficient loss of circulation to cause temporary or permanent loss of some brain function. Delayed pupillary constriction is not necessarily a bad sign as it can be seen in patients that eventually achieve normal neuronal function.

B. Mannitol is the drug of choice initially. It reduces cerebral swelling by its osmotic effect and may have some free radical scavenging properties. Free radicals have been implicated in causing tissue damage after circulation has been restored. A dose of 0.25 to 1.0 g per kilogram is given slowly intravenously. Renal activity is necessary for drug excretion. Alternatively, give furosemide in order to reduce cerebral swelling. Corticosteroids in high doses (dexamethasone phosphate 2 to 4 mg per kilogram, prednisolone sodium succinate 10 to 15 mg per kilogram) may also help to protect the brain against further damage from cells with unstable membranes. Carbon dioxide is involved in the control of the cerebral circulation, and a reduction in $PaCO_2$ helps to prevent an excessive rise in intracranial pressure. A sleep state induced with pentobarbital controls seizures and permits intubation and ventilation. Institute hyperventilation, and lower $PaCO_2$ levels to 20 to 25 mm Hg.

C. Seizures must be treated. Diazepam 0.25 to 1.0 mg per kilogram may give temporary relief, but in the postcardiac arrest patient, it is unlikely to be enough. Add phenobarbital in a fluid drip, or the animal can be anesthetized with pentobarbital (3 to 5 mg per kilogram initially, then to effect). The aim with pentobarbital is to produce a state close to anesthesia since seizure activity is poorly controlled at low doses.

D. Keep blood pressure within close limits since hypotension can result in further reductions in cerebral circulation, and hypertension may increase the degree of damage. Treat mean blood pressure below 80 mm Hg using a vasopressor such as norepinephrine 0.6 to 6.0 µg per kilogram IV, methoxamine 0.1 to 0.4 mg per kilogram IV, or phenylephrine 0.01 to 0.15 mg per kilogram IV. If the blood pressure is elevated (>120 mm Hg) use acepromazine (0.05 mg per kilogram) or nitroglycerin (¼ to ¾ inches [6 to 20 mm] of cream topically).

E. Following cardiac arrest, some patients have very unstable thermoregulation. The rectal temperature (T) should be monitored, and the animal maintained at a slightly subnormal temperature (37 to 38° C). Treat hyperthermia with surface wetting and a blower to create evaporative cooling. Ice cold saline enemas may aid in reducing an elevated body temperature. If the temperature is subnormal, place the animal in a warm environment, and gently warm using a warming blanket and/or a heat lamp. Withdraw this heating as soon as the temperature reaches 37°C in order to prevent an overshoot.

F. Maintain the PaO_2 in the normal range. If it is low, an increase in inspired oxygen tension may be all that is required, but in animals with pulmonary damage, it may be necessary to ventilate and add positive end expiratory pressure (PEEP) as well. If the inspired oxygen tension (FiO_2) is too high (>80 percent), there is a risk of oxygen toxicity, and so the inspired gas should be diluted with air or nitrogen.

G. If recovery has not occurred within 24 hours, the prognosis becomes worse, but patients have returned to normal function with longer periods of coma or cerebral malfunction. Treatment, if continued, should be carried out as carefully as during the initial period. If the animal recovers, but is blind, sight may return by 4 to 6 weeks.

References

Bleyaert AL, Sands PA, Safar P, et al. Augmentation of postischemic brain damage by severe intermittent hypertension. Crit Care Med 1980; 8:41.

Gilroy BA, Rockhoff MA, Dunlop BJ, Shapiro HM. Cardiopulmonary resuscitation in the nonhuman primate. JAVMA 1980; 177:867.

Shapiro HM. Barbiturates in brain ischemia. Br J Anesth 1985; 57:82.

ADEQUATE CIRCULATION

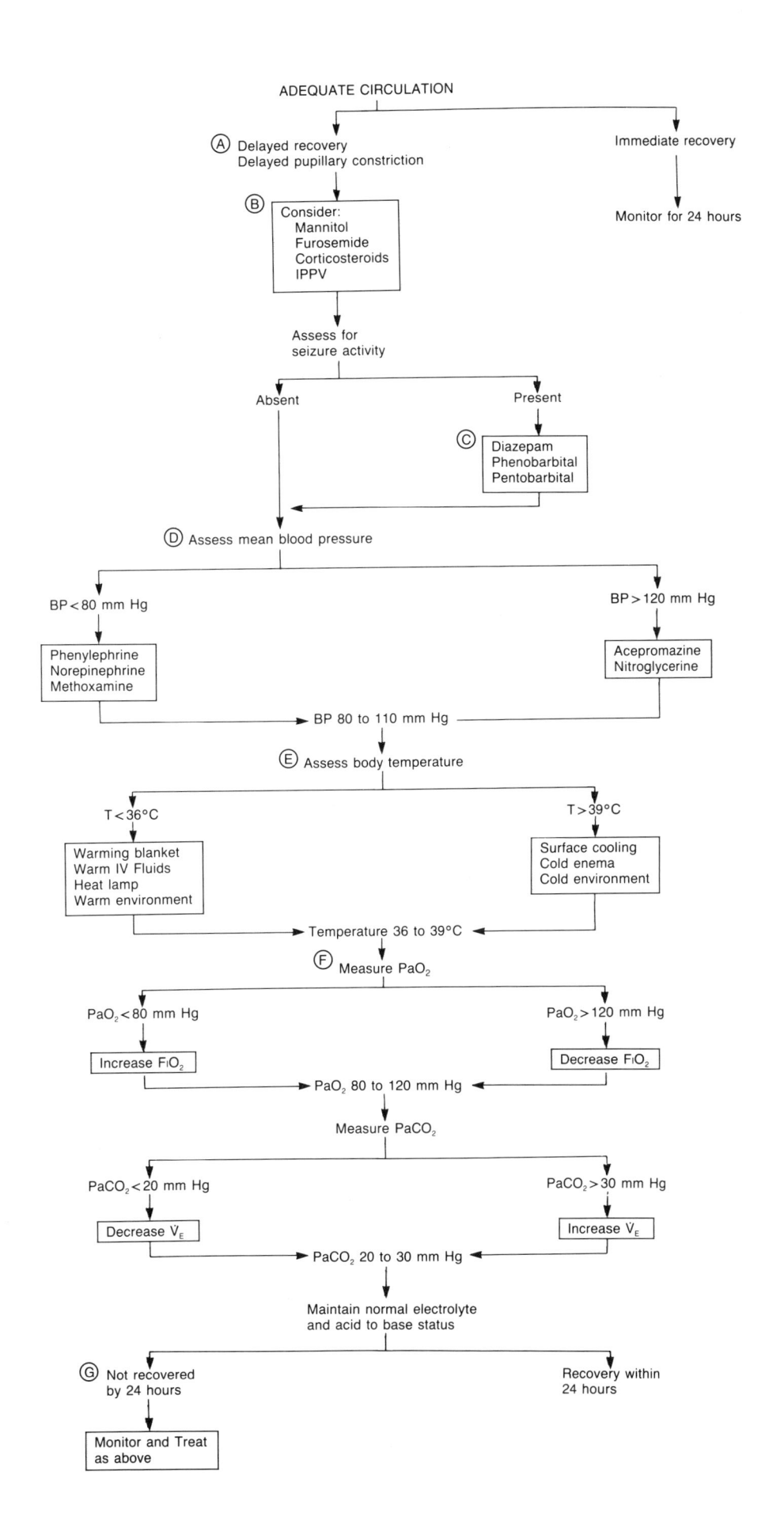

- (A) Delayed recovery / Delayed pupillary constriction
- Immediate recovery → Monitor for 24 hours

(B) Consider:
- Mannitol
- Furosemide
- Corticosteroids
- IPPV

Assess for seizure activity

- Absent
- Present → (C) Diazepam / Phenobarbital / Pentobarbital

(D) Assess mean blood pressure

- BP < 80 mm Hg → Phenylephrine / Norepinephrine / Methoxamine
- BP > 120 mm Hg → Acepromazine / Nitroglycerine
- BP 80 to 110 mm Hg

(E) Assess body temperature

- T < 36°C → Warming blanket / Warm IV Fluids / Heat lamp / Warm environment
- T > 39°C → Surface cooling / Cold enema / Cold environment
- Temperature 36 to 39°C

(F) Measure PaO_2

- PaO_2 < 80 mm Hg → Increase F_IO_2
- PaO_2 > 120 mm Hg → Decrease F_IO_2
- PaO_2 80 to 120 mm Hg

Measure $PaCO_2$

- $PaCO_2$ < 20 mm Hg → Decrease $\dot{V}_E$
- $PaCO_2$ > 30 mm Hg → Increase $\dot{V}_E$
- $PaCO_2$ 20 to 30 mm Hg

Maintain normal electrolyte and acid to base status

- (G) Not recovered by 24 hours → Monitor and Treat as above
- Recovery within 24 hours

NEOPLASIA

Elizabeth J. Laing

Neoplastic disorders are common in pets and the risk increases with age. In dogs, the most common sites for tumor development are the skin and mammary glands. In cats, the hemolymphatic system is most frequently affected.

A. Historic signs suggestive of neoplastic disorder include a persistent swelling or mass, lameness, chronic bleeding or discharge, weight loss, anorexia, difficulty in eating or breathing, loss of stamina, and a change in bladder or bowel habits.

B. A complete physical examination is the first step in localizing the problem. Palpate regional lymph nodes and compare them to the contralateral side. Ancillary diagnostic procedures, such as radiography and ultrasonography, may further define the lesion once it has been localized to an area of the body.

C. Laboratory work-up varies with the age and condition of the patient. Complete blood count (CBC), serum biochemical profile, and urinalysis are recommended if the patient is to be anesthetized, shows signs of systemic illness, or if a paraneoplastic syndrome is suspected.

D. If the biopsy result may alter the treatment plan or prognosis, an incisional or fine-needle biopsy is indicated. Otherwise, an excisional biopsy is preferred. Biopsy margins should be examined for residual tumor, as both benign and malignant tumors may recur following incomplete excision.

E. Nonneoplastic conditions that mimic tumors include granulomas, abscesses, and fungal disease. However, tumors may also have an inflammatory component or be secondarily infected. Therefore, if the clinical presentation suggests neoplasia and the biopsy is nondiagnostic, rebiopsy is indicated.

F. Benign tumors do not spread to distant sites and are rarely locally invasive. They generally have a good prognosis following local tumor therapy.

G. Malignant tumors should be staged prior to therapy in order to determine the extent of disease. Both carcinomas and sarcomas spread hematogenously, especially to the lungs and liver. Carcinomas also spread along lymphatic channels. Biopsy regional lymph nodes if they are enlarged. Chest radiographs should include three views (ventrodorsal, right lateral, and left lateral) in order to screen for pulmonary involvement. Abdominal radiographs may reveal lymphadenopathy or hepatomegaly. Bone marrow aspirates are indicated in order to detect metastatic hemolymphatic tumors.

H. Malignant tumors without the biologic potential or clinical signs of metastasis are treated with local therapy. Invasive tumors, or those with a high metastatic potential, may warrant adjuvant systemic therapy despite the absence of detectable metastatic disease.

I. Surgical excision is the most common form of local therapy. A minimum of 1 cm of tumor-free tissue should be included along all borders. Malignant tumors may require wider margins. All surgical margins should be checked histologically for residual tumor cells. If present, further therapy is indicated. Cryosurgery is useful in areas not amenable to conventional surgery, such as the eyelid or oral cavity. The tumor and, if possible, a 1 cm tumor-free margin should be frozen to $-20°$ C by means of two to three rapid freeze-slow thaw cycles. Radiotherapy may be used as the primary therapy or as an adjuvant to surgical excision. Generally, a dose of 40 to 45 Grey is delivered in ten fractions, over a 3 week period. Hyperthermia and chemotherapy have been used both alone and in combination with radiotherapy in order to increase the response rate of various tumors.

J. Treatment of tumors with nodal or diffuse metastases usually involves two phases. First, local therapy is used to decrease the primary tumor volume. Second, systemic therapy is given to control any metastatic disease. Combination chemotherapy and immunotherapy have been used both to treat and to prevent metastatic disease. Solitary metastatic lesions may also be removed surgically. The success of these treatments varies with the histologic tumor type.

K. As an alternative to aggressive systemic therapy, palliative therapy is used to improve the patient's quality of life without attempting tumor cure. Therapy varies with the patient's signs and may include local excision of irritating masses, antibiotic therapy to control secondary infections, and analgesics or other medication to control paraneoplastic symptoms.

References

Allen SW, Prasse KW. Cytologic diagnosis of neoplasia and perioperative implementation. Comp Cont Ed 1986, 8:72.

Goldstein RS, Hess PW. Cryosurgical treatment of cancer. Vet Clin North Am 1977; 7:51.

Withrow SJ, Lowes N. Biopsy techniques for use in small animal oncology. JAAHA 1981; 17:889.

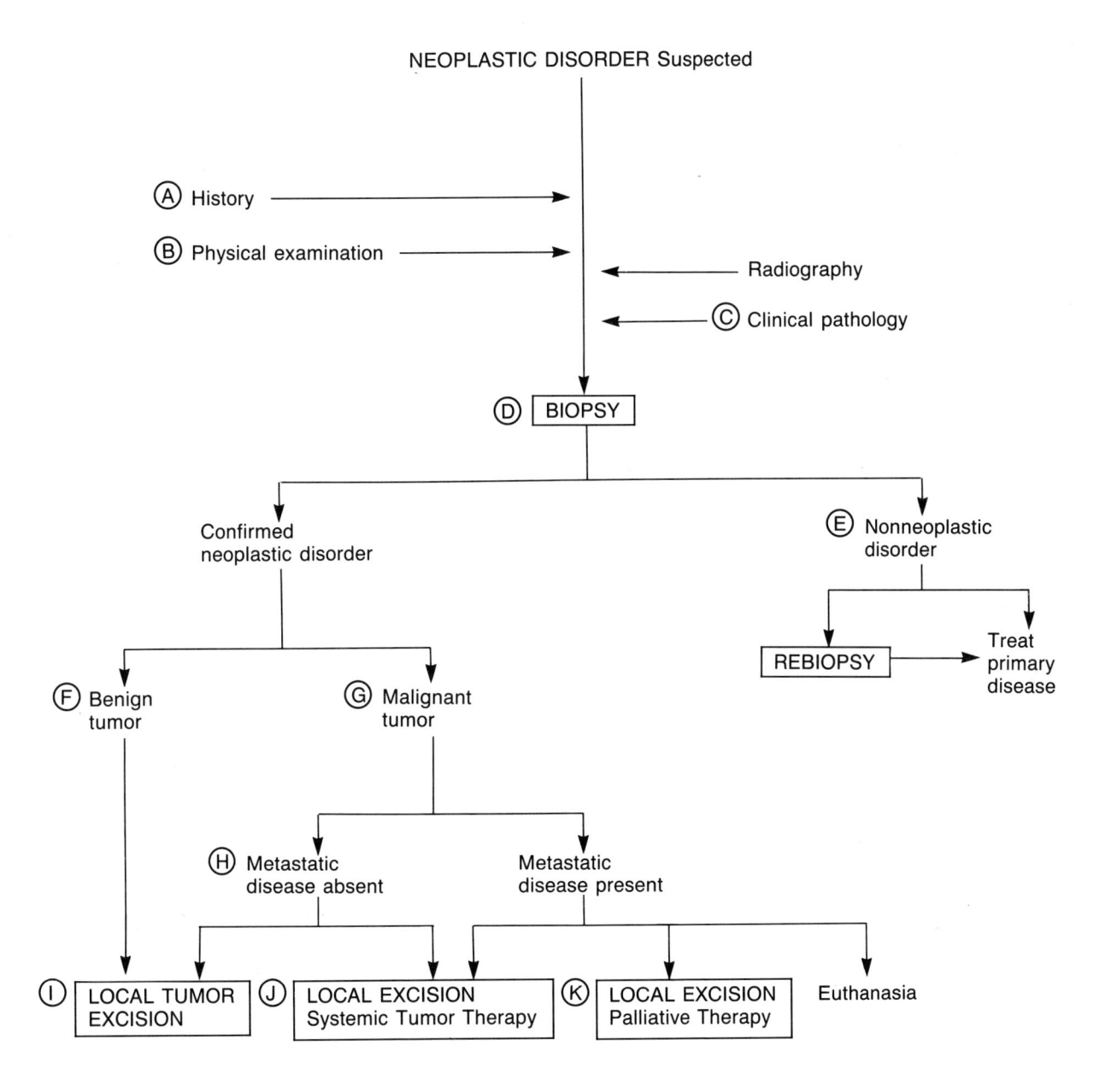

NEOPLASTIC DISORDER Suspected

- Ⓐ History
- Ⓑ Physical examination
- Radiography
- Ⓒ Clinical pathology

→ Ⓓ **BIOPSY**

- Confirmed neoplastic disorder
- Ⓔ Nonneoplastic disorder → **REBIOPSY** → Treat primary disease

From confirmed neoplastic disorder:
- Ⓕ Benign tumor → Ⓘ **LOCAL TUMOR EXCISION**
- Ⓖ Malignant tumor
  - Ⓗ Metastatic disease absent → Ⓙ **LOCAL EXCISION Systemic Tumor Therapy**
  - Metastatic disease present → Ⓚ **LOCAL EXCISION Palliative Therapy** or Euthanasia

201

CHOOSING A SUTURE MATERIAL

Cindy L. Fries

The wide variety of suture materials available reflects the fact that no one suture material is ideal for all situations. While certain general principles apply, the final selection is largely dependent on individual preference.

A. Sutures decrease a wound's ability to combat infection; therefore, their placement in a contaminated environment should be avoided. Multifilament, nonabsorbable sutures (silk, polyester) are contraindicated as they tend to harbor bacteria within fiber interstices. In the case of contaminated wounds, synthetic, absorbable suture materials (polyglycolic acid, polyglactin 910, polydioxanone) are associated with lower infection rates than is catgut. Monofilament, nonabsorbable sutures (polypropylene, polyethylene, polyamides) are the least likely to propagate wound infections.

B. Delayed healing may be observed with chronic corticosteroid administration and in a number of disease conditions; these conditions include hypoproteinemia, uremia, hypothyroidism, and hyperadrenocortism. Catgut degrades prematurely in hypoproteinemic states and consequently should be avoided. The use of multifilament, absorbable sutures in conditions of delayed healing is best avoided because of their rapid loss of tensile strength. For these reasons, the monofilament suture materials (polypropylene, polyethylene, nylon, polydioxanone) are recommended.

C. Minimal tissue reaction in the skin is desirable in order to ensure rapid healing with good cosmetic results. Monofilament, nonabsorbable sutures are suggested. Monofilament stainless steel is generally avoided because of the difficulty in handling and the trauma created by the knot ends. Although metal staples allow good cosmetic results and rapid closure, economic factors limit their use.

D. Use nonabsorbable suture materials for the ligation of large diameter vessels. Absorbable suture is generally sufficient to ligate vessels less than 3 mm in diameter.

E. The natural sutures (silk and catgut) induce a significant inflammatory reaction. They may be used in situations such as herniorrhaphy and repair of chronic luxation wherein increased fibrosis is desirable.

F. Multifilament, nonabsorbable sutures should not be placed within the lumen of a hollow viscus as they may serve as a nidus of infection. They may also potentiate calculus formation in the urinary tract and gallbladder. Avoid catgut in gastric surgery as it is prematurely absorbed in an acidic environment. Polyglycolic acid is rapidly dissolved upon exposure to urine, especially if an infection is present. For this reason, it should be used with caution in urinary tract surgery.

G. Prolonged support is necessary in the repair of tendons and ligaments as they are slow to regain functional strength. A nonabsorbable suture material is recommended.

References

Bellenger CR. Sutures. Part I: the purpose of sutures and available suture materials. Comp Cont Ed 1982; 4:507.

Bellenger CR. Sutures. Part II: the use of sutures and alternative methods of closure. Comp Cont Ed 1982; 4:587.

Boothe HW. Suture materials and tissue adhesives. In: Slatter DH, ed. Textbook of small animal surgery. Philadelphia: WB Saunders, 1985:334.

Crane SW. Suture materials. In: Bojrab MJ, ed. Current techniques in small animal surgery. Philadelphia: Lea & Febiger, 1983:3.

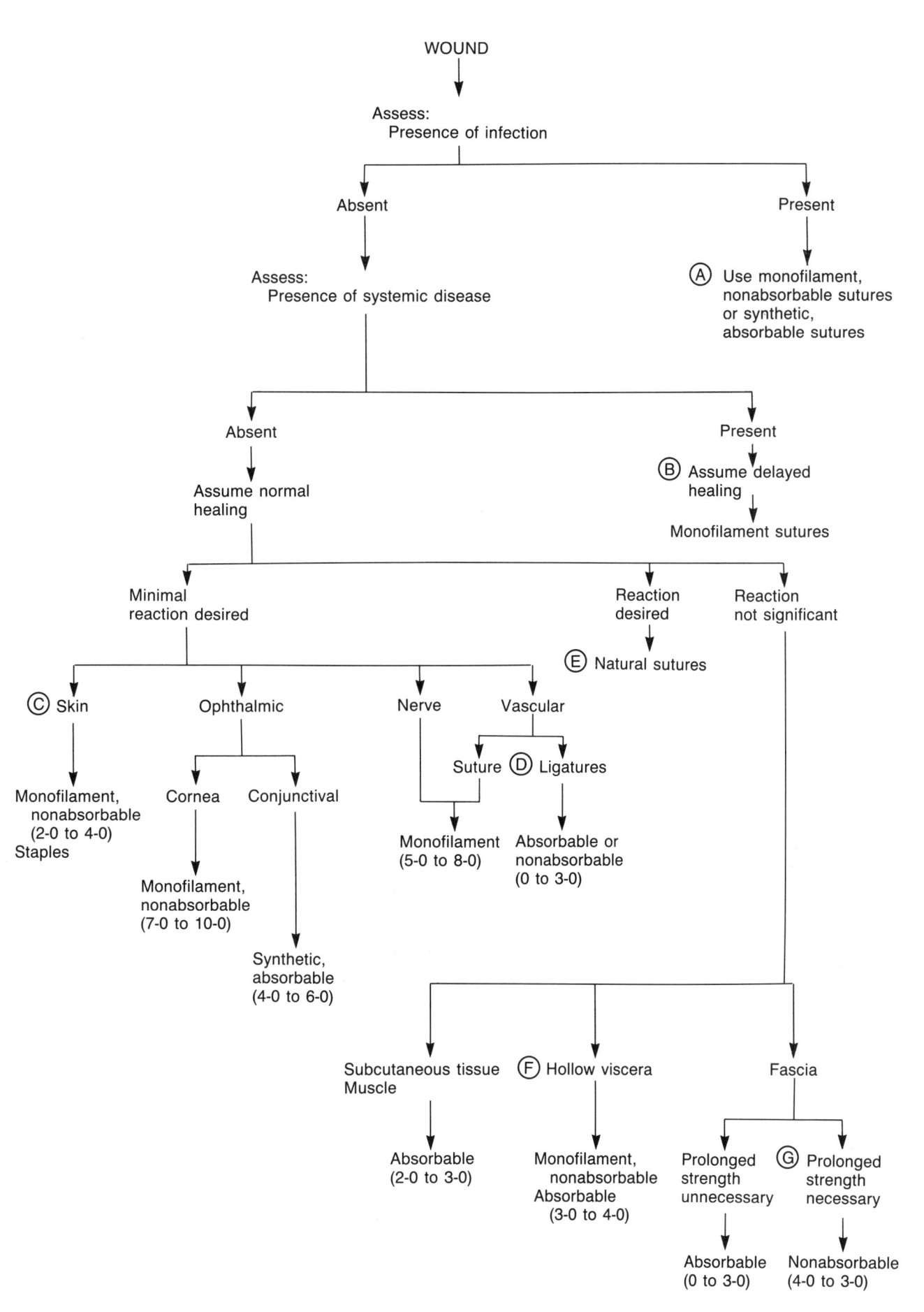

```
WOUND
  │
  ▼
Assess:
Presence of infection
  ├─────────────────────────────────────┐
  ▼ Absent                              ▼ Present
Assess:                            Ⓐ Use monofilament,
Presence of systemic disease          nonabsorbable sutures
  ├──────────────────┐                 or synthetic,
  ▼ Absent           ▼ Present         absorbable sutures
Assume normal    Ⓑ Assume delayed
healing             healing
                    │
                    ▼
                 Monofilament sutures
```

From "Assume normal healing" / "Monofilament sutures":

- **Minimal reaction desired**
  - Ⓒ **Skin** → Monofilament, nonabsorbable (2-0 to 4-0) Staples
  - **Ophthalmic**
    - Cornea → Monofilament, nonabsorbable (7-0 to 10-0)
    - Conjunctival → Synthetic, absorbable (4-0 to 6-0)
  - **Nerve** → Monofilament (5-0 to 8-0)
  - **Vascular**
    - Suture → Monofilament (5-0 to 8-0)
    - Ⓓ Ligatures → Absorbable or nonabsorbable (0 to 3-0)
- **Reaction desired**
  - Ⓔ Natural sutures
- **Reaction not significant**
  - Subcutaneous tissue / Muscle → Absorbable (2-0 to 3-0)
  - Ⓕ Hollow viscera → Monofilament, nonabsorbable / Absorbable (3-0 to 4-0)
  - Fascia
    - Prolonged strength unnecessary → Absorbable (0 to 3-0)
    - Ⓖ Prolonged strength necessary → Nonabsorbable (4-0 to 3-0)

ABDOMINAL FLUID

Karol A. Mathews

A. The history of a patient with abdominal fluid varies from one of acute trauma to that of a chronic, insidiously developing problem. Palpation of a fluid-filled abdomen generally reveals a tense abdomen, often with organs that cannot be discretely palpated, but that can be ballotted.

B. Free abdominal fluid imparts a hazy, opaque, "ground glass" appearance to radiographs, and as recognition of specific abdominal organs may not be possible, little specific information is obtained in most instances. Further radiographic evaluation may be indicated following abdominal drainage. However, this depends on abdominocentesis results.

C. Frequently, the physical examination unequivocally indicates free fluid within the abdominal cavity; however, hepatomegaly, splenomegaly, obesity, abdominal muscle flaccidity (Cushing's syndrome), malignant neoplasms, pyometra, pregnancy, atonic bladder, urethral obstruction with bladder enlargement, gastric dilation, and advanced obstipation may all be mistaken for ascites.

D. Abdominocentesis is indicated on the basis of physical examination and radiographic findings. The differential diagnosis is based on the cytologic, biochemical, bacteriologic, and fungal analysis of the abdominal fluid.

E. The mechanisms of transudation are lowered plasma osmotic pressure, increased capillary hydrostatic pressure, and lymphatic obstruction. The abdominal fluid characteristics are of a colorless, clear fluid with a protein concentration of less than 3.0 g per deciliter, and a cell count of less than 500 per μl, which consist of nondegenerative neutrophils, monocytes, and basophilic mesothelial cells.

F. A modified transudate occurs by transudative mechanisms and is modified by the addition of protein or cells that originate from a hyperplastic mesothelial lining, neoplasms that communicate with the abdominal cavity, congested venules, or obstructed lymphatics. The transudate characteristics vary according to the underlying pathologic process.

G. In congestive heart failure, the fluid is pink to red, sometimes slightly turbid, with a protein concentration of 2.5 to 5.0 g per deciliter. The cell count is usually 300 to 5,500 per μl with variable numbers of erythrocytes, nondegenerative neutrophils, basophilic mesothelial cells, macrophages, and occasionally, eosinophils (dirofilariasis), and lymphocytes.

H. In chylous ascites, the fluid is turbid and white to pink, or occasionally tan in color. The protein values are greater than 3.0 g per deciliter or 50 percent of the plasma protein concentration. The cell count is usually less than 10,000 per μl; small lymphocytes predominate with a variable number of nondegenerative neutrophils. The lymphocyte count may be low if the ascites is chronic. Sudanophilic droplets may be present, and the fluid may clear with alkalinization and ether extraction, but the results vary with the nutritional status of the patient. An effusion triglyceride concentration of greater than 90 mg per deciliter and a cholesterol:triglyceride ratio of less than 1.0 is highly suggestive of a chylous effusion. Lipoprotein electrophoresis may be necessary in equivocal cases.

I. Pseudochylous effusions are usually white and turbid with a variable protein and cell count. The fluid triglyceride levels are lower than the serum levels. Lymphomas may result in a pseudochylous effusion with a cell count of less than 10,000 per μl of predominantly immature lymphocytes.

J. Carcinomas may cause lymphatic obstruction, which results in an effusion high in protein (3.0 to 6.0 mg per deciliter), but with a cell count of less than 10,000 per μl. Neoplastic cells are not commonly observed; however, clusters of hyperplastic basophilic mesothelial cells may be present.

K. In the case of mesotheliomas, clusters of malignant tumor cells are observed; these are difficult to distinguish from basophilic mesothelial cells.

L. Exudative effusions are a consequence of increased vascular permeability and inflammation. They are characterized by a white, yellow, or pink turbid fluid with a protein concentration greater than 3.0 g per deciliter and a cell count greater than 3,000 per μl of which neutrophils predominate.

M. A nonseptic exudate may be caused by nonmicrobial irritants, such as bile urine, or pancreatic enzymes, may develop from a modified transudate. The neutrophils are nondegenerative.

N. Septic exudates are caused by microorganisms, but the causative organism is not always visible in cytologic preparations. The neutrophils are usually degenerative. Bacteria or vegetable fibers are indicative of hollow viscus rupture.

O. In feline infectious peritonitis, the neutrophils are nondegenerative. Exudates caused by *Nocardia* or *Actinomyces* show degenerative neutrophils when associated with colonies and nondegenerative neutrophils when distant from colonies. Therefore, smears of fluid without colonies have a nonseptic cytologic appearance. A septic exudate may exhibit nondegenerative neutrophils if the patient is receiving antibiotic therapy.

P. Recent hemorrhage (within hours) is characterized by a packed cell volume (PCV) greater than 5 percent as obtained by peritoneal lavage, a free-flow of nonclotting blood with a PCV similar to peripheral blood, protein and white cell values of less than peripheral blood values, and a cellular morphology and distribution similar to those in peripheral blood. Platelets and platelet aggregates are also present, but lyse rapidly. Upon standing, the supernatant is clear with red sediment.

Q. Long-standing or resolving hemorrhage is characterized by a red to purple-brown fluid, which contains distorted erythrocytes and hypersegmented leukocytes. Macrophages contain phagocytized erythrocytes and blood pigment. Platelets are absent. Upon standing, the supernatant is xanthochromic or pink.

References

Crowe DT Jr, Crane SW. Diagnostic abdominal paracentesis and lavage in the evaluation of abdominal injuries in dogs and cats: clinical and experimental investigations. JAVMA 1976; 168:700.

Duncan JR, Prasse KW. Cytology in veterinary laboratory medicine and clinical pathology. 2nd ed. Ames, IA: Iowa State University Press, 1986:201.

Ettinger SJ. Ascites, peritonitis and other causes of abdominal enlargement. In: Ettinger SJ, ed. Textbook of veterinary internal medicine. Philadelphia: WB Saunders, 1983:121.

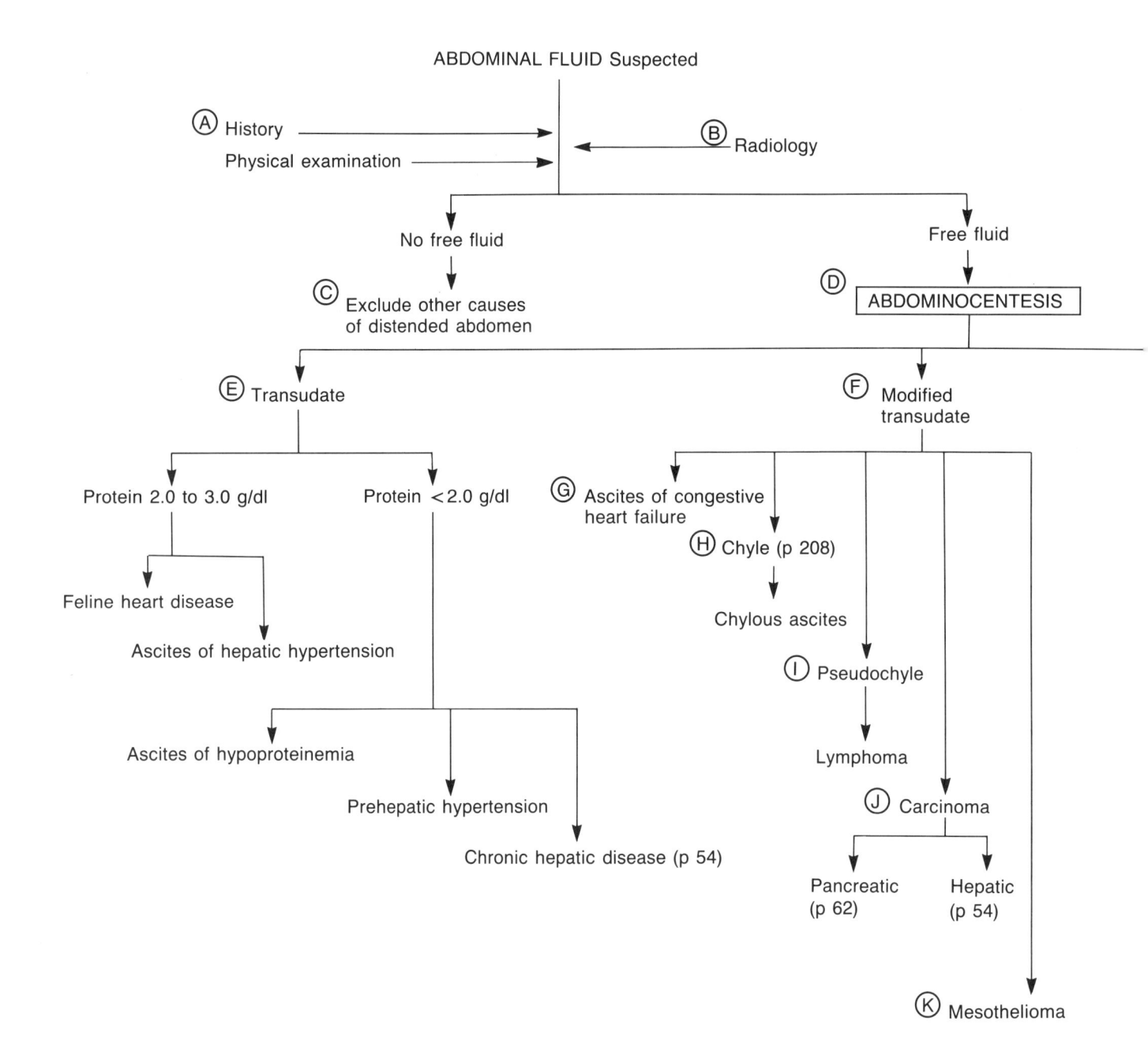

ABDOMINAL FLUID Suspected

- (A) History
- (B) Radiology
- Physical examination

No free fluid → (C) Exclude other causes of distended abdomen

Free fluid → (D) ABDOMINOCENTESIS

(E) Transudate
- Protein 2.0 to 3.0 g/dl
  - Feline heart disease
  - Ascites of hepatic hypertension
- Protein <2.0 g/dl
  - Ascites of hypoproteinemia
  - Prehepatic hypertension
  - Chronic hepatic disease (p 54)

(F) Modified transudate
- (G) Ascites of congestive heart failure
- (H) Chyle (p 208)
  - Chylous ascites
- (I) Pseudochyle
  - Lymphoma
- (J) Carcinoma
  - Pancreatic (p 62)
  - Hepatic (p 54)
- (K) Mesothelioma

- Ⓛ Exudate
  - Ⓝ Degenerative neutrophils, odiferous (septic)
    - Septic peritonitis (p 210)
  - Ⓜ Nondegenerative neutrophils (nonseptic)
    - Ⓞ Possible septic peritonitis (p 210)
      - Septic peritonitis (p 210)
    - Sterile foreign body
    - Chemical peritonitis
      - Urine peritonitis (p 114)
      - Pancreatitis (p 60)
      - Bile peritonitis (p 56)
      - Gastric rupture (fasting animal)
- Hemorrhage
  - Ⓟ Recent hemorrhage
    - Tumor
      - Spleen (p 212)
      - Liver (p 54)
      - Kidney (p 108)
      - Gastrointestinal
    - Trauma
      - Spleen (p 212)
      - Liver (p 52)
      - Kidney (p 108)
      - Gastrointestinal
    - Bleeding disorders
      - Thrombocytopenia
      - Warfarin toxicity
  - Ⓠ Long-standing or resolving hemorrhage
    - Tumor
      - Spleen (p 212)
      - Liver (p 54)
      - Kidney (p 108)
    - Trauma
      - Spleen (p 212)
      - Liver (p 52)
      - Kidney (p 108)

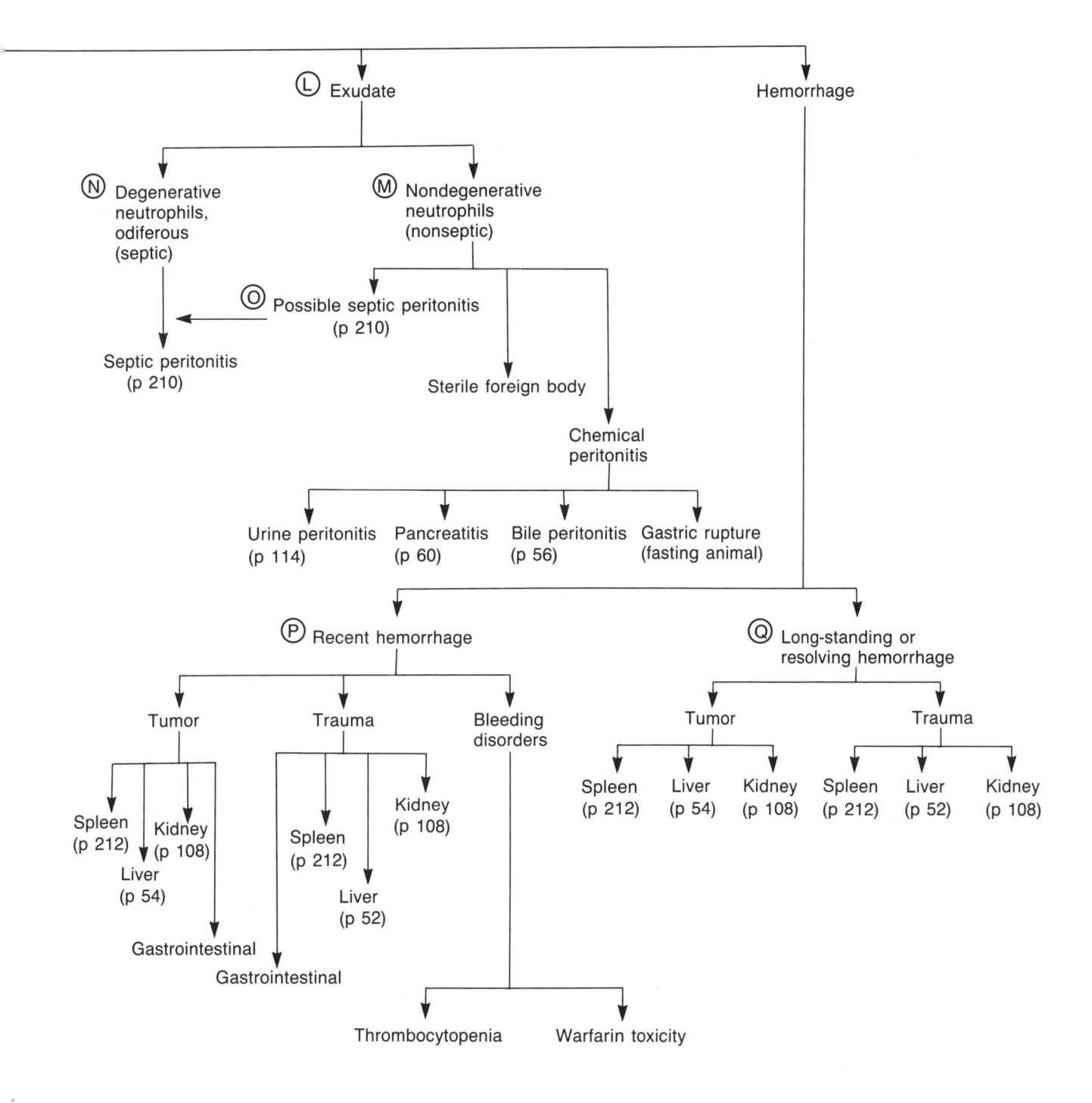

CHYLOUS ASCITES

Karol A. Mathews

A. When associated with trauma or recent abdominal surgery, rupture of the cisterna chyli or abdominal lymphatics may not become evident for several days, during which time the patient may become moderately depressed with a reduced exercise tolerance. There is a gradual enlargement of the abdomen and generalized muscle wastage. Should abdominal distension become severe, vomiting and dyspnea may be reported. Frequently, there is no history of trauma or associated illness; the chylous effusion appears to occur spontaneously. If this is associated with intestinal lymphangiectasia, diarrhea may be observed.

B. Physical findings usually consist of dehydration; poor body condition, with or without dependent edema; or a fluid-filled abdomen, with or without pain. An abdominal mass may be palpable. Dyspnea and tachycardia may be present.

C. The most significant hematologic and biochemical findings are lymphopenia, hypoalbuminemia, hypoproteinemia, and hypocalcemia. Iron deficiency anemia may also be present. The serum triglyceride level is less than that of the abdominal fluid.

D. A milky white to pink fluid with a triglyceride level greater than 90 mg per deciliter is highly suspicious of chylous ascites.

E. Following removal of all abdominal fluid, survey radiography may reveal an abdominal mass or intestinal obstruction. As afferent lymphatics of the pelvic limb drain into the cisterna chyli, lymphangiography, which is carried out by means of water-soluble contrast material via a dorsal pedal lymphatic vessel, may reveal a lymphatic or cisterna chyli leak.

F. Pancreatitis, lymphoma, dirofilariasis, cardiovascular disease, nephrotic syndrome, and thoracic duct pathology have been associated with chylous ascites and should be ruled out.

G. Conservative management is recommended initially in those cases of recent abdominal surgery, in which there are no palpable or radiographic abnormalities and no evidence of septic peritonitis. Absolute cage rest, with periodic abdominocentesis to allow easier breathing, is essential. A strict diet that consists of low-fat cottage cheese, rice, and medium-chain triglyceride (MCT) oil with a multivitamin supplement should be tried for approximately 1 week.

H. Rarely does chylous ascites resolve with conservative therapy, and laparotomy is necessary to identify the cause of leakage. Two hours prior to surgery, give the patient vegetable oil, 3 ml per kilogram of body weight; give additional vegetable oil, 1 ml per kilogram, immediately prior to induction of anesthesia. The oil is transformed into triglycerides, which enter the lymphatics. The lymphatic vessels then appear white and distended, which allows for easy identification of any leaks.

I. Tumors should be removed if possible. Chemotherapy may be instituted following tumor identification. If the tumor is not resectable and is resistant to chemotherapy, euthanasia should be considered.

J. If a ruptured cisterna chyli is identified, attempt primary repair. However, as this could be difficult because of fragility of the vessel wall, omentum may be sutured over the defect in an attempt to seal the leak. Ligate the ruptured lymphatic vessel on each side of the defect. A strict diet (G) should be instituted for 1 week postoperatively. A normal diet should be introduced slowly, while monitoring for recurrence of chylous ascites.

K. Mesenteric lymph node, duodenal, and jejunal biopsies should be obtained if no gross lesion can be seen or if lymphangiectasia is suspected.

L. Definitive treatment is based on biopsy, and fungal and bacterial culture results. If a specific etiology cannot be identified, a strict diet (G), as well as a regimen of an anti-inflammatory dose of steroids, should be instituted.

M. The long-term prognosis is poor where the chylous effusion does not resolve following the initial treatment. In these cases, steroids should be discontinued and strict diet continued. Total parenteral nutrition or a peritoneovenous shunt may be an alternative. Euthanasia should also be considered.

References

Asch MJ, Sherman NJ. Management of refractory chylous ascites by total parenteral nutrition. J Pediatr 1979; 94:260.

Fossum TW, Jacobs RM, Bischard SJ. Evaluation of cholesterol and triglyceride concentrations in differentiating chylous and non-chylous pleural effusions in dogs and cats. JAVMA 1986; 188(1):49.

Sherding RG. Diseases of the small bowel. In: Ettinger SJ, ed. Textbook of veterinary internal medicine. Diseases of the dog and cat. Philadelphia: WB Saunders, 1983:1278.

Staats BA, Ellefson RD, Budahn LL, et al. The lipoprotein profile of chylous and nonchylous pleural effusions. Mayo Clin Proc 1980; 55:700.

Walshaw R. Surgical diseases of the liver and biliary system. In: Slatter DH, ed. Textbook of small animal surgery. Philadelphia: WB Saunders, 1985:798.

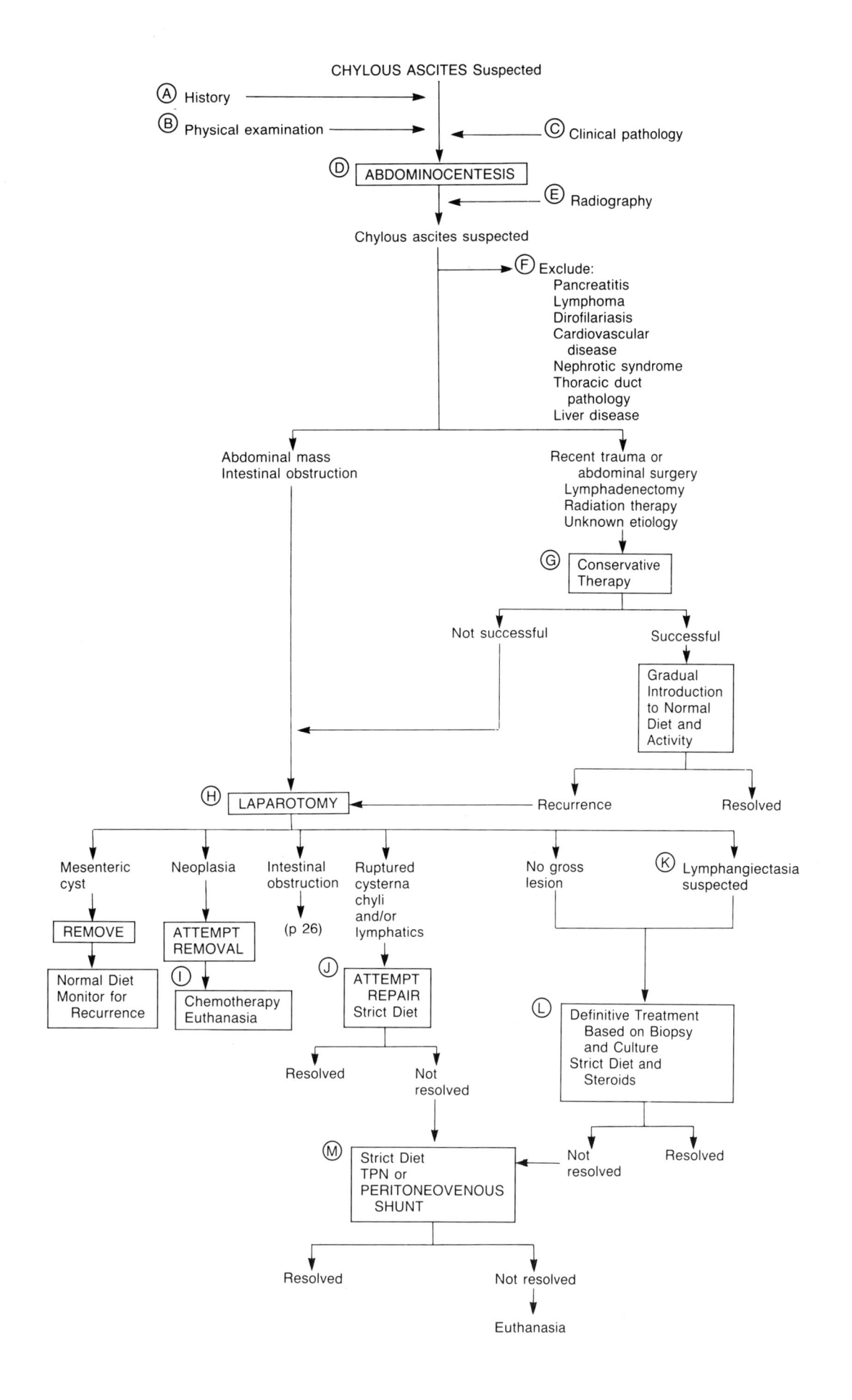

```
                              CHYLOUS ASCITES Suspected
          Ⓐ History ─────────────────→         │
                                                │
          Ⓑ Physical examination ──────→        │ ←────── Ⓒ Clinical pathology
                                                ↓
                                       Ⓓ  ABDOMINOCENTESIS
                                                │ ←────── Ⓔ Radiography
                                                ↓
                                      Chylous ascites suspected
                                                │
                                                │─────────→ Ⓕ Exclude:
                                                │              Pancreatitis
                                                │              Lymphoma
                                                │              Dirofilariasis
                                                │              Cardiovascular
                                                │                disease
                                                │              Nephrotic syndrome
                                                │              Thoracic duct
                                                │                pathology
                                                │              Liver disease
                              ┌─────────────────┴─────────────────┐
                   Abdominal mass                      Recent trauma or
                   Intestinal obstruction              abdominal surgery
                              │                        Lymphadenectomy
                              │                        Radiation therapy
                              │                        Unknown etiology
                              │                                   │
                              │                            Ⓖ  Conservative
                              │                                Therapy
                              │                          ┌────────┴────────┐
                              │                    Not successful      Successful
                              │                          │                 │
                              │                          │            Gradual
                              │                          │            Introduction
                              │                          │            to Normal
                              │                          │            Diet and
                              │                          │            Activity
                              │                          │          ┌─────┴──────┐
                              ↓←─────────────────────────┘      Recurrence    Resolved
                    Ⓗ  LAPAROTOMY ←──────────────────────────────────┘
           ┌──────┬────────┬──────────┬──────────┬──────────┬──────────┐
      Mesenteric  Neoplasia Intestinal Ruptured   No gross   Ⓚ Lymphangiectasia
      cyst                  obstruction cysterna  lesion       suspected
           │        │       (p 26)      chyli       │            │
       REMOVE   ATTEMPT                 and/or      │            │
           │    REMOVAL                 lymphatics  │            │
           │        │                      │       │            │
      Normal Diet  Ⓘ                   Ⓙ ATTEMPT   │       Ⓛ Definitive Treatment
      Monitor for  Chemotherapy          REPAIR    │          Based on Biopsy
      Recurrence   Euthanasia          Strict Diet │          and Culture
                                      ┌────┴────┐  │          Strict Diet and
                                  Resolved   Not   │          Steroids
                                             resolved         ┌─────┴─────┐
                                                │          Not        Resolved
                                                ↓         resolved
                                        Ⓜ Strict Diet ←────┘
                                          TPN or
                                          PERITONEOVENOUS
                                          SHUNT
                                       ┌──────┴──────┐
                                   Resolved      Not resolved
                                                     │
                                                  Euthanasia
```

SEPTIC PERITONITIS

Karol A. Mathews

A. The history is usually vague unless the owner reports recent trauma or abdominal surgery. In primary peritonitis, a progression of general depression, anorexia, vomiting, or abdominal distension for several days to weeks may be noted. Acute abdominal pain with a "tucked-up" appearance, depression, and vomiting are more likely with secondary peritonitis. Occasionally, owners report that the animal assumes a "praying position."

B. Injected mucous membranes, a slow capillary refill time, gastrointestinal ileus, and accumulation of abdominal fluid are frequent symptoms of peritonitis. The patient may be febrile; however, in the old or debilitated animal, or as a state of hypodynamic shock ensues, the temperature may be normal or subnormal. Pain or vomiting may be elicited on palpation of the abdomen.

C. A markedly elevated neutrophilic leukocytosis with left shift is frequently seen. Occasionally, a mild leukocytosis with a degenerative left shift occurs; this is indicative of massive consumption of neutrophils. Diffuse peritonitis may lead to dehydration and consequently to metabolic acidosis, azotemia, and electrolyte imbalance.

D. Free gas may be visible if there is a rupture of the gastrointestinal tract, presence of gas-forming organisms, or a penetrating injury. Air may remain in the abdomen for up to 1 week following abdominal surgery. Generalized intestinal adynamic ileus is a frequent observation. Barium or hyperosmolar iodinated contrast material should not be given if gastrointestinal perforation is suspected.

E. The abdominal fluid white blood cell (WBC) count and differential provide the most useful and rapidly available diagnostic information. The leukocyte count in normal animals is generally <1,000 per μl. A WBC count >3,000 per μl with >50 percent degenerative neutrophils is strongly suggestive of a septic peritonitis, as is the presence of degenerative neutrophils with intracellular bacteria or significant numbers of extracellular bacteria. If a needle abdominocentesis is negative when there is a high level of suspicion for peritonitis, a diagnostic peritoneal lavage should be performed. It is considered positive if the fluid is grossly bloody or opaque in appearance, with degenerative neutrophils present on cytological examination. Perform a Gram's stain and culture and sensitivity testing for aerobic and anaerobic bacteria and fungi.

F. Primary (spontaneous or idiopathic) peritonitis is rare. Usually only one organism is cultured, or a viral infection may be the cause (e.g., feline infectious peritonitis). If the history is consistent with a primary peritonitis and no surgical lesion can be identified on physical, radiologic, or cytologic examination, the lesion should be managed as a primary peritonitis.

G. Secondary peritonitis, which requires exploratory laparotomy, should be suspected if radiologic, cytologic, biochemical, or physical findings support a surgically correctable lesion. If the patient has received antibiotic therapy, the cytologic findings may erroneously suggest a nonseptic process as organisms may not be seen and the neutrophils may be nondegenerative.

H. If no surgically correctable lesion is found on laparotomy, primary peritonitis should be suspected and managed accordingly.

I. Definitive therapy is based on the results of the bacterial culture. Intermittent peritoneal lavage and administration of appropriate antibiotics may be beneficial. Patients with primary peritonitis that undergo exploratory laparotomy have an increased morbidity and mortality, which is caused by wound infection and poor healing.

J. Continued drainage is important and may be by continuous or intermittent lavage of the peritoneal cavity or by creating a free-draining (open) peritoneal cavity that is protected from evisceration by a sterile bandage. Broad-spectrum antibiotics should be instituted immediately, followed by definitive therapy based on culture and sensitivity.

References

Crowe DT, Bjorling DE. Peritoneum and peritoneal cavity. In: Slatter DH, ed. Textbook of small animal surgery. Philadelphia: WB Saunders, 1985:571.

Duncan JR, Prasse KW. Cytology in veterinary laboratory medicine. Clinical pathology. 2nd ed. Ames, IA: Iowa State University Press 1986:201.

Hunt CA. Diagnostic peritoneal paracentesis and lavage. Comp Cont Ed 1980; 11(6):449.

Lee AH, Swaim SF, Henderson RA. Surgical drainage. Comp Cont Ed 1986; 8(2):94.

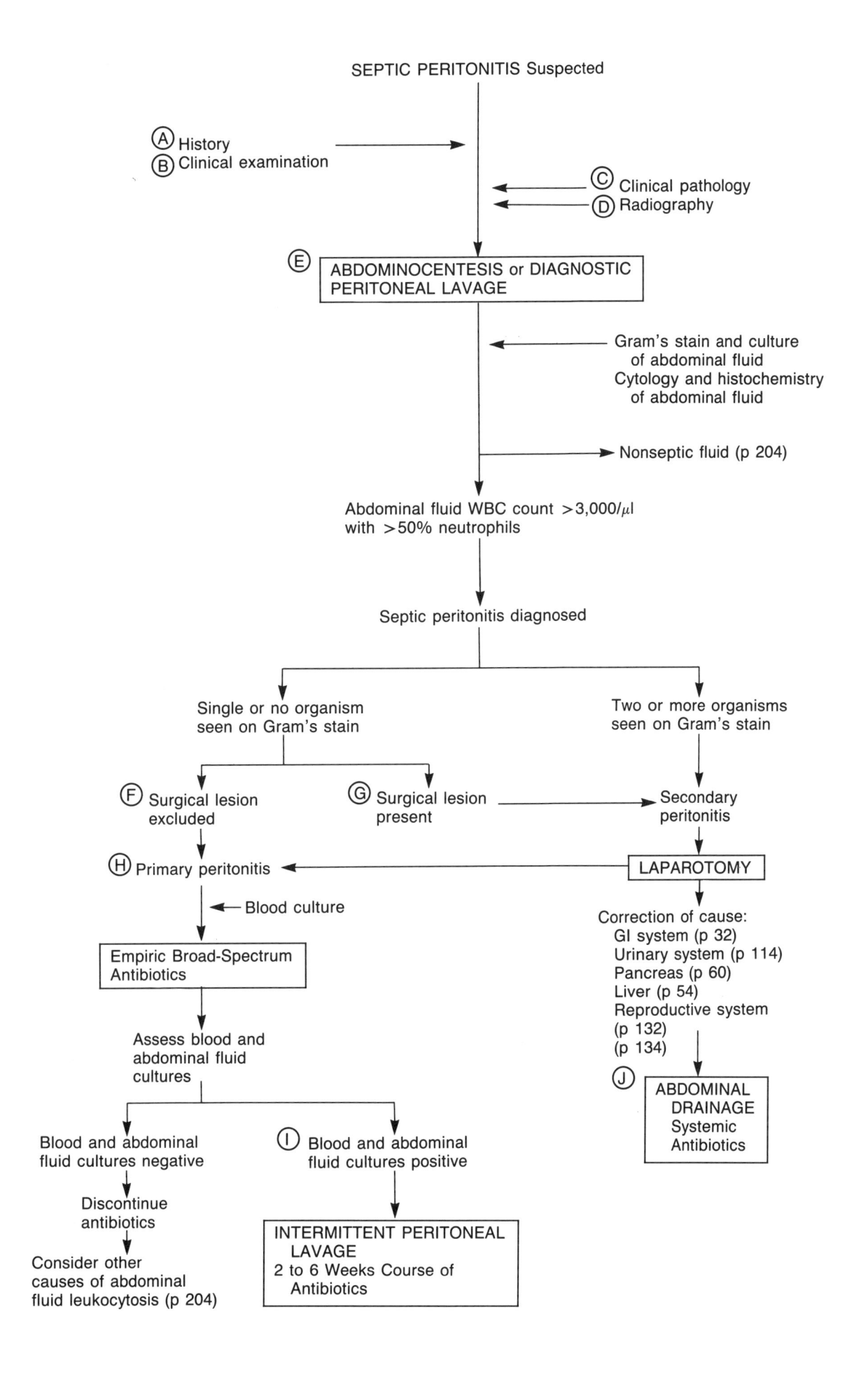

SEPTIC PERITONITIS Suspected

- Ⓐ History
- Ⓑ Clinical examination
- Ⓒ Clinical pathology
- Ⓓ Radiography

↓

Ⓔ **ABDOMINOCENTESIS or DIAGNOSTIC PERITONEAL LAVAGE**

- Gram's stain and culture of abdominal fluid
- Cytology and histochemistry of abdominal fluid

→ Nonseptic fluid (p 204)

↓

Abdominal fluid WBC count >3,000/µl with >50% neutrophils

↓

Septic peritonitis diagnosed

- Single or no organism seen on Gram's stain
- Two or more organisms seen on Gram's stain

Ⓕ Surgical lesion excluded → Ⓗ Primary peritonitis

Ⓖ Surgical lesion present → Secondary peritonitis → **LAPAROTOMY**

← Blood culture

Empiric Broad-Spectrum Antibiotics

↓

Assess blood and abdominal fluid cultures

- Blood and abdominal fluid cultures negative → Discontinue antibiotics → Consider other causes of abdominal fluid leukocytosis (p 204)
- Ⓘ Blood and abdominal fluid cultures positive → **INTERMITTENT PERITONEAL LAVAGE** 2 to 6 Weeks Course of Antibiotics

Correction of cause:
- GI system (p 32)
- Urinary system (p 114)
- Pancreas (p 60)
- Liver (p 54)
- Reproductive system (p 132) (p 134)

↓

Ⓙ **ABDOMINAL DRAINAGE** Systemic Antibiotics

211

SPLENIC DISORDER

Cindy L. Fries

Whereas the spleen may be affected by a wide variety of disease processes, it has a limited number of ways by which it may respond. Therefore, splenomegaly is a nonspecific clinical finding rather than a diagnosis. The underlying disease must be determined before an appropriate course of action may be selected.

- A. The history of an animal presenting with splenic disease is generally vague and nonspecific. The course may be acute, chronic, or intermittent. Depending on the primary disease, the historical findings can vary from sudden collapse or abdominal pain to vomiting, weight loss, or nonspecific malaise.

- B. Abdominal palpation frequently reveals splenomegaly. Careful palpation is used to differentiate asymmetrical enlargement of the spleen from other cranial abdominal masses. Other abnormalities detected on physical examination may help determine the underlying disease.

- C. Splenomegaly may be confirmed radiographically by the enlargement of the splenic shadow, the presence of a soft tissue mass in the area of the spleen, or the appropriate displacement of adjacent organs. Should the plain films be inconclusive, specialized procedures such as ultrasonography and pneumoperitonography may be performed.

- D. Congestive splenomegaly may follow the administration of certain drugs such as barbiturates, phenothiazines, and butyrophenones. This must be considered when splenic size is evaluated in the anesthetized animal.

- E. Torsion of the spleen may occur in conjunction with gastric volvulus or as a single disease entity. Whereas the onset of clinical signs is usually acute, an animal with torsion of the spleen may present with a prolonged or intermittent history. Anemia occasionally accompanies this syndrome.

- F. Fine-needle aspiration is useful in the diagnosis and staging of neoplastic conditions. It is contraindicated if hemangiosarcoma or clotting disorders are suspected. As most neoplasms that cause symmetrical splenomegaly are diffuse myelo- or lympho-proliferative disorders, systemic anticancer therapy is the treatment of choice. Feline systemic mastocytosis is an exception to this rule as prolonged remissions have been observed with splenectomy alone.

- G. Immune-mediated conditions, such as immune-mediated hemolytic anemia, immune-mediated thrombocytopenia, and systemic lupus erythematosus, which have not responded to an adequate regimen of immunosuppressive drugs, may show some improvement with splenectomy. As the results vary from good to temporary, splenectomy is only recommended when the medical options have been exhausted.

- H. The most common primary splenic tumor is hemangiosarcoma. This highly malignant tumor has generally metastasized by the time of diagnosis. While the long-term prognosis is poor, a palliative splenectomy may provide a good quality of life for several months.

- I. Although a splenectomy is to be avoided whenever possible, it may be necessary in cases of diffuse splenic trauma. Splenic function may be preserved by placing healthy remnants within omental pouches.

References

Feldman BF, Zinkl JG. Diseases of the lymphnodes and spleen. In: Ettinger SJ, ed. Textbook of veterinary internal medicine, 2nd ed. Philadelphia: WB Saunders, 1983:2067.

Lipowitz AJ, et al. The spleen. In: Slatter DH, ed. Textbook of small animal surgery. Philadelphia: WB Saunders, 1985:1204.

Stevenson S. Surgical techniques of the spleen. In: Bojrab MJ, ed. Current techniques in small animal surgery. 2nd ed. Philadelphia: Lea & Febiger, 1983:486.

SPLENIC DISORDER Suspected

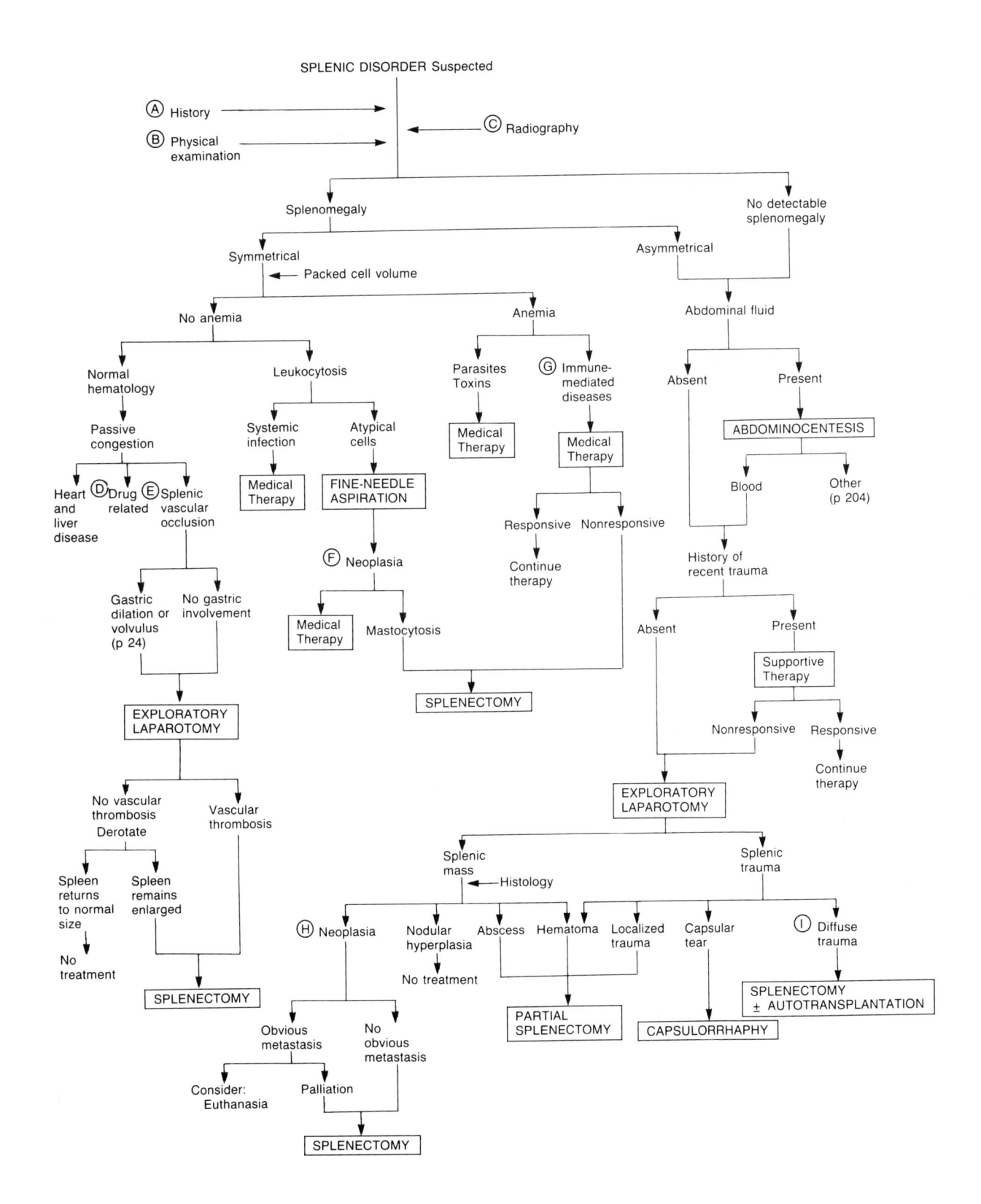

- Ⓐ History
- Ⓑ Physical examination
- Ⓒ Radiography

Splenomegaly

Symmetrical ← Packed cell volume

No anemia

- **Normal hematology** → Passive congestion
  - Heart and liver disease
  - Ⓓ Drug related
  - Ⓔ Splenic vascular occlusion
    - Gastric dilation or volvulus (p 24)
    - No gastric involvement → **EXPLORATORY LAPAROTOMY**
      - No vascular thrombosis → Derotate
        - Spleen returns to normal size → No treatment
        - Spleen remains enlarged
      - Vascular thrombosis → **SPLENECTOMY**

- **Leukocytosis**
  - Systemic infection → Medical Therapy
  - Atypical cells → **FINE-NEEDLE ASPIRATION**
    - Ⓕ Neoplasia
      - Medical Therapy
      - Mastocytosis → **SPLENECTOMY**

Anemia
- Parasites / Toxins → Medical Therapy
- Ⓖ Immune-mediated diseases → Medical Therapy
  - Responsive → Continue therapy
  - Nonresponsive → **SPLENECTOMY**

No detectable splenomegaly

Asymmetrical
- Abdominal fluid
  - Absent
  - Present → **ABDOMINOCENTESIS**
    - Blood
      - History of recent trauma
        - Absent
        - Present → Supportive Therapy
          - Nonresponsive
          - Responsive → Continue therapy
      - → **EXPLORATORY LAPAROTOMY**
        - Splenic mass ← Histology
          - Ⓗ Neoplasia
            - Obvious metastasis → Consider: Euthanasia
            - No obvious metastasis → Palliation → **SPLENECTOMY**
          - Nodular hyperplasia → No treatment
          - Abscess → **PARTIAL SPLENECTOMY**
          - Hematoma → **PARTIAL SPLENECTOMY**
        - Splenic trauma
          - Localized trauma → **PARTIAL SPLENECTOMY**
          - Capsular tear → **CAPSULORRHAPHY**
          - Ⓘ Diffuse trauma → **SPLENECTOMY ± AUTOTRANSPLANTATION**
    - Other (p 204)

PINNA DISCOMFORT

Geoff Sumner-Smith

A. Most conditions of the ear are manifested by the animal either holding its head tilted to one side or by shaking it frequently.

B. Inflammation is a common cause of pinna discomfort. Vigorous scratching by the animal may result in a hematoma. Particular care must be taken to obliterate dead space following extirpation of a resulting blood clot; various suturing techniques or compression bandaging methods may be employed.

C. Dermatologic conditions of the edge of the pinna are common and may take many forms. Particularly severe or chronic cases may be treated surgically by partial amputation.

D. Neoplasia of the pinna may also be associated with neoplasia of the vertical ear canal. An early diagnosis is imperative; even nonmalignant tumors can be locally destructive, and necrosis of the mass occurs more quickly than elsewhere on the skin. The results of the biopsy govern the treatment.

E. The complications of minor lacerations of the pinna vary according to the breed characteristics of the animal injured. A large pendulous ear can often be further traumatized by scratching or violent shaking of the head. Ear wounds should always be taken seriously, otherwise, they may progress to chronic ulceration, infection, or hematoma formation. Suturing through the cartilage is often necessary if the cartilage is split. The top of the cranium acts as an excellent splint and aids compression bandaging of the ear. Exercise care to ensure that the animal's airway is not impeded by the bandage.

F. Major trauma to the pinna is particularly common following a dog fight. Swelling and infection of the area follows soon after the traumatic incident, and therefore repair should not be delayed. Neglected wounds may not respond to either parenteral or topical antibiotic therapy; surgical repair or partial amputation may be necessary.

References

Bostock DE, Owens LN. Neoplasia in the cat, dog and horse. Chicago: Year Book Medical Publication, 1975.

Cowley F. Treatment of hematoma of the canine ear. Vet Med (Small Anim Clin) 1976; 71:283.

Wilson JW. Treatment of aural hematoma using a teat tube. JAVMA 1983; 182:1081.

PINNA DISCOMFORT

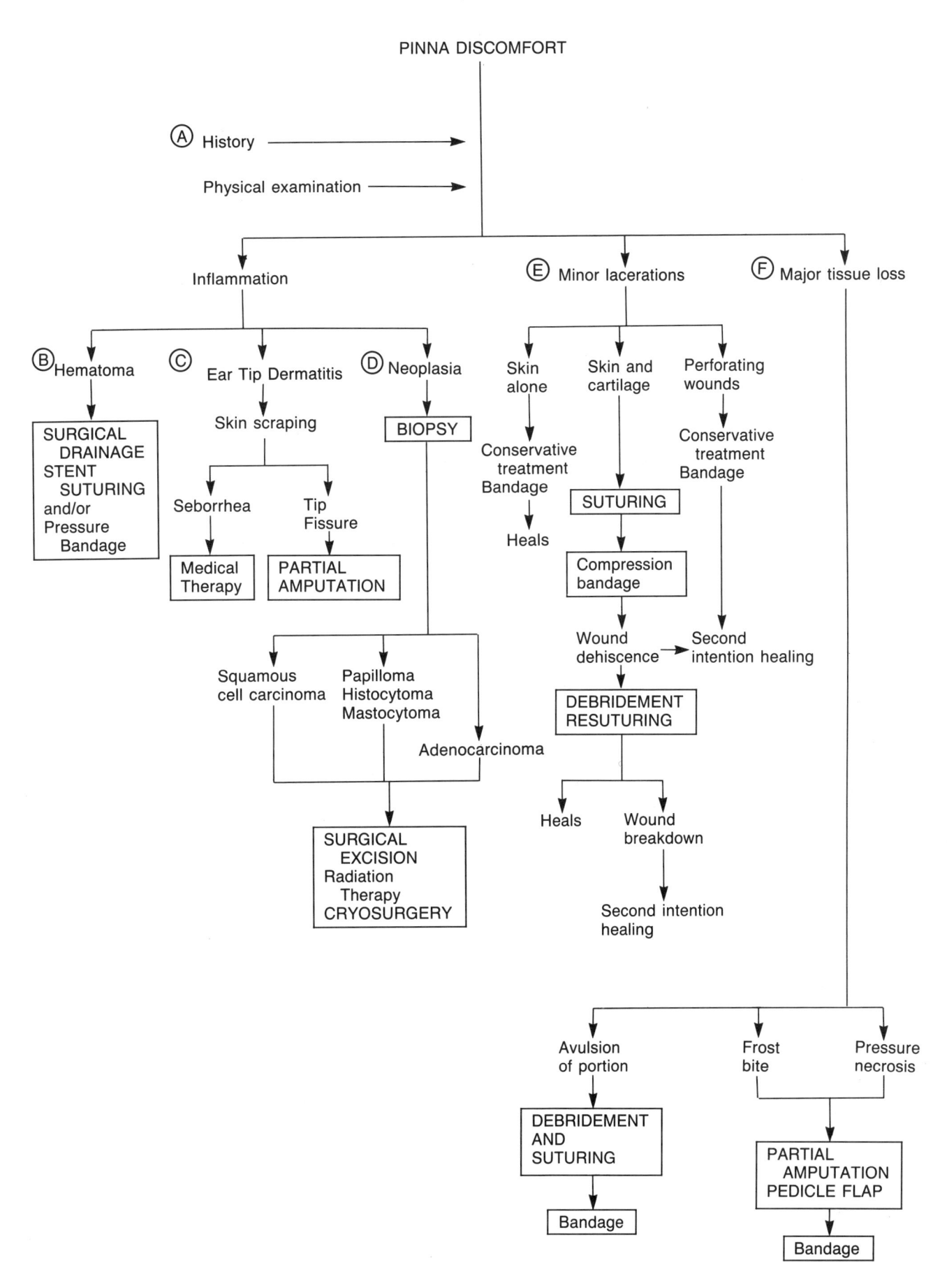

A History →
Physical examination →

Inflammation

- **B** Hematoma → SURGICAL DRAINAGE STENT SUTURING and/or Pressure Bandage
- **C** Ear Tip Dermatitis → Skin scraping
  - Seborrhea → Medical Therapy
  - Tip Fissure → PARTIAL AMPUTATION
- **D** Neoplasia → BIOPSY
  - Squamous cell carcinoma
  - Papilloma / Histocytoma / Mastocytoma
  - Adenocarcinoma
  → SURGICAL EXCISION / Radiation Therapy / CRYOSURGERY

E Minor lacerations

- Skin alone → Conservative treatment Bandage → Heals
- Skin and cartilage → SUTURING → Compression bandage → Wound dehiscence → DEBRIDEMENT RESUTURING
  - Heals
  - Wound breakdown → Second intention healing
- Perforating wounds → Conservative treatment Bandage → Second intention healing

F Major tissue loss

- Avulsion of portion → DEBRIDEMENT AND SUTURING → Bandage
- Frost bite → PARTIAL AMPUTATION PEDICLE FLAP → Bandage
- Pressure necrosis → PARTIAL AMPUTATION PEDICLE FLAP → Bandage

EXTERNAL EAR CANAL DISEASE

Geoff Sumner-Smith

A. The dog may be presented with a history of ear pain, ear scratching, ear odor or discharge, or head tilt.

B. Examination of the auditory canal with an otoscope often determines the etiology of the otitis externa. Otitis externa is usually caused by a bacterial or yeast infection, especially in the case of dogs with pendulous ears; however, foreign bodies, neoplasia, and ear mites must also be considered. Sedation or general anesthesia are generally required for a thorough otoscopic examination.

C. In mild cases, biweekly irrigation with a detergent and antiseptic solution may be sufficient treatment. Topical antibiotics and steroids produce satisfactory results in most cases, with water soluble preparations being preferred over those with an oil base. Perform culture and sensitivity in persistent cases.

D. Early removal of foreign bodies is essential in order to prevent mucosal irritation and subsequent infection. Usually sedation or general anesthesia is necessary.

E. Small neoplasms of the vertical and horizontal canal may be removed by either electrosurgery or cryosurgery. Histologic examination of the tissue removed is mandatory. Removal of larger tumors may require resection of the lateral wall of the vertical canal, or total ablation.

F. A "state of balance" may exist between the mite infestation and the ear canal dermis; the animal suffers irritation and responds by scratching the ear and shaking the head. The local use of ceruminolytics and acaricides usually overcome the infestation, but in more severe cases, infection may also be present and require therapy. Prolonged antimite treatment (3 to 4 weeks) is essential; treatment should include the entire body of the animal as well as others in contact with it.

G. Nonresponsive otitis externa usually requires resection of the lateral wall of the vertical canal in order to obtain proper drainage and ventilation. Many different techniques have been described. Ulceration of both the vertical and horizontal canal are more effectively treated by topical medication and, if necessary, by cauterization.

H. Severe proliferation of the vertical canal may not respond to topical therapy. Perform ablation of the vertical canal in such cases.

I. Care must be taken to ensure that all of the horizontal canal and lining of the auditory meatus are removed. Failure to do so permits the remaining glands within the dermis to continue to secrete. The material accumulates and becomes infected; abscesses and fistulae develop under and through the skin. If the tympanic membrane is destroyed or otitis media is present, a lateral bulla osteotomy is performed concurrently. The lining of the bulla is removed and the bulla flushed with an antibiotic solution prior to closure (p 218).

References

Dallman MJ, Bojrab MJ. Ear canal ablation. In: Bojrab MJ, ed. Current techniques in small animal surgery. Philadelphia: WB Saunders, 1983:99.

Grono LR. The external ear canal. In: Slatter DH, ed. Textbook of small animal surgery. Philadelphia: WB Saunders, 1985:1906.

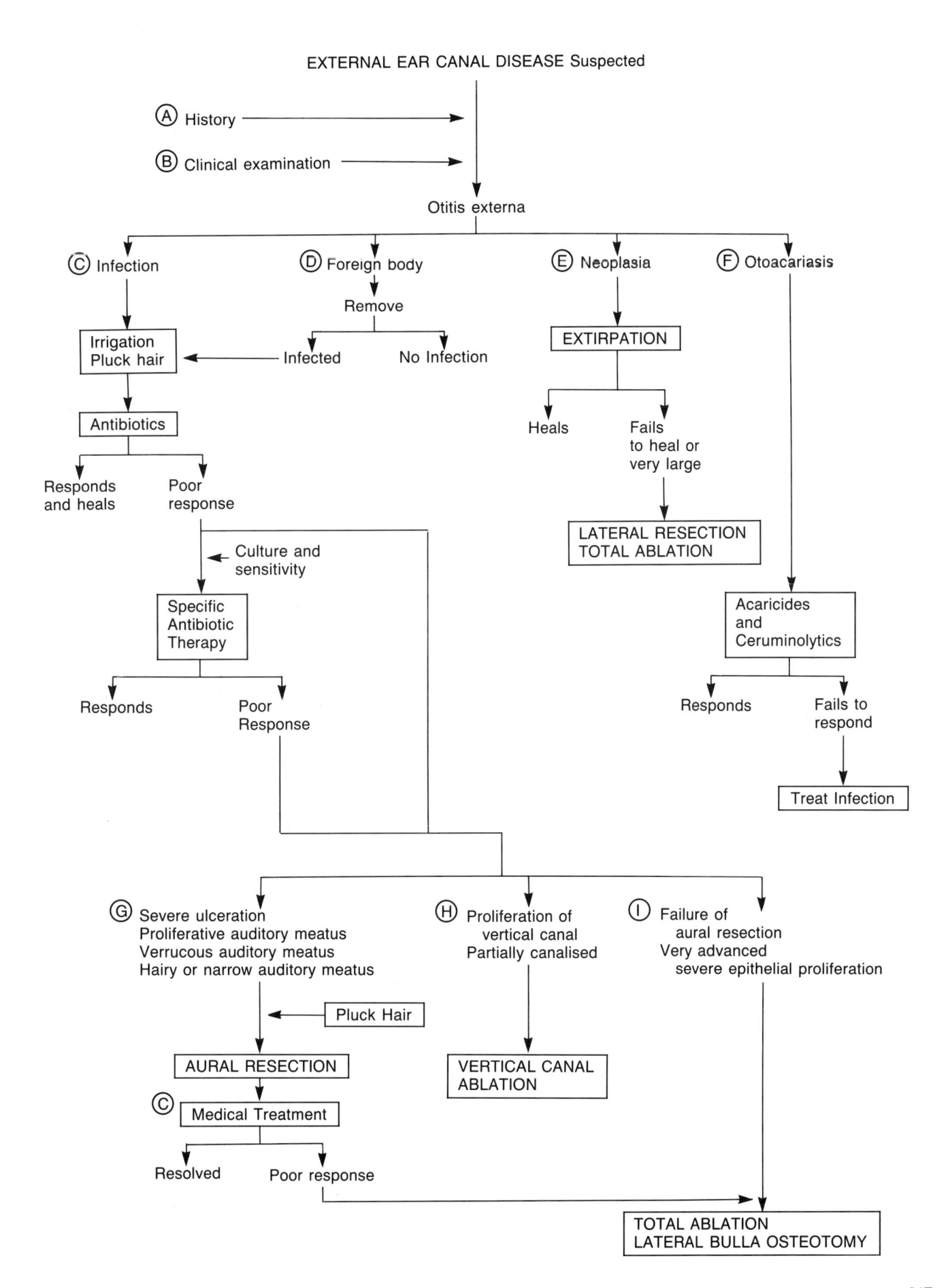

EXTERNAL EAR CANAL DISEASE Suspected

- **A** History
- **B** Clinical examination

↓

Otitis externa

- **C** Infection
  - Irrigation / Pluck hair
  - Antibiotics
    - Responds and heals
    - Poor response
      - Culture and sensitivity
      - Specific Antibiotic Therapy
        - Responds
        - Poor Response

- **D** Foreign body
  - Remove
    - Infected → (Irrigation Pluck hair)
    - No Infection

- **E** Neoplasia
  - EXTIRPATION
    - Heals
    - Fails to heal or very large → LATERAL RESECTION / TOTAL ABLATION

- **F** Otoacariasis
  - Acaricides and Ceruminolytics
    - Responds
    - Fails to respond → Treat Infection

- **G** Severe ulceration / Proliferative auditory meatus / Verrucous auditory meatus / Hairy or narrow auditory meatus
  - Pluck Hair
  - AURAL RESECTION
  - **C** Medical Treatment
    - Resolved
    - Poor response

- **H** Proliferation of vertical canal / Partially canalised
  - VERTICAL CANAL ABLATION

- **I** Failure of aural resection / Very advanced severe epithelial proliferation

→ TOTAL ABLATION / LATERAL BULLA OSTEOTOMY

MIDDLE EAR DISEASE

Geoff Sumner-Smith

Otitis media may arise from infection that ascends the eustachian tube or from blood-borne pathogens; however, the most common etiology is secondary to otitis externa.

A. The animal may be presented because of head shaking, pawing or rubbing of the affected ear, ear pain, or a head tilt with the involved ear lower. There may be a history of chronic ear discharge or chronic otitis externa that has failed to respond to treatment.

B. On examination, signs of otitis externa are noted. Facial nerve involvement may be manifested by a decreased palpebral reflex, an enlarged palpebral fissure, and drooping of the ear and lips. Damage to the sympathetic nerve may cause Horner's syndrome. Under general anesthesia, the bulla can be palpated per os; in chronic otitis media, the surface may be irregular and roughened. The tympanic membrane is examined with an otoscope or rigid fibre optic scope. The membrane may be intact or ruptured. The membrane is usually transparent, is a pearl grey color, and is slightly concave in shape. Bulging or alteration in color are indications of otitis media.

C. Radiography is often helpful in establishing a diagnosis of otitis media. Lateral, oblique, and open mouth views may demonstrate changes in and around the bulla. The bulla may have a fluid or soft tissue density, or sclerosis of the bulla may be noted.

D. A culture is taken from the middle ear by myringotomy if necessary. Examine culture material for aerobic bacteria, fungus, and yeast, and perform sensitivity testing. Biopsy any abnormal tissue in the external or middle ear.

E. Trauma to the osseous bulla or auditory bones usually responds to topical and systemic antibiotics.

F. Neoplastic growths include polyps, fibromas, squamous cell carcinomas, and primary bone tumors. In the cat, inflammatory polyps may develop secondary to otitis media.

G. Common yeast and fungal agents include *Pityrosporon* species, *Candida* species and *Aspergillus* species.

H. Common bacterial agents include *Staphylococcus* species, *Streptococcus* species, *Pseudomonas* species, *Escherichia coli*, and *Proteus mirabilis*.

I. In most cases, the concurrent otitis externa must be treated. Both otitis media and externa require removal of inflammatory debris in order to provide an exit for discharge and proper ventilation of the external and middle ear. Myringotomy may be necessary in order to allow flushing or curettage of the middle ear via the external canal. A lateral ear resection may be necessary (p 216). Use astringents to dry the ear canal. In most cases, both otitis externa and otitis media benefit from corticosteroids applied topically.

J. Nystatin is effective only against *Candida* species, whereas thiabendazole and miconazole topically are broad-spectrum antifungals. In the case of aspergillosis, the addition of ketoconazole (10 mg per kilogram three times daily by mouth) may be of benefit.

K. Topical antibacterials (neomycin, polymycin, gentamycin, chloramphenicol) show good activity against most otitis media pathogens. Ototoxicity, although rare, can occur with the aminoglycosides. Systemic antibiotics should also be given.

L. Nonresponsive otitis media requires exploration and drainage of the osseous bulla. A lateral ear canal resection or total ear canal ablation may be necessary for treatment of the concurrent otitis externa. If an ablation is performed, a lateral bulla osteotomy should be performed at the same time. In the case of a primary otitis media, or where no ablation is contemplated, perform a ventral bulla osteotomy. In either approach, the bulla is curetted of all debris, the lining removed, and the cavity thoroughly flushed. Placement of drainage tubes is advisable for at least 3 to 5 days postoperatively. In the cat a transverse septum divides the bulla into two compartments. It must be broken down to allow adequate treatment.

References

Bojrab MJ, Robertson JJ. Surgical treatment for middle and inner ear infection. In: Bojrab MJ, ed. Current techniques in small animal surgery. 2nd ed. Philadelphia: WB Saunders, 1983:106.

Harvey CE. Diseases of the middle ear. In: Slatter DH, ed. Textbook of small animal surgery. Philadelphia: WB Saunders, 1985:1915.

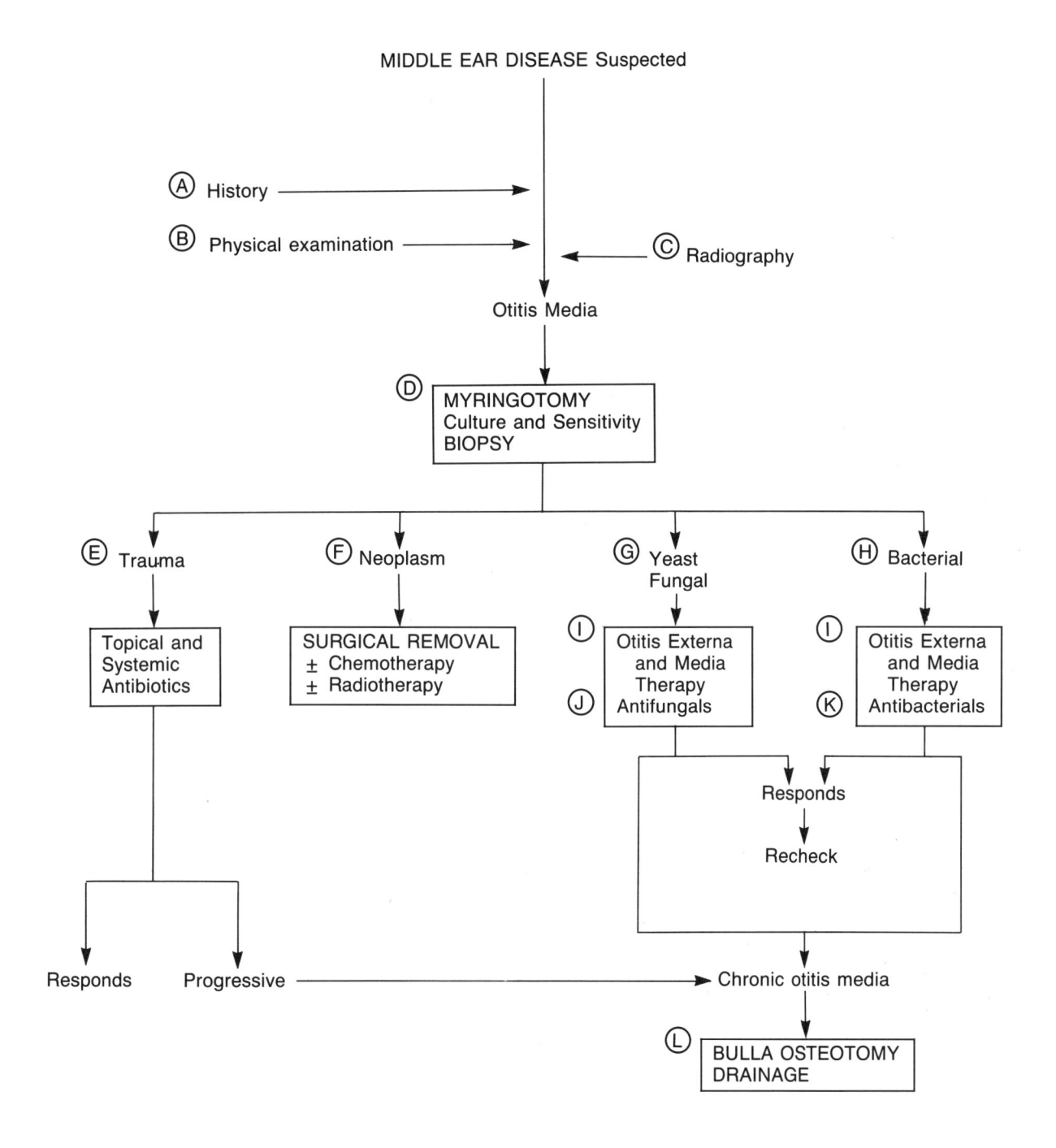

MIDDLE EAR DISEASE Suspected

- Ⓐ History
- Ⓑ Physical examination
- Ⓒ Radiography

↓

Otitis Media

↓

Ⓓ MYRINGOTOMY
Culture and Sensitivity
BIOPSY

- Ⓔ Trauma → Topical and Systemic Antibiotics → Responds / Progressive
- Ⓕ Neoplasm → SURGICAL REMOVAL ± Chemotherapy ± Radiotherapy
- Ⓖ Yeast Fungal → Ⓘ Otitis Externa and Media Therapy / Ⓙ Antifungals
- Ⓗ Bacterial → Ⓘ Otitis Externa and Media Therapy / Ⓚ Antibacterials

→ Responds → Recheck

Progressive → Chronic otitis media

↓

Ⓛ BULLA OSTEOTOMY DRAINAGE

219

CONDITIONS OF GROWING TEETH

Geoff Sumner-Smith

Growing teeth may suffer from conditions that are the result of abnormal eruption or that occur following normal eruption of either the deciduous or permanent dentition.

A. Abnormal eruption of the teeth may result in malocclusion (p 222), which is considered to be "normal" in some breeds (e.g., Bulldog, Pekinese). Various abnormalities of eruption may require treatment in order to prevent development of a painful condition within the mouth or to improve the function of the teeth. Treatment should not be employed to correct abnormal occlusion that has no effect on the animal's health.

B. Hypoplasia of the enamel may be the result of embryonic edema of the pulp or hypoplasia of the enamel organ. If the dog suffers a severe febrile illness during eruption of the teeth, particularly at 4 to 5 months of age when mineralization of the crowns is occurring, multiple enamel hypoplasia may occur, with associated discoloration of the enamel and dentine.

C. Normal eruption is usually followed by the formation of arcades of normal teeth. However, such normal teeth may be discolored a yellow-orange if the animal has received tetracycline during puppyhood. Enamel that is apparently normal may be very thin and quickly develop a hypoplastic appearance, possibly on account of early malnutrition. Inflammation of the pulp capillary may result in grey discoloration and death of a tooth. Root canal therapy may be indicated in such circumstances (p 226).

D. Supernumerary permanent teeth may vary in number from a single "extra" tooth to a total second set of teeth. Careful examination should confirm that the extra teeth are not retained deciduous elements. Carry out surgical extraction if the extra teeth cause problems, such as impaction of food and malalignment that causes trauma to the tongue and buccal mucosa.

E. Treat hypoplasia of enamel in order to prevent further deterioration. Following proper grinding and preparation of the area, minor defects are treated with a filling by means of an amalgam or composite material. (Fig. 1). This technique should only be used in animals that are not inclined to "chew everything in sight." More severe defects may be treated by flat filling or by crowning. Severe hypoplasia of the canine teeth should be treated by amputation, followed by flat filling.

F. Neoplasia of teeth is not common in the canine patient; when it does occur, it is usually teratogenic.

G. Loose deciduous teeth may adhere to the gingiva and rotate into the transverse position. Deciduous teeth, especially the canines, are commonly retained; this is particularly the case in the toy breeds. The retention of teeth may or may not have an effect on the eruption of subsequent permanent teeth. Extraction of retained teeth is recommended, particularly if the puppy has attained the age of 6 months. Impacted teeth are seen rarely in dogs and require surgical exposure and realignment, provided that the retained tooth is radiographically normal. Otherwise, they should be extracted. Impacted teeth may give the impression of oligodontia. They are often an incidental finding on radiography.

H. Ameloblastomas behave as locally invasive malignant tumors, which cause pressure atrophy of the surrounding soft tissue and bone with loosening and displacement of adjacent teeth. The condition may not be diagnosed until it is well advanced as proliferation is towards the oral cavity and is covered by ulcerating mucosa. Extraction of the teeth is necessary, and the operation should also include radical resection of the surrounding bone to ensure all portions of the tumor have been removed.

I. Odontomas are tumors of the dental papilla and contain cement and enamel, whereas cementomas are tumors of the cement alone, which commence during the embryonic development of the tooth.

J. Surgical intervention depends upon the particular condition involved and varies from extraction to resection of the surrounding gingiva and bone, with orthodontic correction of the malalignment as the impacted tooth erupts.

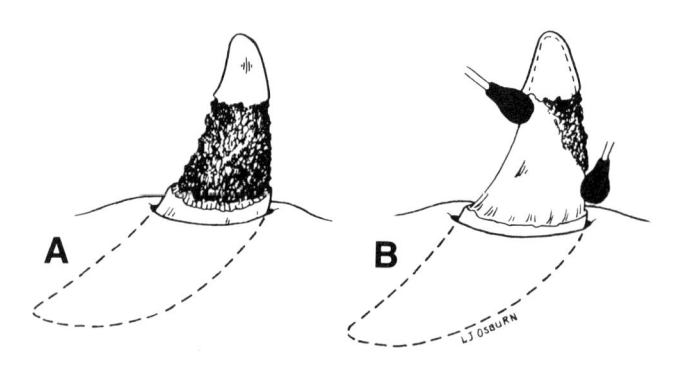

Figure 1 Treatment of enamel hypoplasia: *A*, the remaining enamel is removed, and *B*, a shallow, circular, rounded groove is cut in the dental neck and the amalgam or composite material is applied.

References

Eisenmenger E, Zetner K. Veterinary dentistry. Philadelphia: Lea & Febiger, 1985:48.

Rossman LE, Garber DA, Harvey CE. Disorders of teeth. In: Harvey CE, ed. Veterinary dentistry. Philadelphia: WB Saunders, 1985:79.

Tholen MA. Concepts in veterinary dentistry. Lenexa, KS: Veterinary Medicine Publication, 1983.

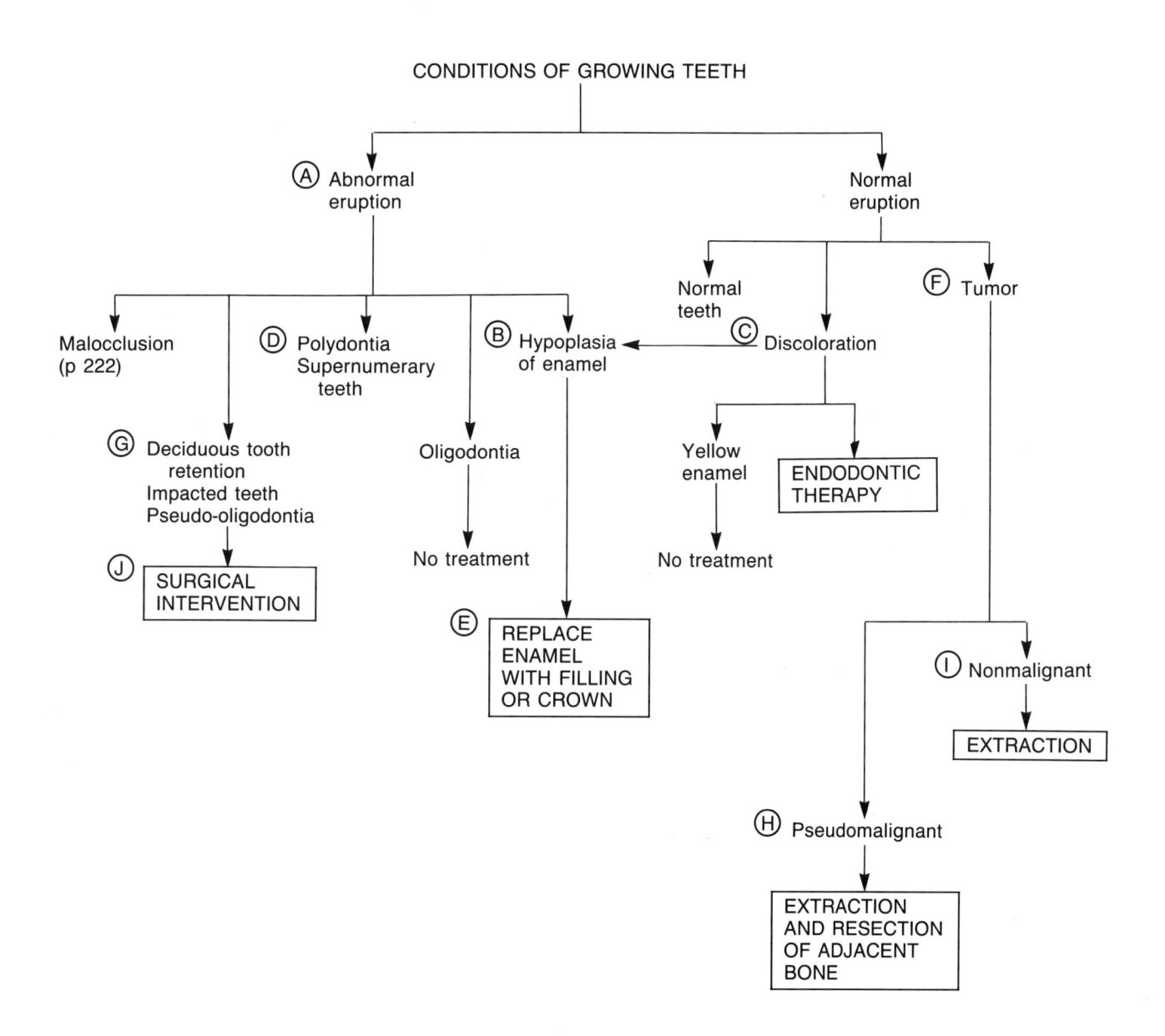

CONDITIONS OF GROWING TEETH

- (A) Abnormal eruption
  - Malocclusion (p 222)
  - (D) Polydontia Supernumerary teeth
    - (G) Deciduous tooth retention
      Impacted teeth
      Pseudo-oligodontia
      - (J) **SURGICAL INTERVENTION**
  - (B) Hypoplasia of enamel
    - Oligodontia
      - No treatment
    - (E) **REPLACE ENAMEL WITH FILLING OR CROWN**
- Normal eruption
  - Normal teeth
  - (C) Discoloration
    - Yellow enamel
      - No treatment
    - **ENDODONTIC THERAPY**
  - (F) Tumor
    - (I) Nonmalignant
      - **EXTRACTION**
    - (H) Pseudomalignant
      - **EXTRACTION AND RESECTION OF ADJACENT BONE**

MALOCCLUSION

Geoff Sumner-Smith

A. Congenital malocclusion is seen in specific breeds in which it is considered "normal," e.g., the prognathism of the Bulldog and Boxer. Treatment is not required unless the malocclusion causes malfunction of the mandible.

B. Malocclusion in breeds that normally have good occlusion may be the result of an autosomal recessive gene inheritance pattern, e.g., prognathism in long-haired Dachshunds.

C. Malocclusion that follows trauma results from a tooth, or teeth, being displaced.

D. Fracture of the supporting bone may take two forms: loss of support on account of alveolar fracture or total fracture of the supporting bone (mandible, premaxilla, or maxilla). Determination of the severity of the fracture plays an important role in deciding upon the line of treatment to be followed.

E. Extraction of individual displaced teeth is the usual method of treating fracture of the supporting bone.

F. If the gingiva is still supporting the fragments of the alveolus and the tooth is still attached within the alveolus, replacement of the elements and wiring of the tooth to adjacent teeth often result in it reseating itself and becoming stable. Careful attention to soft diet is essential until the tooth is firm. Malocclusion caused by more extensive fractures of the supporting bone requires orthopaedic repair in order to reestablish proper dental occlusion. Whichever method is employed to correct fractures of the dental segments of the skull, it may be necessary to extract or repair damaged teeth. A careful assessment of the area should be made; too hasty a decision to extract may result in loss of supporting elements that are needed to return the occlusion to normal or to anchor implants, which are employed in stabilizing extensive fractures.

G. If the malocclusion is not severe, wiring to reposition the teeth may be attempted. Alternatively, burring, with associated filling of exposed dentine, may make it possible to attain a satisfactory occlusion.

H. Should the malocclusion be observed early in the development of the teeth, extraction of specific individual teeth, prior to their eruption, often permits the remaining teeth to grow into place without overcrowding.

I. The remaining displaced fragments of the tooth should be removed. The remaining portion of the tooth is then filled or, alternatively, the crown may be built up or a prosthesis manufactured.

J. Extraction is a simple remedy for the treatment of malocclusion caused by fracture accompanied by displacement, but this may not be acceptable to the owner, particularly if the animal is a show specimen.

References

Grunberg H, Lea AJ. An inherited jaw anomaly in long-haired dachshunds. J Genet 1940; 39:285.

Leighton RL. Surgical correction of prognathous inferia in the dog. Vet Med Small Anim Clin 1977; 72:401.

Weigel JP, Dorn AS. Diseases of the jaw and abnormal occlusion. In: Harvey CE, ed. Veterinary dentistry. Philadelphia: WB Saunders, 1985:106.

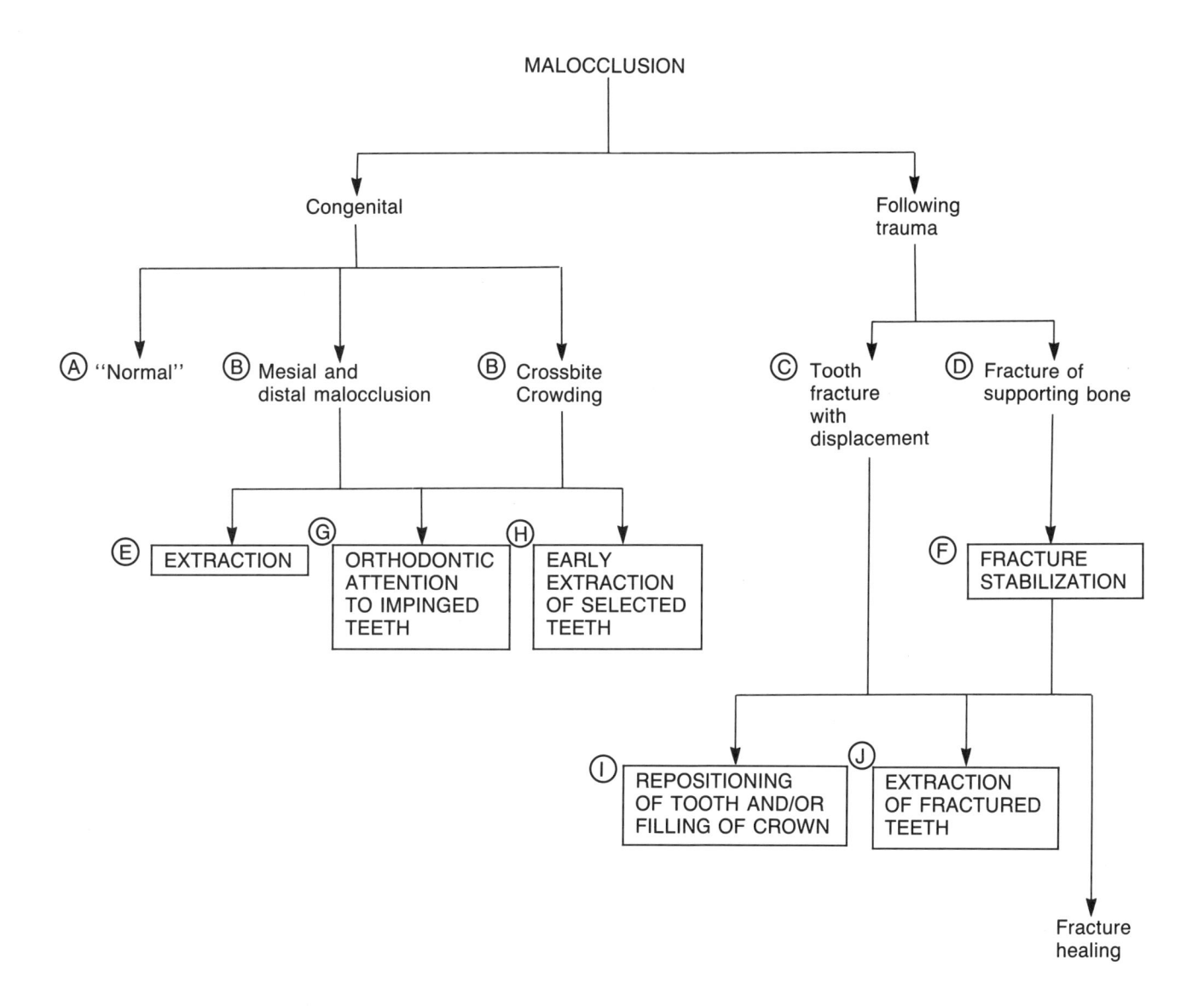

```
                              MALOCCLUSION
                                   │
                   ┌───────────────┴───────────────┐
                Congenital                      Following
                                                  trauma
         ┌─────────┼─────────┐             ┌────────┴────────┐
      Ⓐ "Normal"  Ⓑ Mesial and  Ⓑ Crossbite   Ⓒ Tooth         Ⓓ Fracture of
                  distal         Crowding      fracture         supporting bone
                  malocclusion                 with
                                               displacement
              ┌──────┬──────┐      │                │              │
              ▼      ▼      ▼      ▼                │              ▼
            Ⓔ ┌──────┐  Ⓖ ┌──────────┐  Ⓗ ┌──────────┐            Ⓕ ┌────────────┐
              │EXTRAC-│   │ORTHODONTIC│   │EARLY     │              │FRACTURE    │
              │TION   │   │ATTENTION  │   │EXTRACTION│              │STABILIZATION│
              └──────┘    │TO IMPINGED│   │OF SELECTED│             └────────────┘
                          │TEETH      │   │TEETH     │                    │
                          └──────────┘   └──────────┘                     │
                                                   ┌──────────────────────┤
                                                   ▼                      ▼
                                              Ⓘ ┌──────────┐       Ⓙ ┌──────────┐
                                                │REPOSITIONING│      │EXTRACTION│
                                                │OF TOOTH AND/│      │OF FRACTURED│
                                                │OR FILLING   │      │TEETH     │
                                                │OF CROWN     │      └──────────┘
                                                └────────────┘
                                                                          │
                                                                          ▼
                                                                      Fracture
                                                                      healing
```

223

DISEASES OF PERIODONTAL TISSUE

Geoff Sumner-Smith

Although separate conditions are described in this chapter, it should be appreciated that they often appear together. Plaque is the primary cause of gingivitis and periodontitis.

A. Inflamed gingivae are very common in the dog. The condition may be primary, or secondary to systemic or local diseases. The animal may not display any signs in the early stages, but the condition rapidly progresses and halitosis develops. The gingivae become swollen and spongy. Usually correction of the diet, cleaning of the teeth, and antibiotics ameliorate the condition.

B. When the inflammation involves not only the periodontium, as seen in gingivitis, but affects deeper tissue, thereby causing detachment of the connective tissues from the root surfaces, it is termed periodontitis. Periodontosis, a primary noninflammatory degenerative periodontal disease, is rare in the dog and unreported in the cat. It causes primary loosening and migration of teeth. However, a mixed form of periodontitis and periodontosis is common.

C. Plaque is the build up of food and debris around the teeth. *Bacteroides asaccharolyticus* and *Fusobacterium nucleatum* are especially important in the development of subsequent periodontal disease. Early attention to plaque is facilitated by the use of a plaque-disclosing agent, such as sodium fluorescein, which adheres to the plaque and fluoresces a bright greenish yellow when illuminated by ultraviolet light.

D. If plaque is allowed to accumulate, it thickens and calcifies as tartar (dental calculus).

E. Mechanical removal of the tartar is necessary. Overzealous use of an ultrasonic scaler may cause etching of the teeth, which predisposes to future plaque formation. Following removal of tartar from the exposed neck or root of the tooth, the tooth surface should be smoothed by planing in order to delay tartar formation. Odontoplasty, removal of the enamel ridge around the margin of the neck, decreases the collection of food debris within the furrow between the ridge and the gingiva, and the teeth self-clean more readily.

F. Depending upon the severity of the periodontitis, various surgical techniques are indicated. Resection of diseased gingivae allows complete removal of subgingival tartar. The procedure is facilitated by the use of an electrosurgical blade. Local gingival recession may occur on account of abnormally strong tension that is caused by a hypoplastic frenulum. Excision of the involved frenulum can relieve this excess tension. Gingival flaps are used to help stabilize teeth, to enhance self-cleaning of the region, to fill gingival pockets, and to replace missing gingiva.

G. Remove plaque by brushing the teeth by hand or mechanical polishing. Heavy mineralized plaque is best removed with manual or ultrasonic scalers.

H. Periodontal prophylaxis may retard or prevent the formation of plaque and tartar and the subsequent development of gingivitis and periodontitis; feeding the animal a hard diet and regularily brushing its teeth is important. Canine toothpaste or precipitated chalk and a child's toothbrush work satisfactorily. Chlorhexidine dental ointment is effective for up to 12 hours in reducing bacterial flora when applied to the gingival margins.

References

Eisenmenger E, Zetner K. Periodontal disease. In: Eisenmenger E, Zetner K. Veterinary dentistry. Philadelphia: Lea & Febiger, 1985:131.

Grove TK. Periodontal disease. In: Harvey CE, ed. Veterinary dentistry. Philadelphia: WB Saunders, 1985:59.

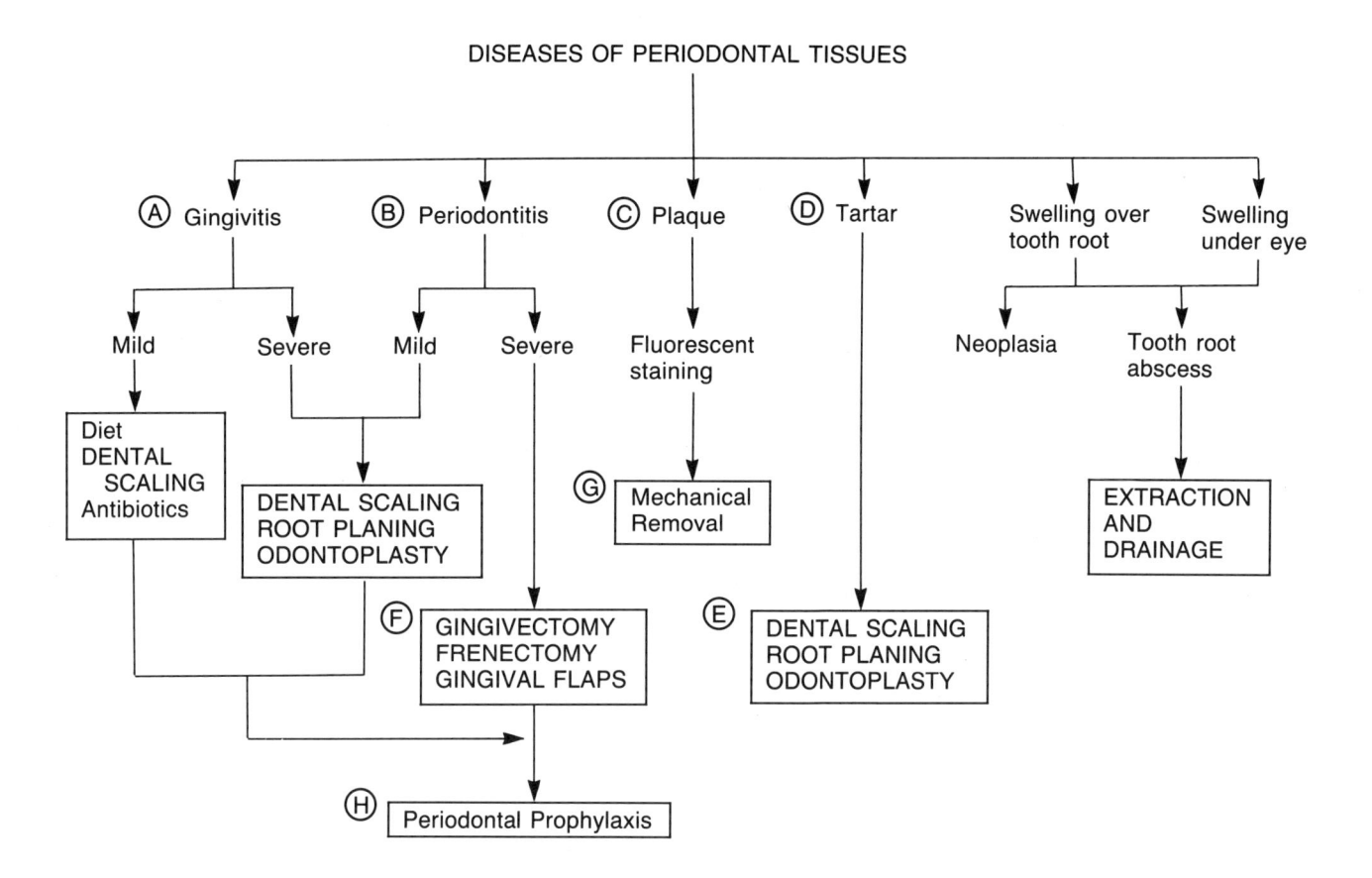

DISEASES OF PERIODONTAL TISSUES

- **(A) Gingivitis**
  - Mild → Diet, DENTAL SCALING, Antibiotics
  - Severe → DENTAL SCALING, ROOT PLANING, ODONTOPLASTY
- **(B) Periodontitis**
  - Mild → DENTAL SCALING, ROOT PLANING, ODONTOPLASTY
  - Severe → **(F)** GINGIVECTOMY, FRENECTOMY, GINGIVAL FLAPS
- **(C) Plaque** → Fluorescent staining → **(G)** Mechanical Removal
- **(D) Tartar** → **(E)** DENTAL SCALING, ROOT PLANING, ODONTOPLASTY
- **Swelling over tooth root** → Neoplasia
- **Swelling under eye** → Tooth root abscess → EXTRACTION AND DRAINAGE

(H) Periodontal Prophylaxis

DISEASES OF THE TEETH

Geoff Sumner-Smith

In examining teeth, a structural protocol sheet is helpful (Fig. 1).

A. Although uncommon, caries does occur in the dog and cat. Approximately 4 percent of small animal patients presented for dental disease have caries in one or more teeth; the molars are most commonly involved, but caries of the neck of the canine tooth is also seen.

B. Fractures of the teeth are common, and result from violent accidents or chewing on very hard objects. Therapy depends on the type and location of fracture. Treatment is not required if the pulp cavity is not exposed. Extraction may be the preferred method if this is functionally and cosmetically acceptable, or if the root is involved.

C. Extensive caries, or tooth fracture with exposure of the pulp, can result in pulp infection that is beyond recovery. Resultant degeneration of the pulp tissue can create an apical inflammatory reaction. This results in apical abscess formation, apical cyst formation, or apical cel-

---

ORAL EXAMINATION AND TREATMENT

General medical findings: _____

_____

1. Habits: Bone chewing-ball fetching-rock chewing-frisbee catching-other
2. Nutrition: a. Staple diet (sugar content) _____
   b. Treats _____
3. Oral cavity:
   a. Lips _____
   b. Cheeks: Mucosa _____
   c. Frenum: Sup. _____ Inf. _____
   d. Palate: Shape _____ Mucosa _____
   e. Maxilla: Palpation _____
   f. Mandible: Palpation _____
   g. Tongue: Dorsum _____ Sides _____ Floor of mouth ____
   h. Lymph glands of head and neck _____
4. Occlusion: Correct _____ Discrepancies _____
   Missing teeth _____ Supernumerous teeth _____
   Retained teeth _____
5. Periodontic findings
   a. Mucous membrane _____
   b. Gingiva: Color _____ Appearance _____ Puffy ____
      Knife sharp edge _____ Depth of pockets _____
      Tooth mobility _____ Bifurcation _____

Services required

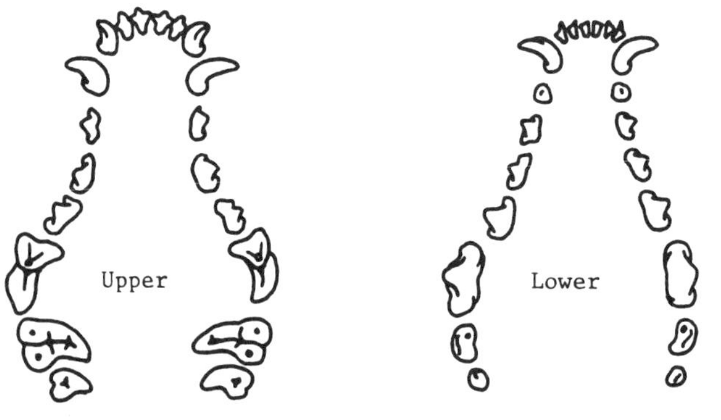

Upper   Lower

Figure 1 Oral examination and treatment

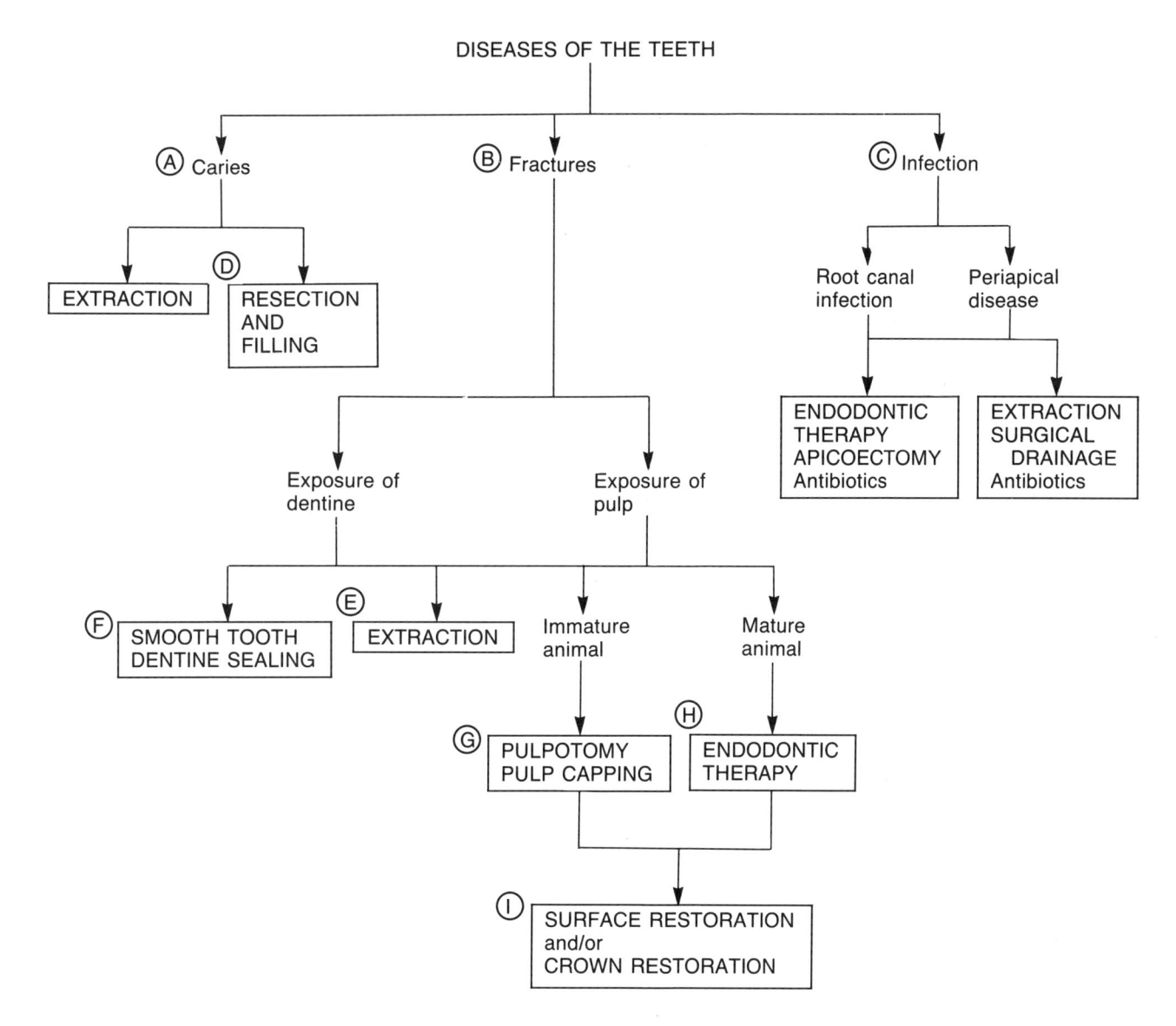

```
                        DISEASES OF THE TEETH
                                │
        ┌───────────────────────┼───────────────────────┐
        ▼                       ▼                       ▼
    Ⓐ Caries                Ⓑ Fractures              Ⓒ Infection
        │                       │                       │
        │                       │                 ┌─────┴─────┐
        │                       │                 ▼           ▼
        │                       │           Root canal    Periapical
        │                       │           infection     disease
        ▼         Ⓓ ▼                             │           │
  ┌──────────┐  ┌──────────┐                      ▼           ▼
  │EXTRACTION│  │RESECTION │                ┌──────────┐ ┌──────────┐
  └──────────┘  │   AND    │                │ENDODONTIC│ │EXTRACTION│
                │ FILLING  │                │ THERAPY  │ │ SURGICAL │
                └──────────┘                │APICOECTOMY│ │ DRAINAGE │
                                            │Antibiotics│ │Antibiotics│
                                            └──────────┘ └──────────┘
                      ┌─────────────────┴─────────────────┐
                      ▼                                   ▼
                 Exposure of                         Exposure of
                  dentine                              pulp
                      │                                   │
              ┌───────┴───┐                    ┌──────────┴──────────┐
              ▼       Ⓔ ▼                    ▼                     ▼
           Ⓕ        ┌──────────┐         Immature              Mature
      ┌──────────┐  │EXTRACTION│          animal                animal
      │  SMOOTH  │  └──────────┘             │                     │
      │  TOOTH   │                           ▼ Ⓖ                Ⓗ ▼
      │ DENTINE  │                      ┌──────────┐        ┌──────────┐
      │ SEALING  │                      │PULPOTOMY │        │ENDODONTIC│
      └──────────┘                      │PULP CAPPING│      │ THERAPY  │
                                        └──────────┘        └──────────┘
                                              │                   │
                                              └─────────┬─────────┘
                                                      Ⓘ ▼
                                              ┌──────────────────┐
                                              │SURFACE RESTORATION│
                                              │      and/or       │
                                              │ CROWN RESTORATION │
                                              └──────────────────┘
```

lulitis, which may involve surrounding tissue (e.g., upper fourth premolar abscess that involves the maxillary recess).

D. Provided that the tooth is not loose, it is preferable to drill it and prepare a cavity, which is then lined and filled with amalgam. If deemed necessary, a "visible" tooth may be filled with a composite the same color as the tooth.

E. A horizontal fracture at the level of the alveolar bone or root, or a longitudinal fracture of the tooth, is best treated by extraction.

F. Fractures that do not enter the pulp cavity are treated by smoothing rough edges in order to prevent mucosal laceration. If enamel loss is extensive, dentine sealing can be performed by the use of calcium hydroxide or composite.

G. When the pulp is exposed and still viable, it can be saved by pulpotomy or pulp capping. This is recommended only in the immature animal in which continued root development is necessary. In the mature animal, or where pulp necrosis has occurred, full endodontic therapy is the treatment of choice. Removal of the dead or infected pulp cavity contents and sealing and filling of the canal leaves a sterile, dead, but functional, tooth for life.

H. Apicoectomy (surgical access to the tooth root apex) is recommended if adequate exposure for endodontic therapy is not obtained through the crown or if a necrotic root is visible radiographically.

I. Sophisticated restorative techniques are not required unless the tooth is functionally or cosmetically important. Restoration may involve the use of amalgam, composite resins, or cements and bases; for crown restoration, posts and cast-metal crowns are used.

References

Eisenmenger E, Zetner K. Veterinary dentistry. Philadelphia: Lea & Febiger, 1983.

Ross DL. Veterinary dentistry. In: Ettinger SJ, ed. Textbook of veterinary internal medicine. Philadelphia: WB Saunders, 1975:1047.

Rossman LE, Garber DA, Harvey CF. Disorders of teeth. In: Harvey CE, ed. Veterinary dentistry. Philadelphia: Lea & Febiger, 1985:79.

INDEX

Note: Page numbers followed by (t) indicate tables; those followed by (f) indicate figures.

A

Abdominal fluid, 204–205
Abscess
  anal sac, 44
  hepatic, 54
  orbital, 164
  prostatic, 134
    drainage of, 134, 134f
Acanthomatous epulis, 2
Acepromazine
  for high blood pressure, 198
  for sedation, 186
  for vascular embolism, 100
Acetaminophen, 186
Acetazolamide, 152
Achalasia, cricopharyngeal, 12, 12f
Acyclic bitch, infertility in, 122
Adenocarcinoma
  of nasal and paranasal sinuses, 66
  pancreatic, 62
  of perianal gland, 40
  prostatic, 134
Adenoma
  hepatocellular, 54
  of perianal gland, 40
Agonal gasps, 192
Airway obstruction, 70, 70f–71, 72
Allergic rhinitis, 66
Ameloblastoma, 2, 220
Anal sac abscess, 44
Anal sac adenocarcinoma, of apocrine glands, 40
Anal sacculectomy, 44, 44f
Anal sacculitis, 44
Anastomosis, esophageal, 20f
Anesthesia
  apnea associated with, 184
  poor recovery from, 188
Anus, imperforate, 42
Aorta, occlusion of, 100
Aortic arch, with right and left ligamentum arteriosum, 92, 92f
Aortic stenosis, 86
Apicoectomy, 227
Apnea, associated with anesthesia, 184
Apocrine glands, anal sac adenocarcinoma of, 40
Arrhythmia
  with gastric dilatation volvulus, 24
  treatment of, 196
Arteriovenous fistula, 98
Ascites, chylous, 208
  fluid in, 204
Aspirin, 186
Ataxia, types of, 136
Atropine
  for bradycardia, 196
  for cardiac arrest, 192
  for uveitis, 152

Azoospermia, 124

B

Bacterial rhinitis, 66
Bacteroides asaccharolyticus infection, 224
Barbiturate anesthesia, 188
Benign prostatic hyperplasia, 134
Bethanechol, 116
Bicarbonate replacement, 190
Bile duct, obstruction of, 58
Biliary tract, trauma to, 56
Bitch. *See also* Canine *entries*
  acyclic, infertility in, 122
  cyclic, infertility in, 120
  cystic endometrial hyperplasia-pyometra complex in, 132
Bladder neoplasia, 106
Bladder-urethral incoordination, 116
Blepharospasm, 160
Blindness, 166
Blood pH, maintenance of, 194
Blood transfusion, 190
Bougienage, for esophageal stricture, 20
Brachial plexus avulsion, 146
Brachycephalic syndrome, 72
Bradycardia, treatment of, 196
Branham's sign, 98
Bruit, orbital, 164
Buphthalmos, 164
Bupivacaine, 186
Burn
  chemical, 10
  thermal, 174, 174f
"Burnt-out" glaucoma, 152

C

Calcium gluconate
  for dystocia, 126
  for hypotension, 182
Calculus (i)
  cystic, removal of, 111
  dental, 224
  urinary tract, 106
Canine dystocia, 126
Canine heartworm disease, 102, 102f
Canine mammary tumor, 178
Canine oral papillomatosis, 2
Canine urethral obstruction, 110, 110f, 111
Carcinoma. *See specific types*
Cardiac arrest, 192
Cardiac arrhythmia. *See* Arrhythmia
Cardiac murmur, 80
Cardiac pacemaker, artificial, 94
Cardiopulmonary bypass, for ventricular septal defect, 88
Caries, 226
Cataract, 154
Catgut sutures, 202
Caustic ingestion, 10
Celiotomy, for intestinal obstruction, 26
Cellulitis, orbital, 164

Cerebellar ataxia, 138
Cerebral resuscitation, 198
Cervical esophageal foreign body, 14
Cervical intervertebral disc disease, 140
Cervical mucocele, 8
Cervical vertebral instability, 140
Cesarean section, for dystocia, 126
Chemicals, ingested, caustic nature of, 10
Chlorhexidine solution, 174
Cholecystoduodenostomy, 58
Cholecystojejunostomy, 58, 58f
Cholecystotomy, 58
Chylous ascites, 208
  fluid in, 204
Chylous effusion, 74
Circulatory resuscitation, 194
Cisterna chyli, rupture of, 208
Cloudy eye, 154
Colon, obstruction of, 34
Congenital heart defect(s)
  aortic stenosis, 86
  common differentials for, 80
  patent ductus arteriosus, 82, 82f
  pulmonic stenosis, 84, 84f
  ventricular septal defect, 88, 88f
Congenital malocclusion, 222
Congestive heart failure, fluid in, 204
Congestive splenomegaly, 212
Conjunctivitis, 156, 162
Continuous murmurs, 80
Corneal endothelial dystrophy, 154
Corneal epidermalization, 154
Corneal erosion syndrome, 158
Corneal haze, 154
Coughing, 64
Cricopharyngeal achalasia, 12, 12f
Cyclic bitch, infertility in, 120
Cyst, pulmonary, 74
Cystic calculus(i), removal of, 111
Cystic endometrial hyperplasia-pyometra complex, in bitch, 132
Cystic hyperplasia, of prostate, 134
Cycstocentesis, 106, 106f, 110
Cystostomy, 110, 110f

D

Dacryocystitis, 162
Dantrolene, for dyssynergia, 116
Debridement, of full-thickness wound, 168, 170
Deciduous teeth, loose, 220
Decompression, treatment of, 24
Deep red eye, 148, 148f
Defibrillation, 192, 192t
Dental calculus(i), 224
Detrusor areflexia, 116
Dexamethasone
  for cardiac arrest, 192
  for cerebral resuscitation, 198
  for thoracolumbar intervertebral disc disease, 142
Diaphragmatic hernia, 76

229

Diaphragmatic muscle patch graft, 16, 20
Diarrhea
  acute, 48
  chronic, 50
Diastolic murmurs, 80
Diazepam
  for pain relief, 186
  for seizures, 198
Diazoxide, 64
Dichlorphenamide, 152
Diethylstilbestrol (DES)
  for hormone-responsive incontinence, 118
  for infertility, 120
  for prostatic disease, 136
  for vaginitis, 130
Dirofilaria immitis infestation, 102
Disc disease
  cervical intervertebral, 140
  thoracolumbar intervertebral, 142
Discharge, nasal, 66
Discospondylitis, 138
Distichiasis, 158, 158f, 160
Dobutamine
  for hypotension, 182
  for increased myocardial contractility, 194
Dopamine, 194
Drainage, peritoneal, of intra-abdominal sepsis, 32
Dyssynergia, treatment of, 116
Dystocia, canine, 126
Dystrophy, corneal endothelial, 154

E

Ear canal disease, external, 216
Effusion
  exudative, 96, 204
  pseudochylous, 75, 204
Effusion tamponade, pericardial, 96
Eisenmenger's syndrome, 88, 90
Embolism, vascular, 100
Emesis, reflex act of, 22
Enophthalmos, 158
Enterotomy, for intestinal obstruction, 26
Entropion, 160
Ephedrine, 182
Epidural analgesia, 186
Epinephrine
  for cardiac arrest, 192
  for red eye, 148
Epiphora, 160
Episcleritis, 148
Episiotomy, 128f
Epistaxis, 68
Epithelioma, 176
Epulides, 2
Eruption, tooth, abnormal and normal, 220
Escherichia coli infection, 132
Esophageal stricture, 20
Esophagotomy, cervical, 14
Esophagus
  foreign body in cervical region of, 14
  foreign body in thoracic region of, 16
Exophthalmos, 164
Exudative effusion, 96, 204
Eye
  cloudy, 154
  protruding, 164
  red, 148, 148f, 150, 152
  wet, 160

F

Feeding, of gastric dilatation volvulus patient, 24
Feline mammary tumor, 180–181
Feline urethral obstruction, 112, 112f
Feline urologic syndrome, 112
Fibromatous epulis, 2
Fibrosarcoma, 176
  of oral cavity, 4
Fistula
  arteriovenous, 98
  perianal, 46
Flail chest, 78, 78f
Fluid, abdominal, 204–205
Fluid therapy, 190
  for cardiac arrest, 192
Foreign body
  bronchial, 74
  esophageal
    in cervical region, 14
    in thoracic region, 16
  linear intestinal, 30
Fracture
  rib, 76
  tooth, 226
Fusobacterium nucleatum infection, 224

G

Gastric dilatation volvulus, 24
Gastropexy, 24, 24f
Gentamicin ointment, 174
Gingiva, inflamed, 224
Glaucoma, 152
  blindness caused by, 166
Glucocorticoid therapy, 144
Glucose therapy, 190
  for dystocia, 146
Goose-honk coughs, 64

H

Head tilt, 146
Heart defect, congenital. *See* Congenital heart defect(s)
Heartworm, canine, 102, 102f
Heller's procedure, modified, 18
Hemangiosarcoma, 176, 212
Hematuria, 108
Hemorrhage
  liver trauma and, 52
  long-standing or resolving, 205
  recent, 205
  retrobulbar, 164
Hemorrhagic effusion, 74
Hemothorax, 76
Heparin, 100
Hepatoma, 54
Hernia, diaphragmatic, 76
Hormone-responsive incontinence, 118
Horner's syndrome, 138, 144
Human chorionic gonadotropin (hCG), 120
Hypercalcemia
  with perianal neoplasia, 40
  treatment of, 194
Hyperemia, 148, 148f
  conjunctival, 156
Hyperkalemia, treatment of, 194
Hyperplasia
  prostatic, benign, 134
  vaginal, 128
Hyperthermia, treatment of, 198
Hypocalcemia, treatment of, 194
Hypokalemia, treatment of, 194
Hypoplasia, of tooth enamel, 220, 220f
Hypotension, 182–183
Hypothermia, after anesthesia, 188
Hypovolemic shock, treatment of, 24

I

Idiopathic effusion, 96
Imperforate anus, 42
Incontinence, urinary, neurogenic, 116
  nonneurogenic, 118
Infertility
  in acyclic bitch, 122
  in cyclic bitch, 120
  in male dog, 124
Ingestion, caustic, 10
Inhalation anesthesia, 188
Innovar-vet analgesia, 188
Insulinoma, 62
  treatment of, 64
Intercostal muscle, rupture of, 78
Intestine
  linear foreign body in, 30
  perforation of, 32, 32f
  small, obstruction of, 26
Intrahepatic shunt, 104
Intraocular pressure, chronic elevation of, 164
Intussusception, 28, 28f
Irreducible intussusception, 28
Islet cell carcinoma, 62

K

Keratitis, ulcerative, 158
Keratoconjunctivitis sicca, 162

L

Lacrimation, 160
Lagophthalmos, 158
Large bowel diarrhea, 50
Laryngitis, 70
Larynx
  paralysis of, 70
  trauma to, 76
  tumors of, 70
Lavage
  peritoneal, for peritonitis, 32
  pressurized, of full-thickness wound, 168, 170
Lid tumors, 160
Lidocaine
  for cardiac arrhythmias, 196
  for ventricular tachycardia, 24
Lipid deposition, in cornea, 154
Liver
  injuries to, acute, 52
  tumors of, 54
Lung, tumors of, 74
Lung lobe torsion, 74
Lymphosarcoma, 176

M

Male dog, infertility in, 124
Malocclusion, 222
Mammary glands, lymphatic drainage of,
  in cat, 180f
  in dog, 178f
Mammary gland tumor
  canine, 178
  feline, 180–181
Mannitol
  for cerebral resuscitation, 198
  for uveitis, 152
Marsupialization
  mucocele, 8
  in treatment of cysts, 137
Mast cell tumors, 176
Megaesophagus, 18
Megaloglobus, 164
Megestrol acetate

for infertility, 120
for prostatic disease, 136
Meibomian gland, infection of, 156
Melanoma
    of oral cavity, 4
    uveal, 164
Membrana nictitans, eversion of, 160
Methoxamine, 198
Metrazolamide, 152
Middle ear disease, 218
Mite infestation, of ear canal, 216
Moist coughing, 64
Mononeuropathy, 144
Morphine, 186
Mucocele, 164
    cervical, 8
    pharyngeal, 8
    salivary, 8
Mucosa, chemical erosion of, 10
Murmur, cardiac, 80
Myotomy, cricopharyngeal, 12, 12f

N

Nasal discharge, 66
Natural sutures, 202
Neck pain, 140
Neoplasia, 200. *See also* Tumor(s)
    bladder, 106
    conjunctival, 156
    with coughing, 64
    oral
        benign, 2
        malignant, 4
    pancreatic, 62, 64
    perianal, 40
    of pinna, 214
Neoplastic effusion, 74
Neuritis, optic, 166
Neuroepithelioma, 138
Neurogenic urinary incontinence, 116
Neuromuscular blocking agents, 188
Nocturnal coughing, 64
Nonabsorbable sutures, 202
Nonclotting bloody effusion, 96
Nonclotting serosanguinous effusion, 96
Nonneurogenic urinary incontinence, 118
Nonseptic exudate, 204
Norepinephrine, 198

O

Obstruction
    airway, 70, 70f, 71, 72
    of bile duct, 58
    of colon, 34
    of small intestine, 26
    tracheal, 72
    urethral
        canine, 110–111, 110f
        feline, 112, 112f
Obstructive effusion, 74
Ocular discharge, chronic purulent, 162
Odontoma, 2, 220
Oligospermia, 124
Optic neuritis, 166
Oral neoplasia
    benign, 2
    malignant, 4
Orbital abscess, 164
Orbital bruit, 164
Orbital cellulitis, 164
Ordontoplasty, 224
Osseous epulis, 2
Otitis externa, 226
Otitis media, 218

Otitis media-interna, 146
Oxymorphone analgesia, 188
Oxytocin
    for fetal expulsion, 126
    for vaginal prolapse, 128

P

Pacemaker, cardiac, artificial, 94
Pain
    intraoperative or postoperative, 186
    neck, 141
Pancreatectomy, partial, 62, 63f
Pancreatic neoplasia, 62, 64
Pancreatitis, 60
Papillitis, 166
Papilloma, 176
Papillomatosis, oral, canine, 2
Paralysis, laryngeal, 70
Paroxysmal coughing, 64
Patent ductus arteriosus, 82, 82f
Pectus excavatum, 78
Pentobarbital, 198
Perforation, intestinal, 32, 32f
Perianal fistula, 46
Perianal neoplasia, 40
Pericardial effusion tamponade, 96
Pericardiocentesis, 96
Periodontal tissue, diseases of, 224
Periodontitis, 224
Periodontosis, 224
Peripheral nerve disease, 144
Peritonitis, septic, 210
Permanent teeth, supernumerary, 222
pH, blood, maintenance of, 194
Pharyngeal mucocele, 8
Phenobarbital, 196
Phenoxybenzamine, 116
Phenylbutazone, 186
Phenylephrine, 198
Phenylpropanolamine, 118
Pinna
    arteriovenous fistula in, 98
    discomfort of, 214
Plaque, 224
Plasmoma, 156
Pleura, filling defects of, 74
Pleural effusion, 74
Pneumothorax, 76
Point of maximal intensity (PMI), of murmur, 80
Polyp(s)
    nasal, 66
    rectal, 38
    vaginal, 128
Portosystemic shunt, 104
Post cardiopulmonary resuscitation, 196
    cerebral resuscitation, 198
    circulatory resuscitation, 194
Postcaval syndrome, 102
Potassium chloride, 194
Prednisolone
    for hypotension, 182
    for insulinomas, 64
Pringle maneuvre, 52
Procainamide
    for cardiac arrhythmias, 196
    for ventricular tachycardia, 24
Prolapse, rectal, 36, 36f
Propranolol
    for cardiac arrhythmias, 196
    for high heart rate, 196
Prostaglandins, 132
Prostate-blood barrier, interruption of, 134, 136
Prostate disease, 134, 134f

Prostatitis, 106
Protruding eye, 164
Pseudochylous effusion, 74, 204
Pudental nerve, loss of function of, 116
Pulmonary artery banding, for ventricular septal defect, 88
Pulmonary cyst, 74
Pulmonary thrombosis, 74
Pulmonic stenosis, 84, 84f
Puppy vaginitis, 130
Pyelonephritis, 116
Pyometra, 132

Q

Quinidine gluconate, 24

R

Ranula, 8
Recovery, poor, from anesthesia, 188
Rectum
    polyps of, 38
    prolapse of, 36, 36f
Red eye
    deep, 148, 148f
    intraocular, 152
    superficial (extraocular), 150
Reducible intussusception, 28
Reflex act, of emesis, 22
Regurgitation, after cricopharyngeal achalasia, 12
Renoliths, 106
Resection, for intestinal obstruction, 26
Retina, elevation or displacement of, 144
Retinitis, 166
Rhinitis, 68
Rib fractures, 80

S

Sacculectomy, anal, 44, 44f
Sacculitis, anal, 44
Sacrococcygeal injury, 144
Salivary mucocele, 8
Schiotz's tonometry, 148
Schirmer tear test, 150
Seizures, treatment of, 198
Septal defect, ventricular, 88, 88f
Septic exudate, 204
Septic peritonitis, 210
Shock, hypovolemic, treatment of, 24
Shunt, portosystemic, 104
Sick sinus syndrome, 94
Silk sutures, 202
Silver sulfadiazine cream, 174
Skin flap, 172, 172f
Skin graft, 172
Skin tumors, 176
Sliding intussusception, 28
Small bowel diarrhea, 50
Small intestine, obstruction of, 26
Sodium bicarbonate, 192
Spinal ataxia, 138
Spinal cord disease, lesion localization in, 138
Spleen, disorders of, 212
Splenomegaly, 212
Squamous cell carcinoma, of oral cavity, 4
Staging, of mammary tumors, 180
Stenosis
    aortic, 86
    pulmonic, 84, 84f
Sternothyroideus muscle patch graft, 14, 20
Stricture, esophageal, 20

Superficial (extraocular) red eye, 150
Suture material, choice of, 202
Systolic murmurs, 80

T

Tachycardia, ventricular, treatment of, 24
Tamponade, effusion, pericardial, 96
Tapered enteric gas bubble, 30
Tartar, removal of, 224
Teeth
   diseases of, 226
   enamel, hypoplasia of, 220, 220f
   growing, conditions of, 220
Tetralogy of Fallot, 90
Thermal burn, 174, 174f
Thoracentesis sites, 76f
Thoracic esophageal foreign body, 16
Thoracic trauma, 76
Thoracic wall disease, 76f, 78
Thoracolumbar intervertebral disc disease, 142
Thoracotomy, intercostal, 16
Thromboembolus, 100
Thrombosis, pulmonary, 74
Tonsillectomy, peroral, 6
Tonsillitis, 6
Tonsils, abnormality of, 6
Torsion
   lung lobe, 74
   of spleen, 212
Trachea
   obstruction of, 70
   trauma to, 76
Transfusion, blood, 190

Transitional cell carcinoma, of bladder, 106
Trauma
   arteriovenous fistula secondary to, 98
   biliary tract, 56
   liver, acute, 52
   thoracic, 76
Traumatic rhinitis, 66
Trichiasis, 160
Tumor(s). *See also* Neoplasia
   benign, 200
   of dental laminar epithelium, 2
   hepatic, 54
   laryngeal, 68
   lid, 160
   malignant, 200
   mammary
      canine, 178
      feline, 180–181
   pulmonary, 74
   skin, 176

U

Ulcerative keratitis, 158
Ureteral ectopia, 118f
Urethral obstruction
   canine, 110, 111, 110f
   feline, 112, 112f
Urethrostomy, 110, 110f
Urinary incontinence
   neurogenic, 116
   nonneurogenic, 118
Urinary tract calculus(i), 106

Urinary tract infection, 106
Uroperitoneum, 114
Uveal melanoma, 164
Uveitis, 152, 154, 166

V

Vaginal hyperplasia, 128
Vaginal polyps, 128
Vaginal protrusion, 128
Vaginitis, 130
Vascular embolism, 100
Vascular ring anomaly, 92, 92f
Ventricular septal defect, 88, 88f
Ventricular tachycardia, treatment of, 24
Vestibular ataxia, 138
Vestibular disease, head tilt in, 146
Volvulus, gastric dilatation, 24
Vomiting, 22

W

Wet eye, 160
Wound
   full-thickness
      acute, 168
      chronic, 170
   reconstruction of, 172, 172f

X

Xylazine analgesia, 188

Z

Zollinger-Ellison syndrome, 62